DATE DUE

4/11/97			
5-14-97			
5/8/98			
3-1-00			
MAR 28 '01			
5-3-21			

Demco No. 62-0549

D1686233

COCAINE PAPERS
By SIGMUND FREUD

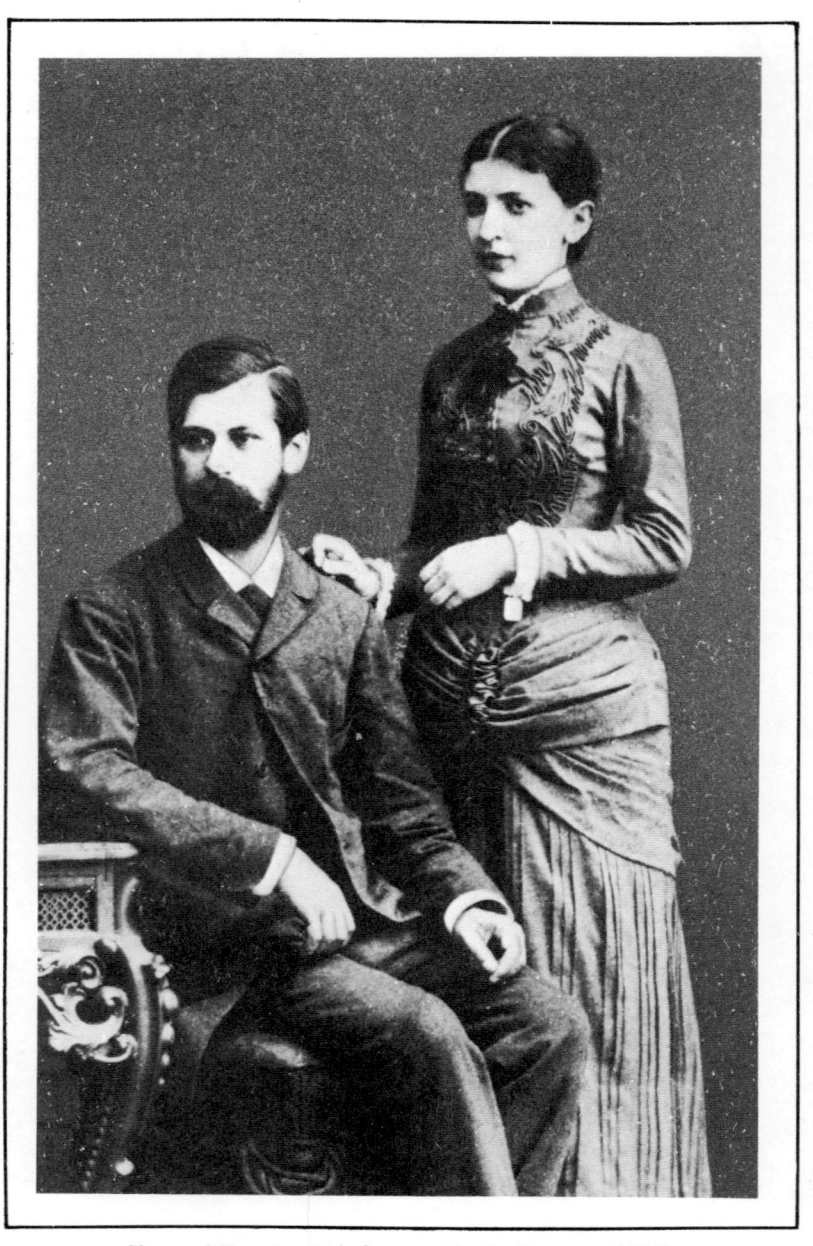

Sigmund Freud and his fiancee, Martha Bernays (1885).

COCAINE PAPERS
By SIGMUND FREUD

NOTES FOR THIS EDITION BY

ANNA FREUD

EDITED AND WITH AN INTRODUCTION BY

ROBERT BYCK, M.D.

STONEHILL

Copyright © 1974 by The Stonehill Publishing Company and Robert Byck.
"The Cocaine Papers" (The Dunquin Press Edition): *Uber Coca,* "Contributions To The Knowledge Of The Effect Of Cocaine," "Addenda To *Über Coca,*" "On The General Effect Of Cocaine," and "Craving For And Fear Of Cocaine." Copyright © 1963 by Sigmund Freud Copyrights, Ltd., London.

No part of this publication may be reproduced or transmitted in any form or by any means without permission in writing from the publisher, except by a reviewer who wishes to quote brief passages in connection with a review written for inclusion in a magazine, newspaper or broadcast.

Illustrations courtesy of The Yale Medical Library, New Haven, Conn. (pp. ii, xxxvii, xxxviii, 14, 19, 27, 48, 84, 124, 148, 240, 361) and Mrs. Hortense Koller Becker (pg. 291).

Library of Congress Catalog Card Number: 73-82134.
ISBN: 0-88373-010-3.

For information address: The Stonehill Publishing Company, 38 East 57 Street, New York, N.Y. 10022.

Book Design by Esther Mitgang.

First Printing

Printed in the USA

Alles, Gordon: "Some Relations Between Chemical Structure and Physiological Action of Mescaline and Related Compounds," from *Neuropharmacology*. Edited by H.A. Abramson. Copyright © 1959 by Josiah Macy, Jr., Foundation, New York. pp. 169-197.

Aschenbrandt, Theodor: "The Psychological Effect and Significance of Cocaine Muriate on the Human Organism," from *Deutsche Medizinische Wochenschrift*, No. 50, December 12, 1883. Translated by Therese Byck. Copyright © 1974 by Robert Byck.

Becker, Hortense Koller: "Carl Koller and Cocaine," from *The Psychoanalytic Quarterly*, No. 32, pp. 304-373. Copyright © 1963 by *The Psychoanalytic Quarterly*.

Bernfeld, Siegfried: "Freud's Studies on Cocaine (1884)," from *The Journal of the American Psychoanalytic Association*, October, 1953, Vol. 1, No. 4, pp. 581-613. Copyright © 1953 by *The Journal of the American Psychoanalytic Association*.

Brecher, Edward, M: *Licit and Illicit Drugs, The Consumer Union Report on Narcotics, Stimulants, Depressants, Inhalants, Hallucinogens, and Marijuana: Including Caffeine, Nicotine, and Alcohol*. Copyright © 1972 by Consumers Union of United States, Inc. Little, Brown & Company, Boston. pp. 33-34.

Freud, Sigmund: *An Autobiographical Study*. Authorized translation by James Strachey. Copyright © 1952 by W.W. Norton & Company, Inc. pp. 24-25.

—*The Interpretation of Dreams*, "The Dream of Irma's Injection" and "The Dream of the Botanical Monograph." Translated by James Strachey. 1961, (Science Editions), Basic Books, Inc. Publishers, New York. pp. 106-121, 292-295 and pp. 169-176.

—*The Letters of Sigmund Freud*, Selected and Edited by Ernst L. Freud, Translated by James and Tania Stern, © 1960 by Sigmund Freud Copyrights Ltd., London.

Gutt(macher, H.): New Medications and Therapeutic Techniques," *Vienna Medical Press*, August, 1885. Translated by Stephen Fleck, Ferenc Gyorgyey, and Robert Byck. Copyright © 1974 by Robert Byck. pp. 1035-1038.

Hoffman, Albert: The Discovery of LSD and Subsequent Investigations of Naturally Occurring Hallucinogens," *Discoveries in Biological Psychiatry*, Edited by F.J. Ayd, Jr. and B. Blackwell. Copyright © 1970 J.B. Lippincott Company pp. 93-94.

Jones, Ernest: *The Life and Work of Sigmund Freud*, chapter VI, "The Cocaine Episode," © 1953 by Ernest Jones, Basic Books, Inc., Publishers, New York.

Musto, David, F.: "Sherlock Holmes and Sigmund Freud: A Study in Cocaine," *The Journal of the American Medical Association*, April 1, 1968. Copyright © 1968, Footnotes © 1974 by David Musto.

—*The American Disease: Origins of Narcotic Control*. Copyright © 1973 by David Musto, Yale University Press, New Haven. p. 7.

Woodley, Richard, A.: *Dealer: Portrait of a Cocaine Merchant*, Warner Paperback Library Edition, reprinted by permission of Holt, Rinehart and Winston, Inc., chapter 5, pp. 52-59. Copyright © 1971 by Richard A. Woodley.

Author's Acknowledgement

This book would not have been possible without the help of many people. In particular, I would like to thank Professor Rosemary Ostwald and Mrs. Hortense Koller Becker for permission to reprint articles by and about their fathers.

Dr. David Musto deserves special thanks, not only for annotating his article on "Sherlock Holmes and Sigmund Freud" but also, for his scholarly help and suggestions. Drs. Stephen Fleck and Frederick C. Redlich were most helpful with additions to and corrections of the translations.

I could never have completed the book without the exceptional generosity and goodwill of The Yale Medical Librarians, in particular, Mr. Ferenc Gyorgyey, Mr. Robert Breedlove, and Ms. Bette Greenberg.

The creative efforts of Mr. Peter Swales were appreciated.

So many people at Yale have been of help and have encouraged me that it is impossible to name them all.

This book was written for my children, Carl, Gillian, and Lucas; to learn about science from history.

Robert Byck

TABLE OF CONTENTS

Chronology   xi

INTRODUCTION   xv

I

Chapter One
"THE COCAINE EPISODE," Part One   3

Chapter Two
FREUD'S SOURCES   13

Chapter Three
"THE COCAINE EPISODE," Part Two   29

Chapter Four
EARLY HOPES   37

Chapter Five
ÜBER COCA by Sigmund Freud (July 1884)   47

Chapter Six
COCAINE AND ITS SALTS by E. Merck   75

Chapter Seven
"COCA"   83

Chapter Eight
PAPERS ON COCAINE AND OTHER PROSPECTS   89

Chapter Nine
CONTRIBUTION TO THE KNOWLEDGE OF THE EFFECT OF COCAINE by Sigmund Freud (January 1885)   95

Chapter Ten
ADDENDA TO *ÜBER COCA*
by Sigmund Freud (February 1885)   105

Chapter Eleven
ON THE GENERAL EFFECT OF COCAINE
by Sigmund Freud (March 1885)   111

Chapter Twelve
PARKE'S UNIVERSAL PANACEA   119

Chapter Thirteen
"THE COCAINE EPISODE," Part Three   151

Chapter Fourteen
COCAINE AS A MEANS TO AN END   159

Chapter Fifteen
CRAVING FOR AND FEAR OF COCAINE
by Sigmund Freud (July 1887)   169

Chapter Sixteen
COCA: ITS PREPARATIONS AND THEIR THERAPEUTICAL QUALITIES, WITH SOME REMARKS ON THE SO-CALLED "COCAINE HABIT"
by W. A. Hammond   177

Chapter Seventeen
"THE COCAINE EPISODE," Part Four   195

Chapter Eighteen
FREUD'S COCAINE DREAMS   203
The Dream of Irma's Injection (July 1895)   205
The Dream of the Botanical Monograph (March 1898)   224

Chapter Nineteen
"COCAINISM" by Louis Lewin — 237

Chapter Twenty
FREUD LOOKS BACK: BIOGRAPHY AND AUTOBIOGRAPHY — 253

II

Chapter Twenty-One
"COCA KOLLER" by Hortense Koller Becker — 261

Chapter Twenty-Two
FREUD'S STUDIES ON COCAINE by Siegfried Bernfeld — 321

III

Chapter Twenty-Three
SHERLOCK HOLMES AND SIGMUND FREUD by David Musto — 355

Chapter Twenty-Four
ILLICIT COCAINE IN AMERICA by Richard Woodley — 371

Chapter Twenty-Five
PROPOSALS FOR THE EVALUATION OF COCAINE — 379

Chapter references — 387
Bibliography — 399
Biographical Notes — 401
Index — 403

A Chronology of Freud and Cocaine

1565—Nicholas Monardes publishes first description of coca in Europe
1855—Gardeke extracts an alkaloid which he calls erythroxylon—the first isolation of cocaine
1856—Freud born in Moravia on May 6th.
1858—The Novarra expedition circles the world and brings coca leaves to Europe
1859—Mantegazza extols the virtues of coca
1860—Albert Niemann describes the isolation of an alkaloid from coca and calls it cocaine
1862—Schroff notes the numbing effect of cocaine on the tongue
1880—Cocaine is an official drug in the United States pharmacopoeia
1880—Bentley and Palmer report the treatment of the morphine habit with cocaine in the *Detroit Therapeutic Gazette*
1880—Von Anrep reports the action of cocaine in animals
1883—Theodor Aschenbrandt tells of his experiments in giving cocaine to soldiers and Sigmund Freud reads the article
1884—In April Freud writes to his fiancée that he is "toying now with a project." He has read American reports and is impressed by Aschenbrandt's article
1884—On April 30 Freud takes cocaine for the first time
1884—In May Freud starts treating his friend Ernst von Fleischl-Marxow, a morphine addict, with cocaine
1884—June 19, Freud writes to his fiancée to say, *"Über Coca* finished last night"
1884—*Über Coca,* Freud's first paper on cocaine, is published.
1884—Carl Koller, a colleague of Freud's, tries cocaine in the eye of frog and man and discovers local anesthesia
1884—September 15th, Joseph Brettauer reads Koller's paper describing local anesthesia to the Heidelberg Ophthalmological Society
1884—October, both Koller and Köenigstein present papers on local anesthesia at the Medical Society of Vienna
1884—In November and December Freud experiments on himself with cocaine
1884—In December a digested translation of Freud's first paper, "On Coca" appears in the *St. Louis Medical and Surgical Journal*
1884—December 6th, Hall and William Halsted report that injection of cocaine into a nerve blocks conduction of sensation, thereby causing local anesthesia

1885—Freud's experimental paper "A Contribution to the Knowledge of the Effect of Cocaine" is released on the 31st of January

1885—A separate reprint of Freud's first paper, *Über Coca,* is published with some additions in February

1885—In March Freud lectures to both the Physiological and Psychiatric Societies. The lecture will be published in August

1885—In April Freud evaluates Parke's cocaine

1885—April 6th, Königstein operates on Freud's father under cocaine anesthesia. Koller is present at the operation

1885—Fleischl, taking increasing amounts of cocaine, has a toxic psychosis with crawling "cocaine bugs"

1885—Louis Lewin attacks Freud's views on the harmlessness of cocaine and its uses in treating morphine addiction. A. Erlenmeyer also joins in the attack on cocaine, calling it the "third scourge of the human race"

1885—July, Freud publishes "Remarks on Craving For and Fear of Cocaine"—he backs off somewhat from his previous position about the harmlessness of cocaine

1888—*The Sign of the Four* by A. Conan Doyle is published and Sherlock Holmes injects cocaine intravenously

1895—Freud takes cocaine and dreams of Irma's injection

1900—*The Interpretation of Dreams* by Sigmund Freud is published in German

1903—Cocaine is removed from Coca Cola

1904—Procaine, a new local anesthetic, is discovered

1924—*Phantastica* by Louis Lewin, the most complete study of drugs that affect the mind, is published

1924—Freud's *Autobiographical Study* is published, and Freud gives credit to Koller for the discovery of local anesthesia

1939—Freud dies in London on September 23rd.

1963—The first publication of the collected Cocaine Papers in any language

1974—Interest in cocaine is reawakened and Freud's articles are rediscovered

INTRODUCTION

Sigmund Freud
and Cocaine

Robert Byck is Associate Professor of Pharmacology in Psychiatry, and Burroughs Wellcome Scholar in Clinical Pharmacology, at the Yale University School of Medicine.

In 1884, some time after the introduction of cocaine in both the United States and Europe, Sigmund Freud became interested in its properties and effects. He reviewed the published literature to discover all that was known about the drug and then proceeded to undertake a series of experimental investigations into its effects in man. He became an enthusiast and user, and attempted to employ cocaine in halting the morphine addiction of a friend, Ernst von Fleischl–Marxow. The disastrous consequences of this experiment and the later controversies—both over the use of cocaine in such treatment and over attribution for the discovery of cocaine as a local anesthetic—prompted him to discontinue further investigations into its central actions, although we know from *The Interpretation of Dreams* that Freud was still using the drug in 1895.

The existence of Freud's writings on cocaine is well-known. Yet, few modern readers have had an opportunity to study any of his papers, despite the many glowing descriptions of his initial review. With the exception of an abstracted translation of *"Ueber Coca"* ("On Coca") which appeared as ("Coca") in *The Saint Louis Medical and Surgical Journal* in December 1884, the papers were unavailable in English and lay scattered in the prolix German literature of the 1880s. In 1963, they were translated into English, read through by Freud's translator, Mr. James Strachey, and published in Vienna by the Dunquin Press.[1] This, as far as I am able to ascertain, was their first appearance in such a form. Because of the obscurity of the edition, however, Freud's cocaine papers were again fated to disappear—even the historical library at the Yale University School of Medicine did not list the Dunquin Press edition, *The Cocaine Papers*, in its catalog.

When first I read the papers, I at once realized that they establish Sigmund Freud as one of the founders of psychopharmacology. I passed on a copy of "On Coca" to Dr. J.M. Ritchie, former Chairman of the Department of Pharmacology at Yale and author of the section on cocaine in the definitive pharmacological textbook, *The Pharmacological Basis of Therapeutics* by Louis Goodman and Alfred Gilman.[2] His immediate reaction was that it is a brilliant review, as up-to-date today as when first published.

Past interest has focused on two aspects of Freud's involvement with cocaine: first, the question of priority in the discovery of local anesthesia and, second, Freud's "mistaken" advocacy of the drug as a catholicon or panacea. Both have been covered thoroughly in Ernest Jones' biography, *The Life and Work of Sigmund Freud,* Siegfried Bernfeld's review, and Hortense Koller Becker's summary, the latter being primarily concerned with the history as it relates to Mrs. Becker's father, Carl Koller, and his discovery of the uses of cocaine as a local anesthetic. These three manuscripts appear in this book along with Freud's personal letters and other writings on cocaine (from *An Autobiographical Study* and *The Interpretation of Dreams*) to provide an integral human and historical backdrop for the scientific papers, all of which are included in full. The relationship between Freud's use of cocaine and the development of psychoanalysis was considered by Vom Scheidt in a recent review.[3]

COCAINE PAPERS, then, is a complete chronicle of Freud's involvement with cocaine and a commentary on a well–known but little– understood segment of medical history. It is also, by necessity, a history of the alkaloid cocaine, since its first isolation from the coca leaf in 1855 to the end of the 19th Century. Past that point, the history of cocaine as a centrally–active drug passes into the realm of law, sociology, and drug abuse. Cocaine has been largely supplanted in medicine today by the synthetic local anesthetics and scientific interest now centers primarily on its biochemical actions and central excitatory effects. Therefore, I would like to here concentrate on Freud's largely unappreciated contribution to psychopharmacology and the continued obfuscation of the central effects of cocaine.

The use of drugs for euphoriant and psychedelic effects has been recorded from the very beginnings of history. The Bible and the heroic myths contain numerous references to psychotropic substances. Two fascinating sources for further reading in this area are the remarkable *Phantastica*[4] by Louis Lewin, a contemporary and adversary of Freud, and the National Institute of Mental Health publication, *The Ethnopharmacological Search for Psychoactive Drugs* (1967).[5]

The history of psychopharmacology (a term coined in 1920 by the American pharmacologist, David Macht) evolved along two paths: research into drugs which could modify normal thinking and behavior, and research into the relief of mental illness by means of drugs. These are of necessity interrelated because both have the physical or biochemical nature of disordered thought as their basic axiom. Until a comprehensive theory of developmental psychology could be synthesized, the idea of "organic" causes of mental illness was the only possible conception. Freud, of course, is best remembered for his monumental contributions to psychological theory but, since it now seems likely that both psychological and biological theories of mental illness will coexist, consideration of Freud's biological contribution is particularly appropriate.

The idea that a sedative drug might be useful in the treatment of mental illness is an old one, and Freud notes this in "On Coca": "It is a well known fact that psychiatrists have an ample supply of drugs at their disposal for reducing the excitation of nerve centers but none which could serve to increase the reduced functioning of the nerve centers." He describes the experiments of Morselli and Buccola in the treatment of melancholia with cocaine, experiments which met with little success, and then states that the "efficacy of coca in cases of nervous and psychic debility needs further investigation." Ninety years later, this statement still holds true.

In 1845, J. J. Moreau de Tours presented a comprehensive theory of psychosis based on a model of hashish intoxication. This work, only recently translated (1973),[6] was the forerunner of the mescaline and LSD "model" psychoses, also advocated as prototypes for an organic or toxic theory of psychosis. Though, at higher dose levels, cocaine can produce a paranoid psychosis, Freud, at least at the time of his studies, missed the importance of this effect. He did note in a letter to Sandor Ferenczi in 1916, that cocaine, "if taken to excess," could produce paranoid symptoms, and that cessation of the drug could have the same effect. (He then added that, altogether, drug addicts were not very suitable for psychoanalysis because every backsliding or difficulty in the therapy led to further recourse to the drug.) Freud was of course interested in finding a treatment for psychosis and depression, this being one reason for his interest in cocaine, but it was left to modern writers, describing amphetamine psychosis, to propose the psychotogenic effect of cocaine as a model for naturally-occurring psychoses. Cocaine is of particular interest because its effects can serve as a model of illness and, also, because it could serve as a model for treatment.

Freud's importance in the history of psychopharmacology does not rest, however, only on his elegant review of the existing literature and his suggestions for therapy, as presented in his paper "On Coca." Most significant of all is his brief paper, published in January 1885, "A Contribution to the Knowledge of the Effect of Cocaine," a study which confirms Freud's role as one of the founders of modern psychopharmacology.

The first point of importance is that Freud, after coming upon a drug with unique pharmacological properties, was not satisfied with merely reviewing the human and animal experimentation which had been done up to that time. Rather, he immediately set out to demonstrate the psychopharmacological properties of the substance. Indeed, the drug had been studied several years earlier. In 1880, von Anrep had investigated the pharmacology of cocaine in experiments with animals. But Freud worked with a purified substance and made careful recordings of his experiments—on himself. He used the most sophisticated measuring instruments available in order to obtain the most accurate possible psychophysiologic measures, and then correlated these simultaneously with carefully-described changes in mood and perception during the course of action of the drug. These experiments established appropriate dosage and a time course of the drug's action—a critical relationship in human experimentation.

A comparison with the reports of any of the modern experiments with psychoactive drugs, including those undertaken with LSD, mescaline, and other psychedelic compounds, shows that Freud's paper established a tradition in the reporting of substances with psychoactive properties. Perhaps the best known of the modern experimenters is Albert Hofmann who, in 1943, discovered the central effects of lysergic acid diethylamide (LSD). After first accidentally ingesting a small amount of LSD, Hofmann then took it deliberately and described the effects as follows:

> I decided to conduct some experiments on myself with the substance in question. I started with the lowest dose that might be expected to have any effect, i.e., 0.25 mg LSD. The notes in my laboratory journal read as follows:

April 19, 1943: Preparation of an 0.5% aqueous solution of d-lysergic acid diethylamide tartrate.
  4:20 P.M.: 0.5 cc (0.25 mg LSD) ingested orally. The solution is tasteless.
  4:50 P.M.: no trace of any effect.
  5:00 P.M.: slight dizziness, unrest, difficult in concentration, visual disturbances, marked desire to laugh ...
At this point the laboratory notes are discontinued: The last words were written only with great difficulty. I asked my laboratory assistant to accompany me home as I believed that I should have a repetition of the disturbance of the previous Friday. While we were cycling home, however, it became clear that the symptoms were much stronger than the first time. I had great difficulty in speaking coherently, my field of vision swayed before me, and objects appeared distorted like images in curved mirrors. I had the impression of being unable to move from the spot, although my assistant told me afterwards that we had cycled at a good pace.... Once I was at home the physician was called.
  By the time the doctor arrived, the peak of the crisis had already passed. As far as I remember, the following were the most outstanding symptoms: vertigo, visual disturbances; the faces of those around me appeared as grotesque, colored masks; marked motoric unrest, alternating with paralysis; an intermittent heavy feeling in the head, limbs and the entire body, as if they were filled with lead; dry, constricted sensation in the throat; feeling of choking; clear recognition of my condition, in which state I sometimes observed, in the manner of an independent neutral observer, that I shouted half insanely or babbled incoherent words. Occasionally I felt as if I were out of my body.
  The doctor found a rather weak pulse but an otherwise normal circulation.... Six hours after ingestion of the LSD my condition had already improved considerably. Only the visual disturbances were still pronounced. Everything seemed to sway and the proportions were distorted like the reflections in the surface of moving water. Moreover, all objects appeared in unpleasant, constantly changing colors, the predominant shades being sickly green and blue. When I closed my eyes, an unending series of colorful, very realistic and fantastic images surged in upon me. A remarkable feature was the manner in which all acoustic perceptions (e.g., the noise of a passing car) were transformed into optical effects, every sound evoking a corresponding colored hallucination constantly changing in shape and color like pictures in a kaleidoscope. At about one o'clock I fell asleep and awoke next morning feeling perfectly well.[7]

If you study this passage you will find many resemblances in style to Freud's descriptions of cocaine effects. Hofmann, like Freud, maintains a careful awareness of what was happening to him, detailing the psychological effects over the course of a precise period of time. Hofmann was, of course, also following J. J. Moreau de Tours' example in the reporting of experimental intoxications. In 1967, Holmstedt described Moreau's 1845 experiments as follows:

> No criticism can be made of his investigative procedures. Moreau took hashish himself. Thanks to the singular property of the substance to keep intact "consciousness and the innermost feeling" of the user, he could analyze all his impressions and in a way be aware of the disorganization of all his mental faculties. In order to complete this internal observation of himself, he also commissioned the persons surrounding him to note carefully his words, acts, gestures and the expression of his face. The results were very characteristic. They fully justified the name of "fantasia" which the Oriental imagination gives to the intoxication with Kief, one of the many names for hashish. Moreau desired, moreover, "controls with other people." He turned to his pupils and with enthusiastic curiosity they lent themselves to experiments with hashish in the most varying doses, giving exact accounts of what they experienced. Moreau observed with scrupulous care every (external) symptom during the course of intoxication. The two series were compared and full conformity was proved.[8]

The discovery of amphetamine, a drug very similar to cocaine in its central actions, bears comparison to Freud's experimentation with cocaine. Gordon Alles, in 1935, was interested in developing an orally–effective compound similar to ephedrine, a drug used in the treatment of allergies. Dr. Alles, again as part of the great tradition, ingested each of the compounds he manufactured to study their central effects. He stated:

> Subjective observations of alertness and antisleep effects upon myself were then being primarily relied upon for central nervous system activity evaluations.... Ephedrine was the primary reference standard for oral sympathomimetic activities. I therefore proceeded to take dosages that were related to the effects I knew of ephedrine upon myself, mainly, that, at that time, I was quite well calibrated with 50 mg doses of ephedrine and with similar doses of amphetamine.[9]

Alles swallowed many compounds related to amphetamine. Here is his account of an experiment with one of them.

To evaluate the effects of 3,4-methylenedioxy-amphetamine, I took 0.4 mg./kg. of the hydrochloride by mouth. This was a total dosage of 36 mg. During the following 2 hours, I observed no noticeable change in blood pressure or heart rate, and, subjectively, I felt nothing comparable to the effects of amphetamine within the same period of time. Consequently, I raised the dosage and proceeded to take, after 2 hours, a dosage of 1 mg./kg., or a total of 90 mg. additionally. Within a few minutes, I realized that a notable subjective response was going to result; I began to feel different quite promptly. Within 20 minutes, the systolic and diastolic blood pressure levels had increased by about 25 mm.; the nose and throat became dry; and I became subjectively attentive. A feeling of "jitteryness" developed, with some muscular tremor, resembling that following an adequate dosage of epinephrine (about 1 mg.), taken intramuscularly.

Forty-five minutes after the second dosage of the methylenedioxy-amphetamine salt, when I was seated in a room by myself, not smoking, and where there was no possible source of smoke rings, an abundance of curling gray rings were readily observed in the environment whenever a relaxed approach to subjective observation was used. Visually, these had complete reality; and it seemed quite unnecessary to test their properties because it was surely known and fully appreciated that the source of the visual phenomena could not be external to the body.

When I concentrated my attention on the details of the curling gray forms by trying to note how they would be affected by passing a finger through their apparent field, they melted away. Then, when I relaxed again, the smoke rings were there. I was as certain they were really there as I am now sure that my head is on top of my body.

Walking required unusual concentration and was accompanied by a subjective awareness of muscular-movement detail and a feeling of unsteadiness. The muscles of my neck became markedly tensed periodically, and I tended to close my jaws tightly and grind my back teeth. Headache was not noted at any time. My gums were white and contracted.

The pupils were markedly dilated, and I could observe details of objects in view at a distance to a remarkable degree. Visual accommodation, however, was slowed. The arteries in the eyegrounds were notably contracted. No hallucinatory colors in any form were observed, nor was there any notable relative change in the observation of colors in the environment. There was a subjective feeling of pressure in the ears. Sound perceptions were most remarkably clear and apparent. Minor sounds, such as the scuffing of shoes as people walked, were clearly distinguishable, even at a great distance and in the presence of a louder background, such as street-car noises and other traffic sounds.

From these descriptions we can see that although Freud may have been one of the earlier investigators to evaluate scientifically the effects of a drug on himself and to describe its central symptoms, he was by no means the last. This method is traditional throughout the scientific study of psychoactive drugs. But, at the same time, Freud was perfectly aware of the weaknesses of some of his experiments. He stated:

> I realize that such self observations have the shortcoming, for the person engaged in conducting them, of claiming two sorts of objectivity for the same thing. I had to proceed in this manner for reasons beyond my control and because none of the subjects at my disposal had such regular reactions to cocaine.

Here, Freud's scientific acumen is apparent by his selection of a *trained* subject to make observations, even though the subject was himself. He must first be an objective reporter of the symptoms and second an objective interpreter of the report. The principle of using trained observers of drug effects is perhaps best exemplified in the series of studies of centrally–active drugs done at the Narcotic Addiction Research Center in Lexington, Kentucky. A familiarity with and a sensitivity to the changes produced by a drug will, in the long run, produce a more accurate description of the complete psychological syndrome that is characteristic of that drug.

Freud shows himself to have been a far more astute observer than many other physicians of his time. He was correct in his prompt classification of cocaine as *both* a central nervous system stimulant and a euphoriant. In contrast to this, Schroff in the 1880s and Louis Lewin in *Phantastica* in 1924, classed cocaine exclusively among the *euphorica,* "sedatives of mental activity . . . substances [which] diminish or even suspend the functions of emotion and perception in their widest sense; sometimes reducing or suppressing, sometimes conserving consciousness, inducing in the person concerned a state of physical and mental comfort." Lewin included morphine, codeine and cocaine in this group, thereby furthering a classification of psychoactive drugs which was used in the original formulation of our narcotics laws. Although cocaine is a euphoriant in low doses, it must, as best we know by all the usual pharmacological tests, be also classed as a stimulant of the central nervous system. Lewin categorized this group as the *exitantia,* or mental stimulants, including caffeine, betel and other substances. Cocaine appropriately belongs in this group and, in a modern classification of psychoactive drugs, is grouped with both amphetamine and caffeine.

Freud's one experimental study is careful in its presentation and contains several significant observations. He accurately states, in discussing the increase in motor power which he observed with cocaine:

> I do not consider the cocaine action itself to be a direct one—possibly on the motor nerve substance or on the muscles—but indirect, effected by an improvement of the general state of well-being. Two facts support this view; muscular energy increases most obviously after taking cocaine when cocaine euphoria has developed but before the total quantity can be absorbed into the circulation; and motor power increases considerably if the cocaine takes effect when the general condition is poor and motor power diminished. In this case, results achieved under the influence of cocaine even exceed the maximum under normal conditions.

The specific observation that cocaine seemed of most effect in a tired person is paralleled by the modern observation that amphetamine increases performance primarily in tired people functioning at a decreased level of performance.

In summary, Freud's paper is lucidly written and pioneers the critical relationship between physiological effect and mental effect, relative to the time course of action of a central nervous system stimulant. "A Contribution to the Knowledge of the Effect of Cocaine" is one of the earliest examples of a scientific paper on a psychoactive drug to clearly make these points. Viewed in this light, Ernest Jones' statement that the paper "is of interest as being the only experimental study Freud ever published," and his further comment that "its rather dilletante presentation shows that this was not his real field. The ideas are all good, but the facts are recorded in a somewhat irregular and uncontrolled fashion that would make them hard to correlate with anyone else's observations" are obviously short-sighted. The paper is of far more interest and significance than he perceived.

But Freud's contribution to pharmacology did not stop with his experimental observations. In a quoted report dated August 9, 1885, giving an opinion on Parke's cocaine, Freud examines the pharmacological equivalence of two different brands of cocaine. To be concerned with generic equivalence in the year 1885 was really quite remarkable. The reasons for his concern were the same as those for similar concern today—the price. He was distressed by the exorbitant cost of the Merck preparation which had been introduced into Europe. In establishing the equivalence of Parke Davis cocaine to Merck cocaine he evaluated their psychoactive equivalence, and did a series of experiments on animals to show that in equal doses the same effects were produced. He comments on the chemical characteristics of the drugs, observing a slight difference in taste between the two preparations. It is significant that this report was the forerunner of the many comparable articles on generic equivalence in the modern pharmacological literature.

Thus, all of Freud's papers on cocaine can be said to be thorough in their review, accurate in their physiological and psychological experimentation, and almost prescient in their consideration of points which have become major issues in modern psychopharmacology. Perhaps the latter is best exemplified by an examination of present–day theories on depression.

It is believed that certain depressions are biologically determined, the result of a biochemical abnormality which is characterized by a deficiency of the hormonal neurotransmitter, norepinephrine, at the nerve endings. This "catecholamine theory of depression," first proposed by Jacobson in 1964, is one of the keystones of modern biological psychiatry. We now know that one way in which cocaine exerts its action and can cause "stimulation" is by preventing the norepinephrine, which is released at nerve endings, from being inactivated, though this does not fully explain the drug's action. One interesting test of the catecholamine theory of depression, therefore, would be to try cocaine in the treatment of depressed patients to determine whether or not it has an antidepressant effect.

Like amphetamine, cocaine can cause euphoria and, as Freud reported, can have an antidepressant effect through this action in mild or neurasthenic depression. Whether or not cocaine has an antidepressant effect in biological depressions has not yet been determined. Only one paper in the modern psychopharmacological literature has examined this possibility; it reported that no antidepressant effects of cocaine were found. If this conclusion is supported by further study, a revision of the catecholamine theory may be required. In this respect, one must consider that, in testing for the biological antidepressant effects of a stimulant and euphoriant agent, Freud was ninety years ahead of his time.

Was Freud unique when, after discovering the pleasurable psychological effects of a drug, he advocated its general use while tending to ignore its inherent dangers? Retrospectively, Freud can be seen as the forerunner of a long line of psychopharmacologists. To experiment with potentially psychoactive agents on oneself, and then proceed to advertise them to friends, is a well–established tradition which continues to this day. It is not, by any means, peculiar to the youth culture but, rather, almost a behavioral norm among scientists working in the area of psychoactive drugs. And making statements which advertise the innocuousness and the pleasures of centrally–active drugs has never been limited to scientists. In *The Doors of Perception,* Aldous Huxley wrote:

> ... to most people mescaline is almost completely innocuous. Unlike alcohol, it does not drive the taker into the kind of uninhibited action which results in brawls, crimes of violence and traffic accidents. A man under the influence of mescaline quietly minds his own business. Moreover, the business he minds is an experience of the most enlightening kind, which does not have to be paid for (and this is surely important) by a compensatory hangover. Of the long–range consequences of regular mescaline taking, we know very little. Indians who consume peyote buttons* do not seem to be physically or morally degraded by that habit. However, the available evidence is still scarce and sketchy.[10]

This was written in 1954, seventy years after "On Coca." But the author's sentiments on the virtues of a centrally–active drug, and its safe use by a native population, echo very clearly Freud's view of cocaine. Initially, Freud may have been alone in Europe in advocating cocaine's virtues, but he had many colleagues of similar persuasion in the United States. An examination of advertisements for coca

---

* Mescaline is the pharmacologically active principle of the peyote cactus.

in the American medical journals gives a fair idea of the acceptance of the drug at that time.

David Musto has described the use of cocaine in the United States of the 1880s as follows:

Cocaine achieved popularity in the United States as a general tonic, for sinusitis and hay fever, and as a cure for the opium, morphine, and alcohol habits. Learned journals published accounts which just avoided advising unlimited intake of cocaine. Medical entrepreneurs such as the neurologist William Hammond, former Surgeon General of the Army, swore by it and took a wineglass of it with each meal. He was also proud to announce cocaine as the official remedy of the Hay Fever Association, a solid endorsement for anyone. Sigmund Freud is perhaps the best-remembered proponent of cocaine as a general tonic and an addiction cure. He wrote several articles in the European medical press on the wonderful substance to which his attention had been drawn by American medical journals.

In the United States the exhilarating properties of cocaine made it a favorite ingredient of medicine, soda pop, wines, and so on. The Parke Davis Company, an exceptionally enthusiastic producer of cocaine, even sold coca-leaf cigarettes and coca cheroots to accompany their other products, which provided cocaine in a variety of media and routes such as a liqueurlike alcohol mixture called Coca Cordial, tablets, hypodermic injections, ointments, and sprays.

If cocaine was a spur to violence against whites in the South, as was generally believed by whites, then reaction against its users made sense. The fear of the cocainized black coincided with the peak of lynchings, legal segregation, and voting laws all designed to remove political and social power from him. Fear of cocaine might have contributed to the dread that the black would rise above "his place," as well as reflecting the extent to which cocaine may have released defiance and retribution. So far, evidence does not suggest that cocaine caused a crime wave but rather that anticipation of black rebellion inspired white alarm. Anecdotes often told of superhuman strength, cunning, and efficiency resulting from cocaine. One of the most terrifying beliefs about cocaine was that it actually improved pistol marksmanship. Another myth, that cocaine made blacks almost unaffected by mere .32 caliber bullets, is said to have caused southern police departments to switch to .38 caliber revolvers. These fantasies characterized white fear, not the reality of cocaine's effects, and gave one more reason for the repression of blacks.[11]

The use of cocaine in conjunction with, or as an alternative to morphine was not limited wholly to America. Sir Arthur Conan Doyle was a reputed user of cocaine, as was his famous detective who used both cocaine and morphine. An extensive comparison of Holmes' and Freud's interests in cocaine is presented in David Musto's "Sherlock Holmes and Sigmund Freud." Holmes' obsession with cocaine is vividly recounted by Watson in the opening paragraphs of *The Sign of Four* (1888):

Sherlock Holmes took his bottle from the corner of the mantelpiece, and his hypodermic syringe from its neat morocco case. With his long, white, nervous fingers he adjusted the delicate needle, and rolled back his left shirt–cuff. For some little time his eyes rested thoughtfully upon the sinewy forearm and wrist, all dotted and scarred with innumerable puncture–marks. Finally, he thrust the sharp point home, pressed down the tiny piston, and sank back into the velvet–lined arm–chair with a long sigh of satisfaction.

Three times a day for many months I had witnessed this performance, but custom had not reconciled my mind to it. On the contrary, from day to day I had become more irritable at the sight, and my conscience swelled nightly within me at the thought that I had lacked the courage to protest. Again and again I had registered a vow that I should deliver my soul upon the subject; but there was that in the cool, nonchalant air of my companion which made him the last man with whom one would care to take anything approaching to a liberty. His great powers, his masterly manner, and the experience which I had had of his many extraordinary qualities, all made me diffident and backward in crossing him.

Yet upon that afternoon, whether it was the Beaune which I had taken with my lunch, or the additional exasperation produced by the extreme deliberation of his manner, I suddenly felt that I could hold out no longer.

'Which is it today,' I asked, 'morphine or cocaine?'

He raised his eyes languidly from the old black–leather volume which he had opened.

'It is cocaine,' he said, 'a seven–per–cent. solution. Would you care to try it?'

'No, indeed,' I answered, brusquely. 'My constitution has not got over the Afghan campaign yet. I cannot afford to throw any extra strain upon it.'

He smiled at my vehemence. 'Perhaps you are right, Watson,' he said. 'I suppose that its influence is physically a bad one. I find it, however, so transcendently stimulating and clarifying to the mind that its secondary action is a matter of small moment.'

'But consider!' I said, earnestly. 'Count the cost! Your brain may, as you say, be roused and excited, but it is a pathological and morbid process, which involves increased tissue–change, and may at last leave a permanent weakness. You know, too, what a black reaction comes upon you. Surely the game is hardly worth the candle. Why should you, for a mere passing pleasure, risk the loss of those great powers with which you have been endowed? Remember that I speak not only as one comrade to another, but as a medical man to one for whose constitution he is to some extent answerable.'

He did not seem offended. On the contrary, he put his finger–tips together, and leaned his elbows on the arms of his chair, like one who has a relish for conversation.

'My mind,' he said, 'rebels at stagnation. Give me problems, give me work, give me the most abstruse cryptogram, or the most intricate analysis, and I am in my own proper atmosphere. I can dispense then with artificial stimulants. But I abhor the dull routine of existence. I crave for mental exaltation. That is why I have chosen my own particular profession, or rather created it, for I am the only one in the world.'

'.... May I ask whether you have any professional inquiry on foot at present?'

'None. Hence the cocaine. I cannot live without brain–work. What else is there to live for? Stand at the window here. Was ever such a dreary, dismal, unprofitable world? See how the yellow fog swirls down the street and drifts across the dun–coloured houses. What could be more hopelessly prosaic and material? What is the use of having powers, Doctor, when one has no field upon which to exert them? Crime is commonplace, existence is commonplace, and no qualities save those which are commonplace have any function upon earth.'[12]

In response to Watson's questions as to how the detective might have benefited from the successful conclusion of the saga, *The Sign of Four*, we find that in the book's last lines Holmes is back to where he had begun the adventure:

'The division seems rather unfair,' I remarked. 'You have done all the work in this business. I get a wife out of it, Jones gets the credit; pray what remains for you?'

'For me,' said Sherlock Holmes, 'there still remains the cocaine–bottle.' And he stretched his long, white hand up for it.

Parallels between the psychotogenic effects of amphetamines and cocaine are frequently drawn. As such, Doyle's paragraphs are often used by modern psychiatric writers to demonstrate the compulsive, intensely curious and preoccupied symptoms common to "speed freaks."

To extend the company in which Freud finds himself, one must consider the case of Dr. William Halsted, the leading surgeon at the Johns Hopkins School of Medicine, and the discoverer of nerve block anesthesia with cocaine. Halsted reversed the pattern which had been followed by Fleischl under Freud's guidance, of attempting to cure morphine addiction with cocaine. A cocaine user and clearly an abuser, he turned to morphine as a cure. Edward Brecher describes his involvement with cocaine:

> Perhaps the most remarkable case was that of Dr. William Stewart Halsted (1852–1922), one of the greatest of American surgeons. Halsted, the scion of a distinguished New York family, and captain of the Yale football team, entered the practice of medicine in New York in the 1870s and soon became one of the promising young surgeons of the city. Interested in research as well as in performing operations, he was among the first to experiment with cocaine—a stimulant drug similar to our modern amphetamines. With a small group of associates, Halsted discovered that cocaine injected near a nerve produces *local anesthesia* in the area served by that nerve. This was the first local anesthetic, and its discovery was a major contribution to surgery.
>
> Unfortunately, Halsted had also injected cocaine into himself numerous times. "Cocaine hunger fastened its dreadful hold on him," Sir Wilder Penfield, another famed surgeon, later noted. "He tried to carry on. But a confused and unworthy period of medical practice ensued. Finally he vanished from the world he had known. Months later he returned to New York but, somehow, the brilliant and gay extrovert seemed brilliant and gay no longer."
>
> What had happened to Halsted during the period of his disappearance? A part of the secret was revealed in 1930, eight years after his death. Then Halsted's closest friend, Dr. William Henry Welch, one of the four distinguished founders of the Johns Hopkins Medical School, stated that he (Welch) had hired a schooner and, with three trusted sailors, had slowly sailed with Halsted to the Windward Islands and back in order to keep Halsted away from cocaine.
>
> In 1969, however, on the occasion of the eightieth anniversary of the opening of the Johns Hopkins Hospital, a "small black book closed with a lock and key of silver" was opened for the first time. This book contained the "secret history" of the Hopkins written by another of its four eminent founders, Sir William Osler. Sir William revealed that Halsted had cured his cocaine habit by turning to morphine.[13]

I have also included an 1887 article by another distinguished proponent of cocaine, Dr. William A. Hammond, retired Surgeon General of the Army, who had previously been court–martialled by Lincoln. In it, he describes, as had Freud, the effects of varying doses of cocaine on himself. He too was clearly resistant to any idea of the dangers of the drug.

Freud, himself, never got into as much trouble with cocaine as some of the other early experimenters with the drug. He was, however, widely accused of attempting to popularize what A. Erlenmeyer at one point called, "the third scourge of mankind." What then can we say about Freud's recommendations for cocaine in the treatment of many diseases, and particularly in the treatment of morphine addiction? We now know, as Louis Lewin knew in 1885, that cocaine is no cure for the morphine (or heroin) habit. Lewin, in an attack on Freud, stated at that time:

> I want to state explicitly that according to all available evidence coca is no substitute for morphine and that a morphine addiction cannot be cured by the use of coca. . . .
> I am convinced that coca cannot be a substitute for morphine for any length of time since the real morphine addict wants the specific morphine effect and since he can very well distinguish the euphoria of other substances. Such an exchange does not suit his special needs. The morphinist wants more than the euphoria which can be brought about in normal man and which Freud experienced himself when taking 0.05–0.1 gr. cocaine hydrochloride.
> However, even if it were possible to treat a morphine addict for a time exclusively with cocaine and even if he were given very large doses producing hallucinations and a pleasant sopor, there would very likely occur a case of what I would like to call double addiction. The man in question would use cocaine in addition to morphine in the same way as many morphine addicts use chloroform, chloralhydrate, ether, etc.[14]

In his last paper, "Craving for and Fear of Cocaine" (1887), Freud attempts to clarify his position. He had, after all, based his original opinions about the efficacy of cocaine as a cure for morphinism on evidence in the American medical literature. In this paper, he lays great emphasis on the dangers of injection of cocaine, despite his earlier advocacy of this method of administration. Here, he had obviously made a judgmental error in not recognizing the abuse potential inherent in cocaine. He could treat "morphinism" with cocaine, but only at the risk of creating what Lewin called a "double addiction." Later, Freud insisted that addiction or abuse of cocaine was never found as a phenomenon in itself but, rather, only occurred among people who had previously been morphine addicts. This defense, untrue as it is, is very reminiscent of a statement made many years later by Frank M. Berger, the discoverer of meprobamate (Miltown), in denying the possibility that meprobamate is an addicting drug:

... Many millions of persons have been taking drugs such as meprobamate for long periods of time. Yet, only very few people have misused these drugs. Invariably, the people who have abused meprobamate or chlordiazepoxide have had a long prior history of dependence on alcohol, barbiturates or the opiates. This indicates that abuse of antianxiety agents when it occurs is more likely to be due to some personality characteristic of the abuser and not to some attributes of these drugs.[15]

As we can see, the continuing hope that a useful centrally–active drug will not be abused did not end with Freud. In fact, it is quite common to find that initial use of a euphoriant drug causes its proponents to make enthusiastic claims that it is either non–addictive or that it will not be abused. Perhaps the two most frightening examples of drugs which were claimed by their discoverers not to have abuse potential are heroin and meperidine (Demerol). Little need be said about heroin; it has now replaced morphine as the leading drug of addiction. Meperidine, similar to morphine in almost all its characteristics, was for a long time thought to be free of morphine's undesirable addicting properties. Because of this misconception, many physicians and nurses became addicted to it. Only recently has meperidine been recognized as having a serious potential for abuse.

In summary then, it can be said that Freud's work on cocaine was pioneering in many respects; that the errors he made in judgment and advocacy of the drug were mistakes that have since been made by many persons who have worked with centrally–active drugs; and that the difficulties he created for himself by his advocacy were relatively minor when compared to the importance of his introduction of a systematic scientific methodology into the study of centrally–active drugs. As Daniel Freedman said in 1969, "I am not sure what [was] meant about Freud being right or wrong since he is always both."

What, then, are the pharmacological effects of cocaine? Strangely enough, there has been almost no recent research into the effects of cocaine on man. Even the literature of recent years on the effect of cocaine as a local anesthetic is sparse. If a search is made for articles about cocaine's psychopharmacological effects, no papers are to be found at all. The most recent edition of *The Pharmacological Basis of Therapeutics* (1970) does not give a single reference in the literature to document the central effects of cocaine in man. And the description of its effects matches Freud's. In 1970, a symposium on psychotomimetic agents ended as follows:

Dr. Larry Stein: "[Cocaine is] almost the perfect tricyclic antidepressant since it has a potent inhibitory effect on reuptake of norepinephrine without any receptor blocking action ... cocaine should theoretically be a good antidepressant, but we heard that from Freud eighty years ago." Dr. Efron: "This will conclude the general discussion...."[16]

The conclusion on this abrupt note may have signified an emotional attitude to cocaine that is worth examining.

The reasons for lack of research are perhaps imbedded in a moralistic viewpoint toward euphoriant drugs which pervades even the most liberal commentators on the drug scene. A fear seems to exist that, if we admit that a drug is pleasure–producing, there will be an epidemic of the drug's use and, because of that, we must take responsibility for any ill–effects caused by the drug. This situation is reminiscent of those events which occurred in Freud's time. Even his sympathetic biographer, Ernest Jones, deplores "The Cocaine Episode," viewing it as a foolhardy adventure, quite lacking in scientific merit. Freud, himself, lent credence to such criticisms by his evasion and confusion of the issue.

Brecher, in discussing cocaine and its control, says about cocaine and amphetamines, "these twin drugs must be considered together. In general, the less said about them the better." In his advice to users he says, "they should be taken orally if at all. The *injection* of amphetamines or cocaine in large doses constitutes one of the most damaging forms of drug use known to man." There is a very familiar ring to these words, written in 1972; they echo those heard in 1884.

What is the evidence for such cautionary statements? High or repeated doses of cocaine almost certainly cause a psychosis similar to that which occurs with amphetamine. Controlled experiments such as have been done with amphetamine have not yet been done with cocaine. Uncontrolled patient reports are common.

There are, however, other drugs which cause psychoses in high doses. Some of these, such as the delirium–inducing drugs (atropine is an example) cause a psychosis which involves a disorientation, an impairment in memory, and a severe impairment in judgment. These psychoses obviously can be dangerous to the individual. There is, however, something peculiar about the amphetamine or cocaine psychosis which makes it particularly frightening because the person under the influence of high doses of cocaine may believe that people are "out to get him" and so lives in a constant fear, ready to attack others or to defend himself. There is a feeling among people working in the field of drug abuse that "speed freaks" and cocaine–users who have been taking large doses represent a danger not only to themselves but to others. The limited literature on drugs and violence does not, as yet, provide support for this otherwise logical notion. We have good reason to suppose that, in high doses, cocaine is a dangerous drug. It shares this property with the amphetamines and, to a lesser extent, with all drugs that can produce a psychosis. But, is there such unusual danger in the use of cocaine that a relatively liberal author on drug abuse writes, "the less we say, the better"? Jaffe states in *The Pharmacological Basis of Therapeutics,* "while it is commonly assumed that the subjective effects of cocaine are more intense and its abuse potential more significant than those of the amphetamines, reliable evidence for this assumption is difficult to obtain."[17] Since no modern study has been undertaken, one can only go by the reports of its users, their doctors, and certain early literature. Louis Lewin's "Cocainism," a text that originally appeared in German in 1924, gives a good impression of the results of cocaine abuse. Apparently, cocaine, when taken in small doses, produces a uniquely pleasureful euphoria. Freud clearly states this in his letters and in his descriptions of the effects of cocaine on himself. It is this euphoria that has led to widespread use of the drug.

An important difference in dosage exists between the chewing of coca leaves and the consumption of pure cocaine. Although the active ingredient is the same, the higher dose can produce a more varied range of effects. A parallel between coca and cocaine can be drawn with wine and cognac. The effects of a bottle of cognac can be far more impressive and different than the effects of a bottle of wine though the active drug, alcohol, is the same in both instances. The consumption of wine with an infusion of coca leaves, a popular habit in the late 1880s, was a way of consuming small doses of cocaine. Coca–Cola contained cocaine until 1903. The early Coca–Cola was a concoction similar to Mariani's wine, which contained wine and coca. W. Golden Mortimer reported in *Peru: History of Coca* (1901) that Pope Leo XIII, "for years . . . has been supported in his ascetic retirement by a preparation of Mariani's coca.[18] An early advertisement (1890) for Mariani's wine and a quote from its inventor are reproduced here with a subsequent disclaimer; after the 1906 drug laws came into effect, the coca was removed as an active ingredient.

If cocaine in small doses is as helpful and pleasant as its users claim, why then does the drug have such a bad name? Some of the reasons have been suggested above. Because of the euphoric qualities of small doses the danger of its continued use and eventual abuse is extraordinary. Users of the drug spread the word with religious fervor. As one cocaine user, quoted by Lewin, stated, "God is a substance!"

Can cocaine be used and not abused? And, if so, can we say that there are appropriate personal uses for euphoriant drugs? Here we come upon an age–old enigma. There is no such thing as a "bad" drug. People can abuse almost any chemical substance ever invented. Some substances are, however, more subject to abuse than others. For example, although the phenothiazine drugs are central nervous system depressants, they are rarely, if ever, abused; they do not cause a euphoria. On the other hand, central nervous system stimulants such as caffeine, cocaine and amphetamine, and depressants such as barbiturates and alcohol, are frequently abused; they cause euphoria. Our society has chosen alcohol, caffeine and nicotine

"*Mariani Bottle*" *showing Shape and Label.*

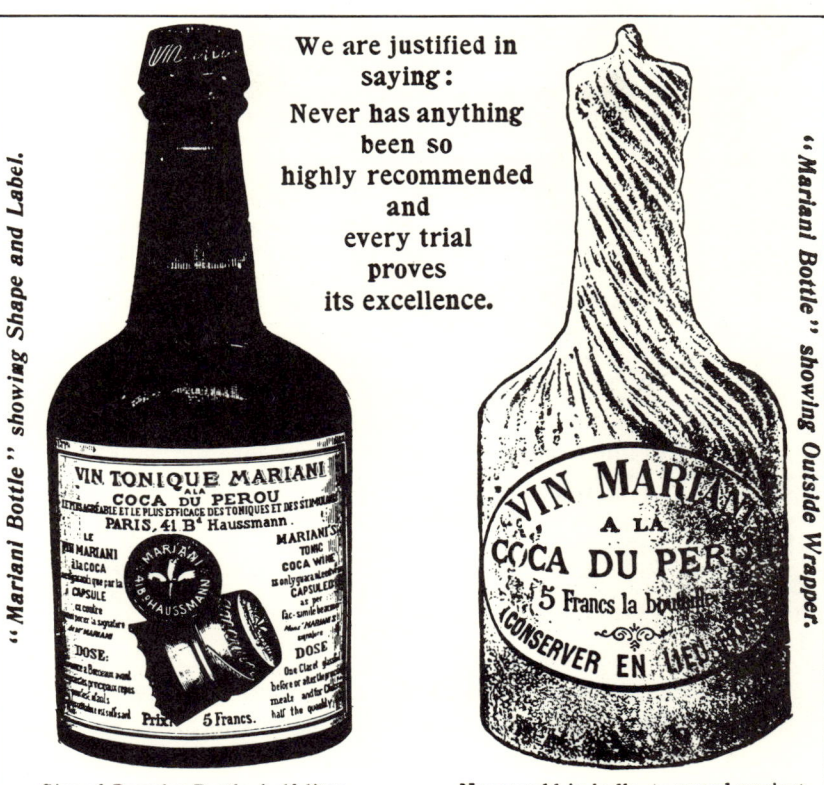

We are justified in saying:

Never has anything been so highly recommended and every trial proves its excellence.

"*Mariani Bottle*" *showing Outside Wrapper.*

Size of Regular Bottle, half litre (about 17 ounces).

Never sold in bulk—to guard against substitution.

VIN MARIANI

Nourishes - Fortifies
Refreshes
Aids Digestion - Strengthens the System.

Unequaled as a tonic-stimulant for fatigued or overworked Body and Brain.

Prevents Malaria, Influenza and Wasting Diseases.

We cannot aim to gain support for our preparation through cheapness; we give a uniform, effective and honest article, and respectfully ask personal testing of **Vin Mariani** strictly on its own merits. Thus the medical profession can judge whether **Vin Mariani** is deserving of the unequaled reputation it has earned throughout the world during more than 30 years.

Inferior, so-called Coca preparations (variable solutions of Cocaine and cheap wines), which have been proven worthless, even harmful in effect, bring into discredit and destroy confidence in a valuable drug.

We therefore particularly caution to specify always " VIN MARIANI," thus we can guarantee invariable satisfaction to physician and patient.

VIN MARIANI NOT A COCAINE PREPARATION.

Regarding the Illinois State Law regulating the sale of Cocaine, it is a pleasure again to have verified in official form, that Vin Mariani is not a cocaine preparation and that the law in no way covers or applies to it. This decision recently rendered is based upon analyses made by Chemists of high professional standing, at request of the Illinois authorities, and confirm former investigations of the Ohio Pure Food Commission, and the Pennsylvania State Board of Health; also conforms with examinations compulsory in Germany, Russia, and with the French Governmental Analysis, a copy of which is attached to each bottle of Vin Mariani, as a guarantee of reliability. Thus the high standard of Vin Mariani established nearly half a century ago, continues unaltered and is a justification for the distinctive and unusual endorsements which physicians everywhere have accorded this unique restorative-tonic.

REWARD OF ONE THOUSAND DOLLARS.

Having learned of certain false statements against the purity of Vin Mariani tending to prejudice and intimidate dealers and users of this preparation, and reflecting upon the intelligence of thousands of reputable physicians who have endorsed Vin Mariani from experience in their practice, we publicly announce that we shall jealously guard and legally protect our interests against all such malicious attacks.

A reward of One Thousand Dollars is offered for information leading to arrest and conviction of any person spreading malicious falsehoods, libelous or defamatory reports intended to discredit the old established reputation of our house or the integrity of Vin Mariana.

41 Boulevard Haussmann, MARIANI & COMPANY,
Paris, France. 52 West Fifteenth St.
  New York

Analysis, Formula and Literature to physicians on request.

as euphoriants—though the alcoholic psychoses are certainly not innocuous. We choose our poisons on the basis of tradition, not pharmacology. Societal attitudes determine which drugs are accepted and the extent to which moral qualities are ascribed to chemicals.

It would be reasonable, though unconventional, to question the strict regulations against the sale and use of cocaine: are they based on its potential for causing dangerous psychosis or are they, in fact, based on a moralistic view towards the enjoyment of chemical substances? Since there are psychotogenic compounds, such as mescaline, which are equally outlawed but not as thoroughly condemned, it seems reasonable to suppose that the attitude of both doctors and lawmakers is to enforce the interdiction of only those substances which, specifically, produce a euphoria. This can either be to prevent overuse and the resultant dangers or, alternatively, to establish a position against the use of any chemical euphoriant other than those which have been specifically sanctioned by our society.

Freud lived at a time when such restrictions were not placed on cocaine. The abuses, which occurred after his studies, were the results of failures in people and the properties of the drug, and not of his popularization of cocaine. I have included some excerpts from a recent book, Richard Woodley's *Dealer: Portrait of a Cocaine Merchant* (1972), which provide an insight into the contemporary world of illicit cocaine. The drug shares effects with many psychedelics that are considered pleasurable by many people. Yet, not only is its use prohibited but there appears to have been a total cessation of investigation into its central effects. This complete lack of responsible experimentation is a striking example of the feelings of moral outrage that have been generated in regard to this substance.

This is another reason why Freud's cocaine papers are pertinent today. In many respects, they are as up–to–date in their review of cocaine as any modern study. Freud's contribution to psychopharmacology thus stands, not only as a pioneering one, but also as one of the most recent studies of the central actions of an extremely important drug.

As I add the last words to this introduction, I have before me a hopeful sign—perhaps one can at last hope for a demystification of cocaine in the years ahead. The National Institute of Drug Abuse has, this week, requested interested investigators to contact them in connection with a proposed series of experiments on the acute effects of cocaine in man. For the reader's interest, I have included the text of this advertisement as an Appendix. Perhaps, ninety years later, Freud's work will be carried forward.

Robert Byck

New Haven
January 1974.

COCAINE PAPERS
By SIGMUND FREUD

I

CHAPTER 1

"The Cocaine Episode,"
PART ONE

From *The Life and Work of Sigmund Freud* by Ernest Jones, M.D.

Ernest Jones was Freud's personally-selected biographer. His three-volume The Life and Work of Sigmund Freud *is a major work, widely considered the definitive Freud biography. Until the publication of the present volume Jones' "The Cocaine Episode" had been the only readily accessible account of Freud's interest in cocaine. Jones' history of this period of Freud's life draws rather heavily on the work of Siegfried Bernfeld and unfortunately repeats many of Bernfeld's errors. Jones' translations of the excerpts from Freud's work are taken from Bernfeld, as are some of the ideas.* Ed.

During the three hospital years Freud was constantly occupied with the endeavor to make a name for himself by discovering something important in either clinical or pathological medicine. His motive was not, as might be supposed, simply professional ambition, but far more the hope of a success that would yield enough prospect of private practice to justify his marrying a year, or possibly two years, earlier than he dared expect in the ordinary course. He must have been very prolific of ideas in his search and in his letters he repeatedly hints at a new discovery which may lead to the desired goal; in the event, none of them did. Unfortunately he gives for the most part only tantalizing glimpses of what the ideas were. The only two he dilates on are the ones that brought him nearest to success: the gold chloride method of staining nervous tissue and the clinical use of cocaine.

As we shall see, the latter case was more than one of the routine efforts and the problems it raises merit the description of it as an episode....

The first we hear of the cocaine topic is in a letter of April 21, 1884, in which he gives news of "a therapeutic project and a hope."

I have been reading about cocaine, the essential constituent of coca leaves which some Indian tribes chew to enable them to resist privations and hardships. A German[*] has been employing it with soldiers and has in fact reported that it increases their energy and capacity to endure. I am procuring some myself and will try it with cases of heart disease and also

---

[*] This refers to an Army doctor, Theodor Aschenbrandt, who had made the observations in question on some Bavarian soldiers during the preceding autumn maneuvers.

of nervous exhaustion, particularly in the miserable condition after the withdrawal of morphium (Dr. Fleischl). Perhaps others are working at it; perhaps nothing will come of it. But I shall certainly try it, and you know that when one perseveres, sooner or later one succeeds. We do not need more than one such lucky hit to be able to think of setting up house. But don't be too sure that it must succeed this time. You know, the temperament of an investigator needs two fundamental qualities: he must be sanguine in the attempt, but critical in the work.[1]

At first he did not expect much would come of the matter: "I dare say it will turn out like the method;* less than I imagined, but still something quite respectable." The first obstacle proved to be the cost of the cocaine he had ordered from Merck of Darmstadt; instead of a gram costing, as he had expected, 33 kreuzer (13 cents) he was dismayed to find it cost 3 gulden 33 kreuzer ($1.27). At first he thought this meant the end of his research, but after getting over the shock he boldly ordered a gram in the hope of being able to pay for it sometime. He immediately tried the effect of a twentieth of a gram; he found it turned the bad mood he was in into cheerfulness and gave him the feeling of having dined well "so that there is nothing at all one need bother about," but without robbing him of any energy for exercise or work. It occurred to him that since the drug evidently acted as a gastric anesthetic, taking away all sense of hunger, it might be useful for checking vomiting from any cause.†

At the same time he decided to offer the drug to his friend Fleischl, who was in the throes of distress in his endeavor to free himself from an addiction to morphia which he had been using to excess because of intolerable nerve pain. It was a decision he bitterly regretted in years to come. The occasion of it was a report he had read in the *Detroit* [Therapeutic] *Gazette* of its use for this purpose. Fleischl clutched at the new drug "like a drowning man"** and within a few days was taking it continually. The rest of the Fleischl story will be told presently.

Freud was now becoming more and more enthusiastic. Cocaine

---
* I.e., the gold chloride method he invented.
† Unpublished letter from Freud to Martha Bernays, dated May 3, 1884.
** Unpublished letter from Freud to Martha Bernays dated May 7, 1884.

was "a magical drug." He had a dazzling success with a case of gastric catarrh where it immediately put an end to the pain.*

If it goes well I will write an essay on it and I expect it will win its place in therapeutics, by the side of morphium and superior to it. I have other hopes and intentions about it. I take very small doses of it regularly against depression and against indigestion, and with the most brilliant success. I hope it will be able to abolish the most intractable vomiting, even when this is due to severe pain; in short it is only now that I feel I am a doctor, since I have helped one patient and hope to help more. If things go on in this way we need have no concern about being able to come together and to stay in Vienna.

He sent some to Martha "to make her strong and give her cheeks a red color," he pressed it on his friends and colleagues, both for themselves and their patients, he gave it to his sisters. In short, looked at from the vantage point of our present knowledge, he was rapidly becoming a public menace. Naturally he had no reason at all to think there was any danger in such proceedings, and when he said he could detect no signs of craving for it in himself, however often he took it, he was telling the strict truth: as we know now, it needs a special disposition to develop a drug addiction, and fortunately Freud did not possess that.†

Some of his colleagues reported success in the use of the drug, others were more doubtful. Breuer, with his characteristic caution, was one of those who was not impressed.

Freud had difficulty in obtaining the literature on this out-of-the-way subject, but Fleischl gave him an introduction to the library of the *Gesellschaft der Ärzte* (Society of Physicians) where he came across the recently published volume of the Surgeon General's catalogue that contained a complete account of it. He was now (June 5) reckoning on finishing the essay in another fortnight and then working on his electrical researches to occupy the remaining four or five weeks before he would be free to go to Wandsbek. He finished it on the

---

* Unpublished letter from Freud to Martha Bernays dated May 25, 1884.
† Jones is in error here since it has been demonstrated that monkeys will press levers and perform hard work to give themselves cocaine. It is unlikely that monkeys have this "special disposition" to which Dr. Jones refers. *Ed.*

eighteenth, and half of it was in print the next day. It appeared in the July number of Heitler's *Centralblatt für die gesammte Therapie*.

The essay, although a comprehensive review of the whole subject—far the best that had yet appeared—might well be ranked higher as a literary production than as an original scientific contribution. It was couched in Freud's best style, with his characteristic liveliness, simplicity, and distinction, features for which he had found little scope when describing the nerves of the crayfish or the fibers of the medulla. It was many years before he again had the opportunity of exercising his literary gifts. There is, moreover, in this essay a tone that never recurred in Freud's writings, a remarkable combination of objectivity with a personal warmth as if he were in love with the content itself. He used expressions uncommon in a scientific paper, such as "the most gorgeous excitement"* that animals display after an injection of cocaine, and administering an "offering"† of it rather than a "dose"; he heatedly rebuffed the "slander" that had been published about this precious drug. This artistic presentation must have contributed much to the interest the essay aroused in Viennese and other medical circles.

He began the essay by going at length into the early history of the coca plant and its use by the South American Indians, then describing it botanically and reciting the various methods of preparing the leaves. He even gave an account of the religious observances connected with its use, and mentioned the mythical saga of how Manco Capac, the Royal Son of the Sun-God, had sent it as "a gift from the gods to satisfy the hungry, fortify the weary, and make the unfortunate forget their sorrows." We learn that the news of the wonderful plant reached Spain in 1569 and England in 1596, how Dr. Scherzer, the Austrian explorer, brought home from Peru in 1859 coca leaves that were sent to Niemann, the assistant of Woehler—the chemist infamous for daring to synthetize urea. It was Niemann who isolated the alkaloid cocaine from the plant.

---

* Jones mistranslates this phrase. The original reads: *freudigsten Aufregung.* *Ed.*

† This is an incorrect translation of the German *Gabe,* in Freud's context meaning a "dose"; clinical usage of the time would not permit a translation of an "offering." *Ed.*

He then narrated a number of self-observations in which he had studied the effects on hunger, sleep, and fatigue. He wrote of the

> exhilaration and lasting euphoria, which in no way differs from the normal euphoria of the healthy person.... You perceive an increase of self-control and possess more vitality and capacity for work.... In other words, you are simply normal, and it is soon hard to believe that you are under the influence of any drug.... Long intensive mental or physical work is performed without any fatigue.... This result is enjoyed without any of the unpleasant after-effects that follow exhilaration brought about by alcohol.... Absolutely no craving for the further use of cocaine appears after the first, or even repeated, taking of the drug; one feels rather a certain curious aversion to it.

Freud confirmed Mantegazza's conclusions about the therapeutic value of the drug, its stimulant and yet numbing action on the stomach, its usefulness in melancholia, and so on. He described a case of his own (Fleischl's) where he had employed cocaine in the process of weaning a morphia addict. The total value of the drug was summed up as applicable in "those functional states comprised under the name of neurasthenia," in the treatment of indigestion, and during the withdrawal of morphine.

As to the theory of its action Freud made the suggestion, since confirmed, that cocaine acts not through direct stimulation of the brain but through abolishing the effect of agencies that depress one's bodily feelings.*

In his final paragraph, written hurriedly, he said:

> The capacity of cocaine and its salts, when applied in concentrated solutions, to anesthetize cutaneous and mucous membranes suggests a possible future use, especially in cases of local infections.... Some additional uses of cocaine based on this anesthetic property are likely to be developed in the near future.

This is the aspect that he subsequently reproached himself with not pursuing, but the view taken here is that this self-reproach was somewhat misplaced. It is not altogether likely that Freud, even with more time at his disposal, would have thought of the surgical appli-

---

* *Gemeingefühl* (coenesthesia).

cation, one foreign to his interests. The local uses he had in mind were concerned only with deadening the pain of cutaneous infections, and when he suggested to his ophthalmological friend Königstein that cocaine could be applied to the eye both of them thought of this in terms of alleviating the pain of trachoma and similar conditions. For Freud cocaine was an analgesic, not an anesthetic, and anyhow he was far more interested in its internal use than in any external application.

Now what evidently fascinated Freud in the coca plant was its extraordinary repute of being able to heighten mental and physical vigor without apparently having any harmful subsequent effect. After all, that had been the whole point of the article by Aschenbrandt which had fired Freud's imagination. But cocaine heightens vigor only when this has been previously lowered; a really normal person does not need the fillip. Freud was not in the latter fortunate position. For many years he suffered from periodic depressions and fatigue or apathy, neurotic symptoms which later took the form of anxiety attacks before being dispelled by his own analysis. These neurotic reactions were exacerbated by the turmoil of his love affair, with its lengthy privation and other difficulties. In the summer of 1884 in particular he was in a state of great agitation before the approaching visit to his betrothed, and by no means only because of the uncertainty about its being possible. Cocaine calmed the agitation and dispelled the depression. Moreover, it gave him an unwonted sense of energy and vigor.

Depression, like any other neurotic manifestation, lowers the sense of energy and virility: cocaine restores it. Any doubt about this being the essence of the matter is dispelled by the following passage from a letter of June 2, 1884, written on hearing that Martha did not look well and had no appetite.

Woe to you, my Princess, when I come. I will kiss you quite red and feed you till you are plump. And if you are froward you shall see who is the stronger, a gentle little girl who doesn't eat enough or a big wild man *who has cocaine in his body.** In my last severe depression I took coca again and a small dose lifted me to the heights in a wonderful

---

* Here italicized.

fashion. I am just now busy collecting the literature for a song of praise to this magical substance.

To achieve virility and enjoy the bliss of union with the beloved, he had forsaken the straight and narrow path of sober "scientific" work on brain anatomy and seized a surreptitious short cut: one that was to bring him suffering in place of success. Within a couple of months another was to attain world fame through cocaine. But that was through a use beneficial to humanity, whereas two years later Freud was to be contemned for having through his indiscriminate advocacy of a "harmless" and wonderful drug introduced what his detractors called the "third scourge of humanity."* Last of all he was to reproach himself for having hastened the death of a dear friend and benefactor by inculcating in him a severe cocaine addiction.

It would be hard not to suffer all these blows without feeling them to be just punishments. For what? The answer to this question we must leave to the psychoanalysts, but at least we can understand why Freud [was later] to associate his self-reproach with the thought of his wife-to-be, and that the excuse he [would later give] of "not being thorough enough" was only a thin hint of what was behind.

All this, however, lay in the future, and Freud, innocent of any inkling of it, went off at the beginning of September to enjoy a happy holiday in Wandsbek. On his return four weeks later he learned that something big had happened.†

---

* The other two being alcohol and morphium.
† This biographical summary is continued in Chapter Three.

CHAPTER 2

Freud's Sources

SPRING 1884

Old Series, Vol. IV.
New Series, Vol. I.   SEPTEMBER, 1880.   No. 9

——— THE ———

Therapeutic Gazette:

A MONTHLY JOURNAL, DEVOTED TO THERAPEUTICS

AND TO

The Introduction of New Therapeutic Agents.

EDITED BY

WM. BRODIE, M. D., and CARL JUNGK, Ph. D.

GEORGE S. DAVIS, Medical Publisher.
P. O. BOX 641, DETROIT, MICHIGAN.

Published on the Fifteenth Day of Every Month.

Erythroxylon Coca in the Opium and Alcohol Habits by W.H. Bentley. *Detroit Therapeutic Gazette.* September 15, 1880.

Erythroxylon Coca as an antidote to the Opium Habit, Editorial. *Detroit Therapeutic Gazette.* June 15, 1880.

Die physiologische Wirkung und Bedeutung des Cocain. muriat. auf den menschlichen Organismus. Klinische Beobachtungen während der Herbstwaffenübungen des Jahres 1883 beim II. Bayer. A.-C. 4. Div. 9. Reg. 2. Bat., gemacht von Dr. Theodor Aschenbrandt in Würzburg, December, 1883.

The Physiological Effect and Significance of Cocaine Muriate on the Human Organism. Clinical Observations during the Fall Maneuvers of the Year 1883 of the II. Bavarian Artillery Company, 4. Division, 9. Regiment, 2. Battalion, by Dr. Theodor Aschenbrandt, Wuerzburg.

Translated by Therese Byck

Although cocaine was yet to be popularized in Europe a considerable literature already existed in both the European and American journals. This chapter presents the critical references which Freud was reading in preparing his new paper, "Über Coca." His reference list was the Index Catalog of the Surgeon General's Office, and his inspiration comes largely from the enthusiasm of Aschenbrandt and Bentley. Ed.

Erythoxylon* Coca in the Opium and Alcohol Habits

By W. H. Bentley, M.D., LL.D., Valley Oak, Ky.[1]

In May, 1878, I wrote an article for *New Preparations* on erythoxylon coca, which was published in the July number of that journal.

The following is the opening paragraph of that article:

A few years since, I procured six or eight pounds of the saturated tincture of erythoxylon coca with a view of testing the virtues of the plant therapeutically. I used all but a single bottle within the course of about fifteen months. All the cases, but one, in which I prescribed it, were those of a chronic character affecting the lungs, and simulating phthisis. The excepted case was one of nervous dyspepsia complicated with uterine troubles and hysteria. The patient was married, the mother of two children, the youngest six months old, while the mother herself was twenty-three years of age. She was greatly emaciated, very despondent, and was, withal, addicted to the "opium habit." It was as a substitute for her accustomed morphine, the use of which I absolutely forbade, that I directed the coca, in drachm doses three times a day. It answered the purpose admirably.

The closing paragraph is as follows: "I shall hereafter give erythoxylon coca a thorough trial in 'wasting diseases,' tardy convalescence from acute maladies, in certain forms of dyspepsia; and carefully test it in the 'opium habit.'"

This promise I have assiduously kept, intending, when I obtained sufficient data, to report, for the benefit of the profession, the results of my observation. To do so, I consider a duty, and this duty I shall now attempt to perform, premising that I have used the fluid extract

---

* This spelling for "Erythroxylon" was used throughout the original article and has been retained here.

of erythoxylon coca from the well known house of Parke, Davis & Co., of which I have prescribed about twenty-five within two years.

Physiologically and pathologically, I consider the opium habit and the "alcoholic habit" or the inability to abstain from drunkenness, (for I do not know that I have seen the term "alcoholic habit" used), as nearly or quite identical.

In the following remarks, I shall use "opium" for that drug and all its preparations, and "alcohol" for all beverages containing alcohol.

Both opium and alcohol in small quantities are stimulant, carried further, hypnotic, and both, when taken in sufficient quantities, become narcotic poisons capable of producing death. The habitual use of one is contracted just as that of the other, and, when carried to a sufficient extent, becomes irresistible. This is the case, at least, with nearly all the victims.

The victims of either take the accustomed drug for the stimulating effect, which, when carried to a certain degree produces a happy—a kind of ethereal—sensation. When this begins to subside there remains a wretched sinking sensation which calls for another dose, and so on *ad infinitum*. A sufficient continuation of either habit will narcotize the brain, destroy the nervous system, and terminate fatally.

Now, if the victim of either opium or alcohol could find a preparation that would produce his accustomed stimulus without leaving a feeling of depression, he could, with the aid of very little exercise of his will, abandon his vice and regain his normal condition.

In the erythoxylon coca we find that very article, for, while in the proper doses it is capable of producing the most exalted mental feeling, far more ecstatic than anything ever experienced from the use of opium or alcohol, its effects pass away gradually after a few hours, leaving a feeling of buoyant serenity, not to be succeeded by any depression. It was this property of erythoxylon, with which I was familiar, that led me to test it in the case referred to at the head of this article. That was in 1874. As I was not soon after called on to especially treat a case of opium habit, the case passed from my mind until 1878, when circumstances again brought it to memory. Since then I have sought opportunities to try its effects frequently, when learning of a case even in other counties I voluntarily recommend the erythoxylon coca.

I subjoin a few cases:

Miss M., a sprightly, intelligent blonde, age thirty. I had been acquainted with her for thirteen years, and for several years of our early acquaintance, when the family lived near me, was her father's family physician. In June 1878, I accidentally met her on a train. Eight years previous she had a protracted attack of pneumonia, during which she contracted the habit of using morphine which she still retained. These facts were well known to me, so I took occasion to ask her if she had left it off. She replied in the negative and told me that she then required 10 grs. twice a day. She had tried nostrums and had visited some advertising quack in another State, to no purpose. I then suggested the erythoxylon, fully explaining its action. The result was I prescribed a pound for her. I received a note from her when she had used this. She was much encouraged and had ordered two pounds more. This quantity completed the cure. I saw her recently when she assured me that she had no desire for morphine.

Case 2: July 1878, was called to a case some fifteen miles distant and nearly all the way "in the hills." I was quite astonished to find about one tenth of an acre in poppies. On inquiry the lady of the house, a widow, age forty, told me that she was an "opium eater," to use her expression, and that she raised her own opium. From what I could learn she used about half a pound of the drug a year. I persuaded her to give up the habit. She declared that she could not. She agreed, however, to try, so I sent her one half–pound fluid extract coca to begin with. When used, she sent for half the quantity, stating that she thought it would complete the cure. I sent her a half pound. She sent me her opium crop that winter, with the message that the medicine had cured her.

Case 3: An old lady, age seventy-two. Had been addicted to the habit for thirty-five years. I persuaded her to try the coca. She was then taking ½-drachm doses of opium three times a day. She said she felt sure she would be unable to leave off the opium, but as she was wealthy and extravagant, she readily consented to try the coca. She procured two pounds on my prescription, and began its use. The progress of the case is rather amusing. She uses one for a time, and then resorts to the other. Sometimes she does not taste opium for a fortnight, using the coca during the time, then she returns to her opium, and thus she alternates. Her doses of opium have been reduced to as little, I think, as 10 grs., and her general health has greatly improved. Before using the coca, she was a great sufferer from duodenal dyspepsia. She has so far improved, in this respect, that she rarely suffers in this particular, and it is a wonder, too, for she is a ravenous feeder and as fond of "cake and pastry" as a child, and withal, uses a great deal of wine.

Case 4: An unmarried man, age twenty-seven. Contracted the "opium habit" five years previous to using the coca. Had become a great slave to morphine. June 1879, I put him upon coca. He ordered three pounds at the beginning. In October following, I met him and he assured me that he was entirely relieved of the habit, and had one pound of his medicine left.

The above are four cases out of eleven treated within a little more than two years. None of the others were so serious, and all were restored except a young lady, who went west immediately after I prescribed for her, and I have not heard from her since. In fact, I have not learned her address.

I have cured three "drunks" of their pernicious habit, but, as I am extending this article, I shall detail but one.

A medical friend with whom I had once been quite intimate, had contracted intemperate habits. He was not a "constant drinker," but was in the habit of "getting on sprees," as he called it, and could not, after tasting spirituous liquors, refrain from getting beastly drunk and remaining so until he broke completely down. He would then get sober and remain so, laboring with much zeal and success at his professional duties for a period, varying from one to two months, when the desire for whisky would seize him with such irresistible force that he "was bound to yield," as he put it.

I had not met him for six years until October 1878. His intemperate habits had been contracted on the mean time. He told me all and appeared much distressed. I recommended the coca. He returned to his home and wrote me, April, 1879: "I am perfectly cured of the whisky habit, thanks to you and erythoxylon coca, but I can scarcely keep from forming a coca habit, becoming a *'coquero,'* as you called it."

One word as to my mode of using coca. As stated above, it is capable of stimulating to any given extent. Now my plan has been to begin with a drachm dose of the fluid extract, *just* when the desire for opium or whisky is quite urgent, giving in a little water. If this does not produce sufficient stimulus to take the place of the accustomed drug, I repeat in thirty minutes and so on. In this way, I soon find the required dose.

I request the patient to substitute the coca for the opiate or liquor, and, if possible, to abstain entirely from his former bane.

I would not think of giving the erythoxylon in a case of acute opium poisoning.

The Therapeutic Gazette

WM. BRODIE, M. D.
CARL JUNGK, Ph. D.
} Editors.

DETROIT, MICH., JUNE 15, 1880.

GEO. S. DAVIS, Medical Publisher, Box 641.

Erythroxylon Coca as an Antidote to the Opium Habit[2]

The article on this subject in the *Louisville Medical News*, by Professor E. R. Palmer, of the University of Louisville, ... will be read with much interest by the profession. Certainly the success which has thus far attended Dr. Palmer's use of coca justifies the hope that this agent may be found to be an efficient means of relief from the thralldom of opium. If subsequent trials of it shall corroborate Dr. Palmer's expression regarding it many will wonder why the article was not sooner recommended, for does not its physiological action clearly indicate it as a remedy in the condition of the nervous system induced by the long continued abuse of opium?

The use of coca in the opium habit suggests an interesting fact connected with the subject of the introduction of new remedies. Necessarily the knowledge of the therapeutic application of a comparatively untried drug is very limited, and it requires experience in its use to develop its possibilities. In some cases the conditions for which a drug is first recommended are found to afford by no means the best illustrations of its therapeutic properties. Take the case of eucalyptus globulus, for instance. This article was introduced as an anti-intermittent, but although the very extensive trial to which it has been put has established its reputation as an antidote to the malarial poisoning, this experience has shown it to be not less efficient as a remedy in other affections, as catarrh of the bronchopulmonary mucous membrane, chronic desquamative nephritis, chronic catarrh of the bladder, as an antiseptic locally applied in chronic ill-conditioned ulcers, etc. Then again in the case of grindelia robusta. This agent was first spoken of as a remedy in spasmodic asthma, but while its usefulness in this affection is now undeniable, it has been ascertained to be scarcely less serviceable in other affections of the respiratory apparatus, as nervous cough, chronic bronchitis, bronchorrhea, etc.

The lessons furnished by these drugs furnish a strong argument in favor of the reception of new remedies by the educated practitioner. He is by education and through his opportunities especially fitted to develop the possibilities of the recent introductions to the materia medica, and in neglecting to turn his education and facilities in this direction he forfeits an opportunity not only of advancing therapeutics, but of connecting his name with this advancement. Therapeutics is the forte of the American medical profession, and year by year the opinion of our practitioners on the therapeutic properties of drugs is becoming more and more respected abroad. This is an additional reason why they should interest themselves in investigation into the possibilities of the newer remedies.

We hope Dr. Palmer's views on the use of coca in the opium habit will be thoroughly tested. And if it relieves the peculiar nervous condition incident to this habit, it may be found useful in other forms of nervous disturbance. The Louisville Medical News says in referring to Dr. Palmer's paper, "One feels like trying coca, with or without the opium habit. A harmless remedy for the blues is imperial." And so say we.

The Physiological Effect and Significance of Cocaine Muriate on the Human Organism

Clinical Observations during the 1883 Fall Maneuvers of the Second Battalion, Ninth Regiment, Fourth Division, Company II, of the Bavarian Artillery by Dr. Theodor Aschenbrandt, of Wuerzburg[3]

In Volume XXI of the Arch. f. ges. Physiol. for 1880, von Anrep published a remarkable article on the physiological effect of cocaine muriate on animals, based on experimental studies. His work had been undertaken at the Pharmacological Institute in Wuerzburg, where von Anrep had been an assistant not long before my own arrival there. It was therefore inevitable that I should discuss this work with Professor Rossbach, Director of the Institute. Von Anrep states at the end of his study that he had also intended to examine the effect of cocaine muriate on human beings, since his experiments with animals did not lead to practical conclusions. It was my intention to take up and continue von Anrep's work, mainly with human beings, but I did not have at that time—as was probably the case with von Anrep and others—the necessary material to allow confirmation of those observations made by Mantegazza, von Bibra and others. The material required would have been strong and healthy people, exposed to the greatest exertion, hunger, thirst, and the like.

E. von Bibra had already experimented on himself with the physiological effects of coca leaves.[4] According to him, homeopathic doses were sufficient to still hunger, to make a man cheerful and more able to work, and to increase his strength over a period of time to such a degree that greater exertion of all kinds became easily possible. Bibra observed the effect on himself of chewing coca leaves while undertaking exhaustive marches. At first he noted a moderately agreeable taste in his mouth and considerable secretion of saliva, but perceived no noticeable effect on the nervous system. Despite the fact that he was fasting, he easily continued through until the evening and then regained his usual appetite. Von Bibra had no answer as to which substance in the coca leaves might be the primary agent of the effect, though his opinion diverges from that of von Gaedeke, Johnston and von Gorup in this respect. Overall they are agreed however, that this effect of the slowing down of the metabolism belongs to narcotic substances such as caffeine.

A very thorough study of coca leaves, classifying psychic and respiratory euphoriants, was done by Dr. P. Mantegazza.[5] He categorizes coca with the narcotic-alkaloid euphoriants, those that have a powerful effect on the heart and nerve centers, almost all of which increase intellectual capacity to a greater or lesser degree but cause a decrease in sensibility. In his account, the physiological effect of coca—no analysis of the leaves existed at that time—consists of a feeling of general well-being, pleasure in intellectual accomplishment, and a beneficial effect on the digestion, the heart and respiration. The effect on the nervous system of chewing coca is very unique: a feeling of warmth pervades the entire body; one gradually becomes aware of greater nervous strength; one feels stronger, more limber and more capable. But the stages of coca intoxication are different from those of liquor intoxication: in the former, the pleasure consists of an increased consciousness of being alive, greater intelligence, and an awareness of a new bodily strength. It is believed in America that alcohol intoxication can be negated, or at least lessened, by coca. Mantegazza, himself, claims to have observed this on more than one occasion. At the end of his study he outlines the physiological effect of coca in a few sentences, one of which I will quote here as being of most relevance to us: In medium doses, coca stimulates the nervous system in such a way that one becomes more capable of muscular exertion, with significant resistance to the interference of external influences.

Schildbach, who had considered Mantegazza's work in great detail, concludes with the opinion that, even if coca were nothing more than a stimulant and not, improbably, a means of nourishing the nervous system, it still seems to surpass all usual stimulants in harmlessness and agreeability; one surely cannot deny it a certain usefulness.

Haller does not have much to say about coca that is worthy of note, but believes that it significantly decreases tissue loss.[6]

Niemann succeeded in isolating from coca leaves an organic base, cocaine, similar to theine and caffeine, and Fronmueller published experiments which he had undertaken with it in several clinical cases.[7] It was not possible, however, to find confirmation of Mantegazza's study in these, nor in the clinical appendices.

Reiss determined that, after taking coca, he experienced an increase in all mental powers, strengthening of the body under exertion, and a decrease of hunger.[8]

A last, highly detailed study is that of von Anrep, mentioned above; at the end of this piece, however, he concludes that the effect of cocaine and that of coca leaves is not the same. Nevertheless, I feel I must stress that von Anrep used too large doses—von Bibra spoke of homeopathic doses. Furthermore, his preparation must also have differed from mine in that his cocaine is difficult to dissolve in water,* while mine is easily soluble.

My study is intended to demonstrate that the alkaloid of the coca leaf, cocaine, is the substance that possesses the "miraculous" quality described by Mantegazza, Moreno y Maiz, Dr. Unanue, von Tschudi, etc.: that, in small doses, cocaine muriate—as was available to me—makes a man more able to bear great exertion, hunger, and thirst—in fact, that cocaine must be regarded as nourishment of benefit to the nerves.

I do not believe one can make such observations with animals kept in cages. What exertion are they exposed to? How would one study their muscular achievements?

During this year's fall maneuvers I had the opportunity I required: a mass of healthy people, exertion of all kinds, dry, hot weather and, above all, the possibility of administering cocaine without anyone being aware of the fact that he was being observed. This, I believe, is the only way in which objective observations can be made, and the only way in which objective descriptions of the behavior of subjects can be achieved. I administered the substance in very small doses to

---

* According to Lossen, one part cocaine to 704 aq.

appropriate cases, and hereby give my results, with a few observations.

I obtained the cocaine, through the local pharmacist, Mr. R. Landauer, from Merck in Darmstadt, and took with me solutions of 0.01, 0.05, 0.1, 0.5 gr. per gr. of water. I must stress here that it was not possible for me to count the drops singly in each individual case; the individual doses varied from fifteen to twenty drops per dose.

Case 1. T., a Volunteer of one year, collapsed of exhaustion directly upon leaving W. on the second day of a march; the weather was extremely hot. I gave him approximately one tablespoon of water with twenty drops of a cocaine solution (0.5/10). A few minutes later (approximately five), he stood up of his own accord and traveled the distance to H., several kilometers, easily and cheerfully and with a pack on his back. T. made the remark along the way that he must have had too much beer back in K. On asking him if he felt completely well again, he answered that he now felt fresher than he had that morning. I observed no unpleasant effects; he did not complain about the taste. T. was reputed to be a smart soldier.

Unfortunately, I had no opportunity during the following brigade exercises to administer cocaine. However, when the battalion reached the bivouac at P., there were a few more appropriate occasions.

Case 2. Private R., severely wounded in the face during a night attack, had to be brought to E. at 11:30 at night. There was no ice, which I needed so badly, nor did I have any other tranquilizing substance on hand. It would also have been impossible for me to determine the entire extent of the wound by the campfire. But R. had lost a great deal of blood and complained, despite his lack of emotion, of great pain, which ceased however as soon as he received a little cocaine. The sleep he fell into a short time later was restless, but his groaning and moaning gradually stopped, as did his excited manner. I lay down at 1:30 A.M., but could not sleep for all the bugs. I therefore went back to the camp at 3:00 in the morning and add, as *Case 3,* an observation made on myself.

The morning was cool, and I felt rather ill as a result of the exertions and sleeplessness of the night. I was really freezing, my head wasn't together, and the prospect of coming maneuvers was not something to cheer me up. In the camp I immediately drank hot coffee with cocaine; during that entire day I felt neither hunger, thirst, nor drowsiness, and was able to hold out without eating until late afternoon with no trouble. I must specifically stress here that I am used to a very routine life and have gotten out of the habit of exerting myself like this.

Case 4. Private A., ill with jaundice for about eight days, had a stubborn constipation after a major dietary error. I gave him Jalappa powder, to which I added 0.01 cocaine so as to strengthen his nervous system. With the exception of one rainy day, the man marched with the other soldiers in full equipment.

Case 5. K., a Volunteer of one year, was administered cocaine in a solution containing tincture of opium for severe diarrhea. He did not accept my offer that he be placed on a baggage cart, but stayed with his company and told me that, in contrast to other occasions when he had diarrhea, he felt cheerful and strong.

Case 6. My servant, V., arrived at J. before me and had drunk a great deal of water with a friend. After he took care of his chores, he gave me a glass of the same water. However, the water smelled and tasted so foul that I spat it out. V. came to me shortly thereafter, complaining of pain in his gut, pressure and dizziness in the head, and general nausea. The other soldier was complaining too, so I gave both of them some opium with spirit of French wine, with no results. They slept badly that night, and by the next morning they were, if anything, sicker than before. So I let the one return but wished to hold on to my servant, whom I told to remain by the carts and not to carry his pack; at worst, he could always get on a cart. I then put 0.01 cocaine in his morning coffee, and the same amount again about two hours later. V. took part in the march, even though it had rained heavily the night before and people were sinking up to their ankles into the deep clayey soil. This was the day on which the division's exercises against the appointed enemy were to take place. In the morning, V. told me on being asked that he felt warmer and better, his weariness was past, and he hoped to be able to hold out.

In addition to these six published cases, I repeatedly used cocaine with people who complained of exhaustion, particularly after diarrhea, which occurred this year with particular frequency due to the late, rich fruit crop; the results were most satisfactory. I believe I have made the overall observation that the influence of cocaine on the body is more benign than that of the alcohols or of cold coffee.

Finally, let me underline the fact that I maintained the best state of health in the division. With the exception of the wounded soldier and another man who had boils, I had not a single soldier sick in quarters during the entire maneuvers.

I do not wish to underestimate the pressure that a superior officer, and especially a physician, can and should exercise on the morale; but one cannot ascribe everything to that. I firmly believe that a part of the success must, as reported in my cases, be ascribed to the stimulating effect of cocaine.

I hope that with this study, which certainly is not complete nor entirely exact as to dosage and which certainly does not claim to be final proof of the properties of cocaine, I have drawn the attention of the military and inspired them to further research. I believe I have given sufficient evidence of its eminent usefulness.

INDEX-CATALOGUE of THE LIBRARY of the SURGEON-GENERAL'S OFFICE,

UNITED STATES ARMY.

VOL. IV.—1883

Erythroxylon *Coca.*

BAIN (J.) De la coca du Pérou et de ses préparatious; faits relatifs à son action physiologique et thérapeutique. 12°. *Paris*, 1877.

DEMARLE (L.-G.) * Sur la coca. 4°. *Paris*, 1832.

GAZEAU (C.) * Nouvelles recherches expérimentales sur la pharmacologie, la physiologie et la thérapeutique du coca. 4°. *Paris*, 1870.

MORÉNO Y MAÏZ (T.) * Recherches chimiques et physiologiques sur l'érythoxylum coca du Pérou et la cocaine. 4°. *Paris*, 1868.

———. The same. 8°. *Paris*, 1868.
Also, transl.: Gac. méd., Lima, 1876, ii, 58; 70; 78; 88; 95; 101; 109; 117; 124; 134; 141.

NIEMANN (A.) * Ueber eine neue organische Base in den Cocablättern. 8°. *Göttingen*, 1860.

NIKOLSKI (M.) * Materijali dlja rieshenija voprosa o vlijanii kokaina na jivotnii organizm. [Iufluence of cocaine in animal organism.] 8°. *St. Petersburg*, 1872.

OTT (I.) Cocain, veratria and gelsemium. Toxicological studies. 12°. *Philadelphia*, 1874.

DE LOS RIOS (J. A.) * Sobre la coca de Perú. 4°. *Lima*, 1868.
Also, in: Gac. méd. de Lima, 1867-8, xii, 26-28.

SEARLE (W. S.) A new form of nervous disease; together with an essay on Erythroxylon Coca. 8°. *New York*, 1881.

SOUDÉE (L.) * Étude synthétique sur le coca. 4°. *Paris*, 1874.

WÖHLER (F.) & HAIDINGER (W.) Ueber das Cocain. 8°. *Wien*, 1860.
Repr. from: Sitzungsb. d. k. Akad. d. Wissensch. Math.-naturw. Cl., Wien, 1860, xl, 7.

von **Anrep** (B.) Ueber die physiologische Wirkung des Cocaïn. Arch. d. ges. Physiol., Bonn, 1870, xxi, 38–77. *Also* [Rev.]: J. de méd., chir. et pharmacol., Brux., 1880, lxx, 373–377.—**Arango** (A.-P.) Note sur la coca. Bull. gén. de thérap., etc., Par., 1871, lxxx, 462-466.—**Bell** (J. A.) The use of coca. Brit. M. J., Lond., 1874, i, 305.—**Bennett** (A.) An experimental inquiry into the physiological actions of theine, guaranine, cocaine, and theobromine. Edinb. M. J., 1873, xix, 323–341. ———. The physiological action of coca. Brit. M. J., Lond., 1874, i, 510.—**Bentley** (W. H.) Erythroxylon coca. Therap. Gaz., Detroit, 1880, n. s., i, 350. ———. Erythroxylon coca in the opium and alcohol habits. *Ibid.*, 253.—**Bernard** (W.) Observations on the effects of coca leaves. Brit. M. J., Lond., 1876, i, 750.—**Bordier** (A.) Coca. Dict. encycl. d. sc. méd., Par., 1875, xviii, 161-170.—**Carter** (W.) The use of coca. Brit. M. J., Lond., 1874, i, 414.—**Cazeau** (C.) Recherches expérimentales sur la propriété alimentaire de la coca. Courrier méd., Par., 1871, xxi, 2-7.—**Christison** (R.) Observations on the effects of the leaves of Erythroxylon coca. Brit. M. J., Lond., 1876, i, 527-531.—**Clemens** (T.) Erfahrungen über die therapeutische Verwendung der Cocablätter. Deutsche Klinik, Berl., 1867, xix, 49.—

Erythroxylon *Coca.*

Coca (La) du Pérou. Bull. gén. de thérap., etc., Par., 1867, lxxii, 458-460.—**Collin** (R.) De la coca et ses véritables propriétés thérapeutiques. Union méd., Par., 1877, 3. s., xxiv, 239.—**Dowdeswell** (G. F.) The coca leaf. Lancet, Lond., 1876, i, 631; 664.—**Frankl** (J.) Mittheilung über Coca. Ztschr. d. k.-k. Gesellsch. d. Aerzte zu Wien, 1860, xvi, 204-206.—**Fristedt** (R. F.) Om cocabladen såsom njutnings- och läkemedel. Upsala Läkaref. Förh., 1867-8, iii, 304–311.—**Fronmüller** sen. Coca und Cat; pharmakologische Studien. Vrtljschr. f. d. prakt. Heilk., Prag, 1863, lxxix, 109-141.—**Garcia** (E.) Erythroxylon coca ó coca del Perú. Gac. de l. hosp., Valencia, 1882, i, 108; 128; 180; 200.—**Gibbs** (B. F.) Report on coca. San. & M. Rep. U. S. Navy 1873-4, Wash., 1875, 675.—**Girtler** (J.) Ueber Coca, Extractum der Coca und Cocain. Wien. mod. Wchnschr., 1862, xii, 423.—**Haller** (C.) Notizen über die Coca. Ztschr. d. k.-k. Gesellsch. d. Aerzte zu Wien, 1860, xvi, 435-438.—**Huse** (E. C.) Cocaerythroxylon; a new cure for the opium habit. Therap. Gaz., Detroit, 1880, n. s., i, 256.—**Jolyet**. Recherches sur l'action physiologique de la cocaïne. Compt. rend. Soc. de biol. 1867, Par., 1869, 4. s., iv, 162.—**Leared** (A.) The use of coca. Brit. M. J., Lond., 1874, i, 272.—**Leebody** (J. R.) The action of coca. *Ibid.*, 1876, i, 750.—**McBean** (S.) Erythroxylon coca in the treatment of typlus and typhoid fevers, and also of other febrile diseases. *Ibid.*, 1877, i, 291.—**Maisch** (J. F.) On coca leaves. Med. & Surg. Reporter, Phila., 1861, n. s., vi, 399.—**Mantegazza** (P.) Sulle virtù igieniche e medicinali della coca, e sugli alimenti nervosi in generale. Ann. univ. di med., Milano, 1859, clxvii, 449-519, 1 pl. *Also* [Abstr.]: Gazz. med. ital. lomb., Milano, 1859, 4. s., iv, 201; 208.—**Marinni** (A.) La coca du Pérou. Rev. de thérap. méd.-chir., Par., 1872, 148–152. *Also*: Monde pharm., Par., 1875, iv, 25.—**Mason** (A. P.) Erythroxylon coca; its physiological effects, and especially its effects on the excretion of urea by the kidneys. [Graduation thesis.] Boston M. & S. J., 1882, cvii, 221-223.—**Motta** (E.) Do Erythroxylon coca. J. Soc. d. sc. med. de Lisb., 1862, 2. s., xxvi, 257; 307; 325.—**Neudörfer** (J.) Dio Coca. Allg. mil.-ärztl. Ztg., Wien, 1870, 377–380.—**Nuñez del Prado** (E.) Estudio sobre la coca. Gac. méd., Lima, 1875, i, 238; 246; 254; 262; 271; 279.—**Ott** (I.) Physiological action of the leaves of the Erythroxylon coca on the excretion of urine. Med. Times, Phila., 1870-71, i, 56. ———. Coca and its alkaloid, cocain. Med. Rec., N. Y., 1876, ii, 586.—**Plass** (H.) Verfügungsversuch durch Cocaïn. Ztschr. f. Med., Chir. u. Geburtsh., Leipz., 1863, n. F., ii, 222-2.7.—**Poinat** (C. H.) The Erythroxylon coca. Med. & Surg. Reporter, Phila., 1881, xlv, 418.—**Rossier** (H.) Sur l'action physiologique des feuilles de coca. Écho méd., Neuchât., 1861, v, 193-198.—**Scagilia**. Le coca et ses applications thérapeutiques. Gaz. d. hôp., Par., 1877, l, 427.—**Schroff** (C.) Vorläufige Mittheilungen über Cocaïn. Wchnbl. d. k. k. Gesellsch. d. Aerzte in Wien, 1862, xviii, 233; 241; 249; 268.—**Scrivener** (J. H.) On the coca leaf, and its uses in diet and medicine. Med. Times & Gaz., Lond., 1871, ii, 407.—**Sieveking** (E. H.) Coca; its therapeutic use. Brit. M. J., Lond., 1874, i, 234.—**Stimmel** (A. F.) Coca in the opium and alcohol habits. Therap. Gaz., Detroit, 1881, n. s., ii, 102.—**Stockwell** (G. A.) Erythroxylon coca. Boston M. & S. J., 1877, xcvii, 399-405.—**Tanner** (W.) Erythroxylon coca. Med. & Surg. Reporter. Phila., 1877, xxxvi, 327.—**Ward** (G. A.) The uses of coca in South America. Med. Rec., N. Y., 1880, xvii, 497.

CHAPTER 3

"The Cocaine Episode,"
PART TWO

From *The Life and Work of Sigmund Freud* by Ernest Jones, M.D.

At this point a new figure enters on the scene: Carl Koller, a man eighteen months younger than Freud, who won the distinction of inaugurating local anesthesia. Koller was at the time an interne in the Department of Ophthalmology, where he aspired to become an Assistant. His thoughts ran so exclusively on the subject of eye diseases that, according to Freud, his monomania became rather tiresome to his colleagues. Rightly perceiving the need for it, he was particularly set on finding some drug that would anesthetize the sensitive surface of the eye; he had already tried various drugs, such as morphine and chloral bromide, but so far in vain. In one of his later lectures, desiring to point a moral, Freud related the following incident.

> One day I was standing in the courtyard with a group of colleagues of whom this man was one, when another interne passed us showing signs of intense pain. [Here Freud told what the localization of the pain was, but I have forgotten this detail.] I said to him: "I think I can help you," and we all went to my room, where I applied a few drops of a medicine which made the pain disappear instantly. I explained to my friends that this drug was the extract of a South American plant, the coca, which seemed to have powerful qualities for relieving pain and about which I was preparing a publication. The man with the permanent interest in the eye, whose name was Koller, did not say anything, but a few months later I learned that he had begun to revolutionize eye surgery by the use of cocaine, making operations easy which till then had been impossible. This is the only way to make important discoveries: have one's ideas exclusively focused on one central interest.[1]

Freud had begun some tests with a dynamometer to ascertain whether the apparent increase of muscular strength obtained by the use of cocaine was a subjective illusion or was objectively verifiable, and in these he cooperated with Koller. They both swallowed some cocaine and, like everyone else, noticed the numbing of the mouth and lips. This meant more to Koller than to Freud.

Koller read Freud's essay when it appeared in July, pondered over it, and early in September, after Freud had left Vienna for Hamburg, appeared in Stricker's Institute of Pathological Anatomy carrying a bottle containing a white powder. He announced to the Assistant there, Dr. Gaertner,* that he had reason to think it would act as a local anesthetic in the eye. The matter was at once easily put to the test. They tried it first on the eyes of a frog, a rabbit, and a dog, and then on their own—with complete success. Koller wrote a "Preliminary Communication" dated early in September, and got Dr. Brettauer to read it and make practical demonstrations at the Ophthalmological Congress that took place at Heidelberg on September 15. On October 17 he read a paper in Vienna before the *Gesellschaft der Ärzte,* which he published shortly afterwards. It contained the sentence: "Cocaine has been prominently brought to the notice of Viennese physicians by the thorough compilation and interesting therapeutic paper of my hospital colleague Dr. Sigmund Freud."

Freud had also called the attention of a closer ophthalmological friend, Leopold Königstein, a man six years older than himself and a Docent of three years' standing, to the numbing powers of cocaine and had suggested that he use it to alleviate the pain of certain eye complaints, such as trachoma and iritis. This Königstein faithfully did, with success, and it was only some weeks later, early in October, that he extended its use to the field of surgery by enucleating a dog's eye with Freud's assistance. He was just a little too late. At the meeting on October 17 he also read a paper describing his experiences with cocaine, but without mentioning Koller's name. It looked like an ugly fight for priority, but Freud and Wagner-Jauregg managed to persuade him reluctantly, to insert in his published paper a reference to Koller's "Preliminary Communication" of the previous month and thus to renounce his own claim. As we shall see, Koller did not reciprocate Freud's chivalrous behavior.

It has generally been assumed that Freud must have been very disappointed and also angry with himself on hearing of Koller's discovery. Interestingly enough, this was not at all so. This is how he reported it:

My second piece of news is pleasanter. A colleague has found a striking application for coca in ophthalmology and communicated it to the Heidelberg Congress, where it caused great excitement. I had advised

---

* The Professor Gaertner who in a dream of Freud's, the night after Stricker's *Festschrift* appeared, disturbed his discussion with Königstein.

Königstein a fortnight before I left Vienna to try something similar. He really discovered something and now there is a dispute between them. They decided to lay their findings before me and ask me to judge which of them should publish first. I have advised Königstein to read a paper simultaneously with the other in the *Gesellschaft der Ärzte*. In any event it is to the credit of coca, and my work retains its reputation of having successfully recommended it to the Viennese.*

Evidently at this time Freud still regarded the province of cocaine as, so to speak, his private property. Its value when taken internally was the main thing, and he kept on experimenting with a variety of diseases he hoped it would cure. So far from being disconcerted by Koller's discovery, he viewed it as one more of the outlying applications of which his beloved drug was capable. It took a long time before he could assimilate the bitter truth that Koller's use of it was to prove practically the only one of value and all the rest dust and ashes.

On the day after hearing of Koller's work, the chemical firm of Merck invited Freud to investigate a new alkaloid, ecgnonin, which had been isolated from cocaine, and sent him 100 grams. Together with Fleischl, whose appearance was very irregular, he experimented with frogs, rabbits, and other animals, and also with himself. It proved to be very toxic with lower animals, but he could take very large doses himself without perceiving much effect.

When the Physiological Club re-opened for the fall session Freud received many congratulations on his cocaine monograph. Professor Reuss, the Director of the Eye Clinic, told him that it had "brought about a revolution." Professor Nothnagel, handing him some of his reprints, reproached him for not having published the monograph in his journal. In the meantime he was experimenting with diabetes, which he hoped to cure with cocaine. If it succeeded he could marry a year earlier and they would be rich and famous people. But nothing came of it. Then his sister Rosa and a friend of his, a ship's surgeon, had favorable experiences in the use of cocaine for averting seasickness, and Freud hoped this was another future for it. He expressed his intention of trying the effect of cocaine after making himself giddy on the swing boats in the Prater, but we hear nothing more of the experiment.

---

* Unpublished letter from Freud to Martha Bernays dated October 10, 1884.

And just then came the discussion between Koller and Königstein at the *Gesellschaft der Ärzte* which opened his eyes somewhat to the importance of what had happened. In describing the meeting he says he got only five per cent of the credit and so came off poorly. If only, instead of advising Königstein to carry out the experiments on the eye, he had believed more in them himself, and had not shrunk from the trouble of carrying them out, he would not have missed the "fundamental fact" (i.e., of anesthesia) as Königstein did.* "But I was led astray by so much incredulity on all sides." It was the first self-reproach. And a little later he wrote to his future sister-in-law: "Cocaine has brought me a great deal of credit, but the lion's share has gone elsewhere."† He had to note that Koller's discovery had produced an "enormous sensation" throughout the world.

The rather unnecessary initial and concluding remarks in Freud's autobiographical account of it suggest that someone ought to be blamed, and there is plenty of evidence that it was himself that Freud really blamed. In another context he wrote: "I had hinted in my essay that the alkaloid might be employed as an anesthetic, but I was not thorough enough to pursue the matter further." In conversation he would ascribe the omission to his "laziness."

So for the second time Freud had missed fame by a hair's breadth. He might have consoled himself with the reflection that his revered master, Brücke, had suffered a similar fate. In 1849 he recognized that the red reflex from the eye came from the retina, but had not the wit to put a lens in front of it so as to focus its vessels. In the following year his friend, Helmholtz, did so, and so was hailed as the discoverer of the ophthalmoscope.

The somewhat disingenuous excuse Freud gave for the failure when writing his autobiography must cover a deeper explanation, since it does not tally very closely with the facts. To begin with, the parting had lasted not two years, but one.** The cocaine essay was finished on June 18, 1884,†† and Martha Bernays had left Vienna for Wands-

---

* Unpublished letter from Freud to Martha Bernays dated October 18, 1884.
† Unpublished letter from Freud to Minna Bernays dated October 29, 1884.
** In a letter to Wittels Freud even said "several years." So in retrospect, as well as at the time, the waiting had seemed terribly long.
†† Letter from Freud to Martha Bernays dated June 19, 1884.

bek only on June 14, 1883.* Nor was there any sudden opportunity for visiting her, as his passage rather suggests. From the very time of her departure he planned to do so in the summer holiday of the following year,† and there are many references in the correspondence to his difficulty in saving up, gulden by gulden, the sum necessary to cover the cost of the journey. As the time approached he planned to leave in the third week of July, and, since he delivered his manuscript to the editor on the date he had promised, June 20, he was hard put to it to find some other distraction to allay his impatience during the five weeks that remained before he could depart for his holiday. As things turned out he was not able to go before September.

The psychology of the self-reproach would seem to be more complex. It is true that Freud hoped to achieve some measure of fame through his study of cocaine, but he could not know that a much greater measure of fame than he had imagined was within the grasp of whoever would apply cocaine in a certain way. When he realized this, which he was slow to do, he blamed himself, but also inculpated his fiancée. The latter irrational feature is, as is usually so, a hint of some unconscious process. There are two further ones. In a letter to Wittels forty years later he wrote: "I know very well how it happened to me. The study on coca was an allotrion which I was eager to conclude." The word "allotrion," with its punitive connotation, was one familiar to Freud from his schoolteachers' use of it to signify anything, such as a hobby, that detracted from the serious fulfillment of a duty. Freud's interest in cocaine, which he termed a "side interest," was of just this nature, taking him far from his serious "scientific" work in neuropathology. A hobby, if intensely pursued, always indicates a very personal interest, often one divorced from a man's main vocation, and the deep sources in the personality from which the interest arises are commonly associated with some sense of guilt.**

---

* Unpublished letter from Freud to Martha Bernays dated June 12, 1885.
† Unpublished letter from Freud to Martha Bernays dated June 16, 1883.
** In Freud's dreams this theme of guilt about his hobbies appears together with a vigorous self-defense.

Part Three of this biographical summary is continued in Chapter Thirteen. *Ed.*

CHAPTER 4

Early Hopes

APRIL–JUNE 1884

From *The Letters of Sigmund Freud,* edited by Ernst L. Freud. Translated by Tania and James Stern.

In his letters to his fiancée, Martha Bernays, Freud describes the beginnings of his cocaine project. He was driven not only by his desire for fame but also by a need to help a friend and colleague, Ernst von Fleischl-Marxow, who had been taking increasing quantities of morphine for the treatment of a painful wound. Ed.

To MARTHA BERNAYS
Vienna, Monday, at the *Journal*
April 21, 1884

You will certainly be surprised, my darling, to hear that I am sitting here again after having written to you as recently as Saturday from the same spot; this is the result of my having been absent through being laid up so long, and rather awkward it is, too. I feel there is something altogether missing at the moment; I cannot work in the laboratory because of the prospering practice; work on the experiments, from which I expect a little recognition, is lying idle.— It gave me quite a turn today when the proofs of my paper on the Method arrived from Leipzig; since then, with the exception of two small discoveries, I have done no work whatever. But otherwise I am very well, feel fitter than ever, I also love you even more than during our best days here, and if I write to you so rarely it is because of the beastly combination of being on duty and work at the *Journal* during these past few days; even yesterday, Sunday, I was in harness. Paneth was here today and told me that I may *perhaps* be summoned to a nervous case in Schwechat. Alois Schönberg has mentioned the prospect of a job in Pest. All these are simply beginnings, which do not necessarily have to materialize, but they are nonetheless beginnings. . . .

I am also toying now with a project and a hope which I will tell you about; perhaps nothing will come of this, either. It is a therapeutic experiment. I have been reading about cocaine, the effective ingredient of coca leaves, which some Indian tribes chew in order to make themselves resistant to privation and fatigue. A German has tested this stuff on soldiers and reported that it has really rendered them strong and capable of endurance. I have now ordered some of it and for obvious reasons am going to try it out on cases of heart disease, then on nervous exhaustion, particularly in the awful condition following withdrawal of morphine (as in the case of Dr. Fleischl). There may be any number of other people experimenting on it already; perhaps it won't work. But I am certainly going to try it and, as you know, if one tries something often enough and goes on wanting it, one day it may succeed. We need no more than one stroke of luck of this kind to consider setting up house. But, my little woman, do not be too convinced that it will come off this time. As you know, an explorer's temperament requires two basic qualities: optimism in attempt, criticism in work.

Now that I have talked out everything concerning myself, I shall come to you, my precious girl. No, I am still here. I don't even consider seeing you in the spring, I would like to have achieved something really good before we meet again. And this is what I am looking forward to more than I can say. . . .

The mailman has just arrived, Marty; he brought very few nice things, but a letter containing twenty-eight florins. It does a man good to have some money, darling; now another ten florins are coming to you; I shall hold onto them for a while, for I have no other money, but they are yours. Now what plans have you for your wardrobe? A jersey jacket? Are they still in fashion?

I am holding onto the money for a while not because I am stingy, but because the cocaine will cost something and because I impoverished myself yesterday by paying ten florins for an electric apparatus. . . .

Now please write to me as much about yourself as I have of myself. And also whether you are well, completely well. Whether the iron is doing you good and whether you are drinking any wine. I shall be angry if you don't say yes to both. . . .

Fondest greetings
Your
Sigmund

Vienna, Thursday
June 19, 1884
My beloved treasure,

I can't remember ever having been so rushed, otherwise I would have answered all your sweet, good letters with long pages of explanation; but as it is I have to be brief today, too; after all, I hope we will soon be able to talk.

"Coca"* wasn't finished till last night; the first half has already been corrected today; it will be one and a half sheets long; the few gulden I have earned by it I had to subtract from my pupil, whom I sent away yesterday and today. Now there is still the correction of a second paper; in addition I have to give electrical treatments, read, and work at the *Journal*, but I am as strong as a lion, gay and cheerful, and you can well imagine that this isn't the mood in which to drop everything and become a male nurse to a mental case.†

My beloved girl, you must utterly banish from your mind gloomy thoughts such as that you are hindering me from earning a living. After all, you know the key to my life: that I can work only when spurred on by great hopes for things uppermost in my mind. Before I met you I didn't know the joy of living, and now that "in principle" you are mine, to have you completely is the one condition I make to life, which I otherwise don't set any great store by. I am very stubborn and very reckless and need great challenges; I have done a number of things which any sensible person would be bound to consider very rash. For example, to take up science as a poverty-stricken man, then as a poverty-stricken man to capture a poor girl—but this must continue to be my way of life: risking a lot, hoping a lot, working a lot. To average bourgeois common sense I have been lost long ago. And now I am supposed not to see you for three months—and this in addition to our uncertain circumstances, and with people as unpredictable as our families! In three months Eli may be in Hamburg, or the situation in my family may prevent me from leaving. In short, I know nothing about the future. I daren't count on it, but what I do know is that I need the refreshment of holding you in my arms again as urgently as I need food and drink; I know perfectly well that I have inflicted upon you enough worry and privation and mustn't rob you of our few happy weeks together, even if you were willing to renounce them yourself. I am going to follow my impulse and continue my

---

* "Über Coca"
† Breuer had offered Freud the well-paid job as companion to a critically ill patient on a journey of several months.

venture; I want to strengthen myself through you and then with renewed strength go on trying to improve my position rather than tear myself away from all work for three months. The latter would have no great advantage; what I would save in money I would lose in time, and not much money would be saved anyway. Could you imagine me having a thousand gulden in the drawer and letting Rosa and Dolfi go hungry? At least half of it I would give to them and the rest would be just sufficient to make up for the time I would have lost. It's true, they will be the losers, but I have to do the one thing that is right for my nature and our situation. I am completely of one mind about this.

Paneth came today, also convinced of course of the necessity of my accepting the job, but I possess the good quality of being able to believe in my own judgment. I have also found a number of people who agree with me. Anyhow, my darling, I know I shall be seeing you again before very long. Keep well; I must stop, for again there is a paper to correct.

Your
Sigmund

My beloved sweetheart

You are quite right. From now on I too will write only about the journey. I can no longer think of anything else. If you really insist on meeting me at the station, I cannot stop you. I was against it because I don't want the station and the luggage to get mixed up with our first kisses. But if you are not embarrassed by the serious Hamburgers and will give me a kiss as soon as I see you, and on our way to Wandsbek a second one, and a third, etc., then I will give in. I won't be tired because I shall be traveling under the influence of coca, in order to curb my terrible impatience.

Do rent a little room for me, very close to you and very modest, otherwise I will grumble that you are not being economical; if possible a little attic, I give you unlimited powers to decide.

My wardrobe won't be very grand, but respectable. I have a gray suit which I am now wearing, and a dark one which is still at the tailor's, a new overcoat and hat. For shirts I am rather badly off; I was going to buy some here, but Father has suggested I buy them in

Hamburg, where everything is better and cheaper, and what's more, you understand what one should buy.

I still haven't got my leave, will have to fight for it, if necessary with the threat to quit altogether, but I have no doubt that I shall get it. I hear that Anna is now leaving [Wandsbek] already on the tenth, in which case I shall come a few days earlier, for my pupil will probably release me on the tenth, certainly not before; perhaps even later if I stay longer, and since each day brings in three florins this cannot be despised.

Cocaine runs to twenty-five pages, ready only today; you will see it before you see me. You know what I have been working on today.

Let us not worry about the weather. If it rains we can sit together and talk and read. I am going to bring a few books on neurology; apart from *this* branch of science I want to forget everything connected with Vienna in your presence. For you I will not bring anything, girl, but you will be having your birthday while I am there. I am very undecided whether to hand over the money and the bookkeeping to you or keep accounts myself. I think I shall save you the trouble and not let the control pass out of my hands too early. For two and occasionally three people the sum is not very impressive. On the contrary, if I can still scrape something together, I shall do so. I have to leave something for my family. Dolfi seems to need a little for herself. Yesterday I took her to the Prater; for the first time I was the rich man of the family. Rosa leaves today for Oberwaltersdorf with Herzig for three weeks. Dolfi and Pauli have jobs starting on the fifteenth. Father is bearing up, but he has a lot of troubles. Oh, girl, I must become a rich man and then when they want something they will all have to come to you.

Your
Sigmund

Vienna, Monday
June 30, 1884
My beloved girl

I am so glad we now see eye to eye and that you won't have to reproach yourself for anything while waiting for me. I am also so happy in anticipation of the beautiful days we are going to spend together. I know that at this point you want to interrupt: I must not anticipate anything so as to avoid disappointment. But, Marty, the beauty of these days depends on ourselves alone and not on the weather, not on the moods of other people, nor on the good or bad news that may come in the meantime. I want to bring back from the journey nothing but the certainty, the final conviction that you are utterly mine—in your attitude, great love, and all the little signs of affection. To take a retrospective glance as you do is quite justified; I really think I have always loved you much more than you me, or, more correctly: until we were separated you hadn't surmounted the *primum falsum* of our love—as a logician would call it—i.e., that I forced myself upon you and you accepted me without any great affection. I know it has finally changed and this success, which I wanted more than anything else, and the prolonged absence of which has been my greatest misery, gives me hope for the other successes which I still need.

....Waiting is as much my fate as yours. To wait in peace and with resignation, or to wait in the midst of struggle and agitation—the difference is not so great, no greater than our different ways of facing the world. Another two weeks—but further I refuse to think. The years beyond are hidden from me as though by a screen. I love you so much and am longing to hear from you that you love me too, and I want to spend four weeks that are not sacrificed to the future, as all time hitherto has been, but which are the future itself.

I trust that you are well again, my sweet child? I have never felt better, and I now miss the work. I must think how best to spend the next two weeks. Probably writing reviews for periodicals and regular daily observation of patients. I am very much respected in the department.

      Your
      Sigmund

Tuesday, July 1, 1884
My sweet treasure

The new month has begun with rain, but in my case with high spirits and good news. And I am hoping to experience so many lovely things before it ends.

My darling, I have been interrupted so many countless times, I must stop, which I do with fondest greetings and happiest expectations. It is even possible that something nice can be acquired for your birthday; a pupil in brain anatomy has been suggested to me; he wants to take a four–week course; I am going to offer him one of only two weeks. If he comes and accepts, it will mean quite a bit of money, and then we will go for a walk through Hamburg and look for something Marty wants. What's more, I may get a free ticket through Franceschini as far as the border, in which case I shall be able to leave a little something for my family. Coca appeared today, but I haven't seen it yet.

I hope there is nothing in this letter that offends you, my sweet Marty? If so, you must tell
                Your
                  Sigmund

CHAPTER 5

Über Coca
by Sigmund Freud

JULY 1884

ÜBER COCA.

Von

DR. SIGM. FREUD

Secundararzt im k. k. Allgemeinen Krankenhause
in Wien.

*Neu durchgesehener und vermehrter Separat-Abdruck aus dem
„Centralblatt für die gesammte Therapie".*

WIEN, 1885.
VERLAG VON MORITZ PERLES

"Über Coca." Von Dr. Sigm. Freud, Secundararzt im k.k. Allgemeinen Krankenhause in Wien. Centralblatt für die ges. Therapie. 2, 289–314, 1884 Juli.

On Coca. By Dr. Sigmund Freud, house officer of the General Hospital of Vienna.

Translated by Steven A. Edminster; additions to the translation by Frederick C. Redlich.

In his vividly written earliest article on the coca plant, Freud offers the reader a wealth of material on the history of its use in South America, its spread to Western Europe, its effects on humans and animals and its manifold therapeutic uses. Investigations by a host of authors are reported in detail. There are, at this stage, various hints towards the anesthetizing property of the drug and promises are held out in this respect, but no specific area of application is advocated.

The author's attitude toward the use of coca is favorable and comes near occasionally to being enthusiastic.

In the later Addenda to the paper, Freud mentions Koller's use of cocaine to anesthetize the cornea in eye operations, a practice which since then has become famous. Anna Freud

I. The Coca Plant

THE COCA PLANT, Erythroxylon coca, is a bush four to six feet in height, similar to our blackthorn. It is cultivated extensively in South America, in particular in Peru and Bolivia. It thrives best in the warm valleys on the eastern slopes of the Andes, 5000–6000 feet above sea level, in a rainy climate free from extremes of temperature.[1] The leaves, which provide an indispensable stimulant for some 10 million people,[2] are egg-shaped, 5–6 cm long, stalked, undivided, and pruinose. They are distinguished by two linear folds, especially prominent on the lower surface of the leaf, which, like lateral nerves, run along the medial nerve from the base of the leaf to its point in a flat arc.* The bush bears small white flowers in lateral clusters of two or three, and produces red egg-shaped fruits. It can be propagated either by seed or by cuttings; the young plants are transplanted after a year and yield their first crop of leaves after eighteen months. The leaves are considered ripe when they have become so stiff that their stalks break upon being touched.

They are then dried rapidly, either in the sun or with the aid of fire, and sewn into sacks (*cestos*) for transport. In favorable conditions a coca bush yields four or five leaf crops annually and will continue to produce a yield for between thirty and forty years. The large-scale

---

* I owe this description to Professor Vogl of Vienna, who has most kindly placed his notes and books about coca at my disposal.

production (allegedly 30 million pounds annually) makes coca leaves an important item of trade and taxation in the countries where they are grown.[3]

II. The History and Uses of Coca in its Country of Origin

When the Spanish conquerors forced their way into Peru they found that the coca plant was cultivated and held in high esteem in that country; and indeed that it was closely connected with the religious customs of the people. Legend held that Manco Capac, the divine son of the Sun, had descended in primeval times from the cliffs of Lake Titicaca, bringing his father's light to the wretched inhabitants of the country; that he had brought them knowledge of the gods, taught them the useful arts, and given them the coca leaf, this divine plant which satiates the hungry, strengthens the weak, and causes them to forget their misfortune.[4] Coca leaves were offered in sacrifice to the gods, were chewed during religious ceremonies, and were even placed in the mouths of the dead in order to assure them of a favorable reception in the beyond. The historian of the Spanish conquest,[5] himself a descendant of the Incas, reports that coca was at first a scarce commodity in the land and its use a prerogative of the rulers; by the time of the conquest, however, it had long since become accessible to everyone. Garcilasso endeavored to defend coca against the ban which the conquerors laid upon it. The Spaniards did not believe in the marvelous effects of the plant, which they suspected as the work of the devil, mainly because of the role which it played in the religious ceremonial. A council held in Lima went so far as to prohibit the use of the plant on the ground that it was heathenish and sinful. Their attitude changed, however, when they observed that the Indians could not perform the heavy labor imposed upon them in the mines if they were forbidden to partake of coca. They compromised to the extent of distributing coca leaves to the workers three or four times daily and allowing them short periods of respite in which to chew the beloved leaves. And so the coca plant has maintained its position among the natives to the present day; there even remain traces of the religious veneration which was once accorded to it.[6]

The Indian always carries a bundle of coca leaves (called *chuspa*) on his wanderings, as well as a bottle containing plant ash (*llicta*).[7] In his mouth he forms the leaves into a ball, which he pierces several times with a thorn dipped[8] in the ash, and chews slowly and thoroughly with copious secretion of saliva. It is said that in other areas a kind of earth, *tonra,* is added to the leaves in place of the plant ash.[9] It is not considered immoderate to chew from three to four ounces of leaves daily. According to Mantegazza, the Indian begins to use this stimulant in early youth and continues to use it throughout his life. When he is faced with a difficult journey, when he takes a woman, or, in general, whenever his strength is more than usually taxed, he increases the customary dose.

(It is not clear what purpose is achieved through the admixture of the alkalis contained in the ash. Mantegazza claims to have chewed coca leaves both with and without *llicta* and to have noticed no difference. According to Martius[10] and Demarle,[11] the cocaine, probably held in compound with tannic acid, is released by the action of the alkalis. A *llicta* analyzed by Bibra consisted of 29% carbonate of lime and magnesia, 34% potassium salts, 3% argillaceous earth and iron, 17% insoluble compounds of argillaceous earth, siliceous earth and iron, 5% carbon and 10% water.)

There is ample evidence that Indians under the influence of coca can withstand exceptional hardships and perform heavy labor, without requiring proper nourishment during that time.[12] Valdez y Palacios[13] claims that by using coca the Indians are able to travel on foot for hundreds of hours and run faster than horses without showing signs of fatigue. Castelnau,[14] Martius,[15] and Scrivener[16] confirm this, and Humboldt speaks of it in connection with his trip to the equatorial regions as a generally known fact. Often quoted is Tschudi's[17] report concerning the performance of a *cholo* (half-breed) whom he was able to observe closely. The man in question carried out laborious excavation work for five days and nights, without sleeping more than two hours each night, and consumed nothing but coca. After the work was completed he accompanied Tschudi on a two-day ride, running alongside his mule. He gave every assurance that he would gladly perform the same work again, without eating, if he were given enough coca. The man was sixty-two years old and had never been ill.

In the *Journey of the Frigate 'Novara'*, similar examples are recounted of increased physical powers resulting from the use of coca. Weddell,[18] von Meyen,[19] Markham,[20] and even Poeppig[21] (whom we have to thank for many of the slanderous reports about coca) can only confirm this effect of the leaf, which, since it first became known, has continued to be a source of astonishment throughout the world.

Other reports stress the capacity of the *coqueros* (coca chewers) to abstain from food for long periods of time without suffering any ill effects. According to Unanuè,[22] when no food was available in the besieged city of La Paz in the year 1781, only those inhabitants survived who partook of coca. According to Stewenson,[23] the inhabitants of many districts of Peru fast, sometimes for days, and with the aid of coca are still able to continue working.

In view of all this evidence, and bearing in mind the role which coca has played for centuries in South America, one must reject the view sometimes expressed, that the effect of coca is an imaginary one and that through force of circumstances and with practice the natives would be able to perform the feats attributed to them even without the aid of coca. One might expect to learn that the *coqueros* compensate for abstention from food by eating correspondingly more during the intervals between their fasts, or that as a result of their mode of life they fall into a rapid decline. The reports of travelers on the former point are not conclusive; as for the latter, it has been denied emphatically by reliable witnesses. To be sure, Poeppig painted a terrible picture of the physical and intellectual decadence which are supposed to be the inevitable consequence of the habitual use of coca. But all other observers affirm that the use of coca in moderation is more likely to promote health than to impair it, and that the *coqueros* live to a great age.[24] Weddell and Mantegazza too, however, point out that the immoderate use of coca leads to a cachexia characterized physically by digestive complaints, emaciation, etc., and mentally by moral depravity and a complete apathy toward everything not connected with the enjoyment of the stimulant. White people sometimes succumb as well to this state, which bears a great similarity to the symptoms of chronic alcoholism and morphine addiction. It is not taken in wholly immoderate quantities, and never from a presumptive disproportion between the amount of nourishment taken and the amount of work performed by the *coqueros.*

III. Coca Leaves in Europe—Cocaine

According to Dowdeswell,[25] the earliest recommendation for coca is contained in an essay by Dr. Monardes (Seville, 1569) which appeared in English translation in 1596. Like the later reports of the Jesuit Father Antonio Julian,[26] and the doctor Pedro Crespo,[27] both of Lima, Monardes' essay extols the marvelous effect of the plant in combating hunger and fatigue. Both of the former authors had great hopes for the introduction of coca into Europe. In 1749 the plant was brought to Europe; it was described by A. L. de Jussieu and classed with the genus Erythroxylon. In 1786 it appeared in Lamarck's *Encyclopédie Méthodique Botanique* under the name of *Erythroxylon coca.* Reports of travelers such as Tschudi and Markham, among others, provided proof that the effect of coca leaves is not confined to the Indian race.

In 1859, Paolo Mantegazza, who had lived for a number of years in South America's coca regions, published his discoveries about the physiological and therapeutic effects of coca leaves in both hemispheres [28] Mantegazza is an enthusiastic eulogist of coca and illustrated the versatility of its therapeutic uses in reports of case histories. His report aroused much interest but little confidence. However, I have come across so many correct observations in Mantegazza's publication that I am inclined to accept his allegations even when I have not personally had an opportunity to confirm them.

In 1859, Dr. Scherzer, a member of the expedition in the Austrian frigate *Novara,* brought a batch of coca leaves to Vienna, some of which he sent to Professor Wöhler for examination. Wöhler's pupil Niemann[29] isolated the alkaloid cocaine from them. After Niemann's death, Lossen,[30] another pupil of Wöhler, continued the investigation of the substances contained in coca leaves.

Niemann's cocaine crystallizes in large, colorless, 4–6-sided prisms of the monoclinic type. It has a somewhat bitter taste and produces an anesthetic effect on the mucous membranes. It melts at a tempera-

54 Cocaine Papers

ture of 98°C, is difficult to dissolve in water* but is easily soluble in alcohol, ether, and dilute acids. It combines with platinum chloride and gold chloride to form double salts. On heating with hydrochloric acid it breaks down into benzoic acid, methyl alcohol, and a little-studied base called ecgonin. Lossen established the following formula for cocaine: $C_{17}H_{24}NO_4$. Because of their high degree of solubility in water, the salts which it forms with hydrochloric acid and acetic acid are particularly suitable for physiological and therapeutic uses.[31]

In addition to cocaine, the following substances have been found in coca leaves: cocatannic acid, a peculiar wax, and a volatile base, hygrine, which has a smell reminiscent of trimethylamine, and which Lossen isolated in the form of a viscous light yellow oil. Judging by reports from chemists, there are still more substances contained in coca leaves which have not yet been discovered.

Since the discovery of cocaine numerous observers have studied the effects of coca on animals as well as on healthy and sick human beings; they sometimes used a preparation described as cocaine, and sometimes the coca leaves themselves, either in an infusion or after the manner of the Indians. In Austria, Schroff senior carried out the first experiments on animals in 1862; other reports on coca have come from Frankl (1860), Fronmüller (1863), and Neudörfer (1870). As for work carried out in Germany, the therapeutic recommendations of Clemens (1867), von Anrep's experiments on animals (1880) and Aschenbrandt's experiments on exhausted soldiers (1883) may be mentioned.

In England A. Bennett carried out the first experiments on animals in 1874; in 1876 the reports of the president of the British Medical Association, Sir Robert Christison, created a considerable stir; and when a correspondent of the *British Medical Journal* claimed that a Mr. Weston (who had astonished scientific circles in London by his remarkable walking feats) chewed coca leaves, coca became, for a time, a subject of general interest. In the same year (1876) Dowdeswell published the results of a completely ineffective experiment carried out in the laboratory of University College, after which coca seems to have found no one in England willing to undertake further

---

* There is very little agreement among authors about the solubility of cocaine in water. It is evident that various preparations of "cocaine" came on the market and were brought into use.

research.*

From the French literature on the subject, the following should be mentioned: Rossier (1861), Demarle (1862), Gosse's monograph on Erythroxylon coca (1862), Reiss (1866), Lippmann's *Etude sur la coca du Pérou* (1868), Moréno y Maïz (1868), who provided certain new facts about cocaine, Gazeau (1870), Collins (1877), and Marvaud in the book *Les aliments d'épargne* (1874), the only of the above essays at my disposal.

In Russia Nikolsky, Danini (1873), and Tarkhanov (1872) concentrated particularly on studying the effects of cocaine on animals. Many reports, all of which have been published in the *Detroit Therapeutic Gazette,* have emerged from North America in recent years on the successful therapeutic use of cocaine preparations.

The earlier of the investigations referred to here led, on the whole, to great disillusionment and to the conviction that effects from the use of coca such as had been reported so enthusiastically from South America could not be expected in Europe. Investigations such as those carried out by Schroff, Fronmüller, and Dowdeswell produced either negative or, at the most, insignificant results. There is more than one explanation for these failures. Certainly the quality of the preparations used was largely to blame.† In a number of cases the authors themselves express doubt as to the quality of their preparations; and to the extent that they believe the reports of travelers on the effects of coca, they assume that these effects must be attributed to a volatile component of the leaf. They base this assumption on the report of Poeppig, among others, that even in South America leaves which have been stored for a long time are considered worthless. The experiments carried out recently with the cocaine prepared by Merk

---

* For the collation of literature, I relied on the article, "Erythroxylon coca" in the Index Catalogue of the Library of the Surgeon-General's office, vol. IV, 1883, which can almost be considered as a complete index of the literature. Because of the inadequacy of our own public libraries, I was able to acquaint myself with a part of the literature which I have referred to on coca only by way of references and second-hand reports; I hope, however, that I have read enough to achieve my aim in this essay: to gather together all the existing information on coca.

† The cocaine content of coca leaves varies, according to Lossen, between 0.2% and 0.02%. 0.05g of *cocaïnum muriaticum* appears to be the minimum dose which is effective in man. According to Lippmann (*Etude sur la coca du Pérou,* Thesis. Strasbourg: 1868), a dried coca leaf weighs 1dg.

[sic] in Darmstadt alone justify the claim that cocaine is the true agent of the coca effect, which can be produced just as well in Europe as in South America and turned to good account in dietetic and therapeutic treatment.

IV. The Effect of Coca on Animals

We know that animals of different species—and even individuals of the same species—differ most markedly from one another in those chemical characteristics which determine the organism's receptivity to foreign substances. We would, therefore, as a matter of course, not expect to find that the effect of coca on animals in any way resembled the effects which it has been described to have on man. We may be satisfied with the results of our inquiry to the extent that we can comprehend the way cocaine affects both man and animals from a unified standpoint.

We are indebted to von Anrep[32] for the most exhaustive experiments regarding the effects of coca on animals. Before him, such experiments were carried out by Schroff senior,[33] Moréno y Maïz,[34] Tarkhanov,[35] Nikolsky,[36] Danini,[37] A. Bennett,[38] and Ott.[39] The majority of these authors introduced the alkaloid either orally or subcutaneously.

The most general result of such experiments is that, in small doses, coca has a stimulating, and in larger doses a paralyzing, effect on the nervous system. In the case of cold-blooded animals the paralyzing effect is particularly noticeable, while in warm-blooded animals symptoms of stimulation are the most apparent.

According to Schroff, cocaine produces in frogs a soporific condition accompanied by paralysis of the voluntary muscles. Moréno y Maïz, Danini, Nikolsky, and Ott made fundamentally the same discovery; Moréno y Maïz alleges that the general paralysis ensuing from moderate doses is preceded by tetanus; under the same conditions Nikolsky describes a stage of excitation of the muscular system, while Danini, on the other hand, never observed any spasms.

Von Anrep likewise reports a paralyzing effect of cocaine on frogs after a short period of excitation. At first the sensory nerve endings and later the sensory nerves themselves are affected; breathing is at first accelerated and then brought to a standstill; and the functioning of the heart is slowed down until the point of diastolic failure is reached. Doses of 2mg suffice to provoke symptoms of poisoning.

According to Schroff's accounts of his experiments with rabbits (which in detail are fraught with contradictions), coca produces multiple spasms in rabbits, increased respiration and pulse rate, dilation of the pupils, and convulsive death. The effectiveness of the poisoning depended to a large extent on the mode of application. According to Danini, cocaine poisoning in warm-blooded animals produces at first agitation, which manifests itself in continuous jumping and running, then paralysis of the muscular functions, and finally spasmodic (clonic) cramps. Tarkhanov discovered an increase of mucous secretion in dogs dosed with coca, and also sugar in the urine.

In von Anrep's experiments, the effect of cocaine, even in large doses, on warm-blooded animals manifested itself first of all in powerful psychic agitation and an excitation of the brain centers which control voluntary movement. After doses of 0.01g of cocaine per kg, dogs show obvious signs of happy excitement and a maniacal compulsion to move. From the character of these movements von Anrep sees evidence that all nerve centers are affected by the stimulation, and he interprets certain swinging motions of the head as an irritation proceeding from the semi-circular canals. Further manifestations of cocaine intoxication are accelerated respiration, a great increase in the pulse rate owing to early paralysis of the N. vagi, dilation of the pupils, an acceleration of intestinal movement, a great increase in blood-pressure, and diminution of secretions. Even after doses large enough to produce eventual convulsions, symptoms of paralysis and death due to paralysis of the respiratory center, the striated muscle substance remains intact. Von Anrep does not establish the lethal dose for dogs; for rabbits it is 0.10g and for cats 0.02g per kg.*

When the spinal cord is severed from the oblongata, cocaine produces neither cramps nor a rise in blood-pressure (Danini); when the dorsal portion of the spinal cord is severed, cocaine spasms occur in the front but not in the rear extremities (von Anrep). Danini and von Anrep assume, therefore, that cocaine affects primarily the vital area of the medulla oblongata.

I should add that only the elder Schroff refers to cocaine as a nar-

---

* Administered in subcutaneous injection.

cotic and classes it with opium and cannabis, while almost everyone else ranks it with caffeine, etc.

V. The Effect of Coca on the Healthy Human Body

I have carried out experiments and studied, in myself and others, the effect of coca on the healthy human body; my findings agree fundamentally with Mantegazza's description of the effect of coca leaves.*

The first time I took 0.05g. of *cocaïnum muriaticum* in a 1% water solution was when I was feeling slightly out of sorts from fatigue. This solution is rather viscous, somewhat opalescent, and has a strange aromatic smell. At first it has a bitter taste, which yields afterwards to a series of very pleasant aromatic flavors. Dry cocaine salt has the same smell and taste, but to a more concentrated degree.

A few minutes after taking cocaine, one experiences a sudden exhilaration and feeling of lightness. One feels a certain furriness on the lips and palate, followed by a feeling of warmth in the same areas; if one now drinks cold water, it feels warm on the lips and cold in the throat. On other occasions the predominant feeling is a rather pleasant coolness in the mouth and throat.

During this first trial I experienced a short period of toxic effects, which did not recur in subsequent experiments. Breathing became slower and deeper and I felt tired and sleepy; I yawned frequently and felt somewhat dull. After a few minutes the actual cocaine euphoria began, introduced by repeated cooling eructation. Immediately after taking the cocaine I noticed a slight slackening of the pulse and later a moderate increase.

I have observed the same physical signs of the effect of cocaine in others, mostly people of my own age. The most constant symptom proved to be the repeated cooling eructation. This is often accom-

---

* Like Aschenbrandt (*Deutsche med. Wochenschrift*, Dec., 1883) I used the hydrochloric preparation of cocaine as described by Merk [sic] in Darmstadt. This preparation may be bought in Vienna in Haubner's Engelapotheke am Hof at a price which is not much higher than Merk's [sic], but which must, nevertheless, be regarded as very high. The management of the pharmacy in question is trying, as they have been kind enough to inform me, to lower the price of the drug by establishing new sources of supply.

panied by a rumbling which must originate from high up in the intestine; two of the people I observed, who said they were able to recognize movements of their stomachs, declared emphatically that they had repeatedly detected such movements. Often, at the outset of the cocaine effect, the subjects alleged that they experienced an intense feeling of heat in the head. I noticed this in myself as well in the course of some later experiments, but on other occasions it was absent. In only two cases did coca give rise to dizziness. On the whole the toxic effects of coca are of short duration, and much less intense than those produced by effective doses of quinine or salicylate of soda; they seem to become even weaker after repeated use of cocaine.

Mantegazza refers to the following occasional effects of coca: temporary erythema, an increase in the quantity of urine, dryness of the conjunctiva and nasal mucous membranes. Dryness of the mucous membrane of the mouth and of the throat is a regular symptom which lasts for hours. Some observers (Marvaud, Collan)[40] report a slight cathartic effect. Urine and feces are said to take on the smell of coca. Different observers give very different accounts of the effect on the pulse rate. According to Mantegazza, coca quickly produces a considerably increased pulse rate which becomes even higher with higher doses; Collin,[41] too, noted an acceleration of the pulse after coca was taken, while Rossier,[42] Demarle,[43] and Marvaud experienced, after the initial acceleration, a longer lasting retardation of the pulse rate. Christison noticed in himself, after using coca, that physical exertion caused a smaller increase in the pulse rate than otherwise; Reiss[44] disputes any effect on the pulse rate. I do not find any difficulty in accounting for this lack of agreement; it is partly owing to the variety of the preparations used (warm infusion of the leaves, cold cocaine solution, etc.), and the way in which they are applied,* and partly to the varying reactions of individuals. With coca this latter factor, as Mantegazza has already reported, is in general of very great significance. There are said to be people who cannot tolerate coca at all; on the other hand, I have found not a few who remained unaffected by 5cg, which for me and others is an effective dose.

---

* For the results obtained from subcutaneous injections see Morselli's and Buccola's work.

The psychic effect of *cocaïnum muriaticum* in doses of 0.05–0.10g consists of exhilaration and lasting euphoria, which does not differ in any way from the normal euphoria of a healthy person. The feeling of excitement which accompanies stimulus by alcohol is completely lacking; the characteristic urge for immediate activity which alcohol produces is also absent. One senses an increase of self-control and feels more vigorous and more capable of work; on the other hand, if one works, one misses that heightening of the mental powers which alcohol, tea, or coffee induce. One is simply normal, and soon finds it difficult to believe that one is under the influence of any drug at all.*

This gives the impression that the mood induced by coca in such doses is due not so much to direct stimulation as to the disappearance of elements in one's general state of well-being which cause depression. One may perhaps assume that the euphoria resulting from good health is also nothing more than the normal condition of a well-nourished cerebral cortex which "is not conscious" of the organs of the body to which it belongs.

During this stage of the cocaine condition, which is not otherwise distinguished, appear those symptoms which have been described as the wonderful stimulating effect of coca. Long-lasting, intensive mental or physical work can be performed without fatigue; it is as though the need for food and sleep, which otherwise makes itself felt peremptorily at certain times of the day, were completely banished. While the effects of cocaine last one can, if urged to do so, eat copiously and without revulsion; but one has the clear feeling that the meal was superfluous. Similarly, as the effect of coca declines it is possible to sleep on going to bed, but sleep can just as easily be omitted with no unpleasant consequences. During the first hours of the coca effect one cannot sleep, but this sleeplessness is in no way distressing.

I have tested this effect of coca, which wards off hunger, sleep, and fatigue and steels one to intellectual effort, some dozen times on myself; I had no opportunity to engage in physical work.

A very busy colleague gave me an opportunity to observe a striking example of the manner in which cocaine dispels extreme fatigue and

---

* Wilder's account of the effects of cocaine on himself coincide most closely with my own observations. (*Detroit Therapeutic Gazette*. Nov., 1882).

a well justified feeling of hunger; at 6:00 P.M. this colleague, who had not eaten since the early morning and who had worked exceedingly hard during the day, took 0.05g of *cocaïnum muriaticum*. A few minutes later he declared that he felt as though he had just eaten an ample meal, that he had no desire for an evening meal, and that he felt strong enough to undertake a long walk.

This stimulative effect of coca is vouched for beyond any doubt by a series of reliable reports, some of which are quite recent.

By way of an experiment, Sir Robert Christison[45]—who is seventy-eight years old—tired himself to the point of exhaustion by walking fifteen miles without partaking of food. After several days he repeated the procedure with the same result; during the third experiment he chewed 2 drams of coca leaves and was able to complete the walk without the exhaustion experienced on the earlier occasions; when he arrived home, despite the fact that he had been for nine hours without food or drink, he experienced no hunger or thirst, and woke the next morning without feeling at all tired. On yet another occasion he climbed a 3000-foot mountain and arrived completely exhausted at the summit; he made the descent upon the influence of coca, with youthful vigor and no feeling of fatigue.

Clemens[46] and J. Collan[47] have had similar experiences—the latter after walking for several hours over snow; Mason[48] calls coca "an excellent thing for a long walk"; Aschenbrandt[49] reported recently how Bavarian soldiers, weary as a result of hardships and debilitating illnesses, were nevertheless capable, after taking coca, of participating in maneuvers and marches. Moréno y Maïz[50] was able to stay awake whole nights with the aid of coca; Mantegazza remained for forty hours without food. We are, therefore, justified in assuming that the effect of coca on Europeans is the same as that which the coca leaves have on the Indians of South America.

The effect of a moderate dose of coca fades away so gradually that, in normal circumstances, it is difficult to define its duration. If one works intensively while under the influence of coca, after from three to five hours there is a decline in the feeling of well-being, and a further dose of coca is necessary in order to ward off fatigue. The effect of coca seems to last longer if no heavy muscular work is undertaken. Opinion is unanimous that the euphoria induced by coca is not followed by any feeling of lassitude or other state of depression. I should be inclined to think that after moderate doses (0.05–0.10g) a part at least of the coca effect lasts for over twenty-four hours. In my own case, at any rate, I have noticed that even on the day after taking coca my condition compares favorably with the norm. I should be inclined to explain the possibility of a lasting gain in strength, such as has often been claimed for coca by the totality of such effects.

It seems probable, in the light of reports which I shall refer to later, that coca, if used protractedly but in moderation, is not detrimental to the body. Von Anrep treated animals for thirty days with moderate doses of cocaine and detected no detrimental effects on their bodily functions. It seems to me noteworthy—and I discovered this in myself and in other observers who were capable of judging such things—that a first dose or even repeated doses of coca produce no compulsive desire to use the stimulant further; on the contrary, one feels a certain unmotivated aversion to the substance. This circumstance may be partly responsible for the fact that coca, despite some warm recommendations, has not established itself in Europe as a stimulant.

The effect of large doses of coca was investigated by Mantegazza in experiments on himself. He succeeded in achieving a state of greatly increased happiness accompanied by a desire for complete immobility; this was interrupted occasionally, however, by the most violent urge to move. The analogy with the results of the animal experiments performed by von Anrep is unmistakable. When he increased the dose still further he remained in a *sopore beato:* His pulse rate was extremely high and there was a moderate rise in body temperature; he found that his speech was impeded and his handwriting unsteady; and eventually he experienced the most splendid and colorful hallucinations, the tenor of which was frightening for a short time, but invariably cheerful thereafter. This coca intoxication, too, failed to produce any state of depression, and left no sign whatsoever that the experimenter had passed through a period of intoxication. Moréno y Maïz also experienced a similar powerful compulsion to move after taking fairly large doses of coca. Even after using 18 drams of coca leaves Mantegazza experienced no impairment of full consciousness. A chemist who attempted to poison himself by taking 1.5g of cocaine[51] became sick and showed symptoms of gastroenteritis, but there was no dulling of the consciousness.

VI. The Therapeutic Uses of Coca

It was inevitable that a plant which had achieved such a reputation for marvelous effects in its country of origin should have been used to treat the most varied disorders and illnesses of the human body. The first Europeans who became aware of this treasure of the native population were similarly unreserved in their recommendation of coca. On the basis of wide medical experience, Mantegazza later drew up a list of the therapeutic properties of coca, which one by one received the acknowledgment of other doctors. In the following section I have tried to collate the recommendations concerning coca, and, in doing so, to distinguish between recommendations based on successful treatment of illnesses and those which relate to the psychological effects of the stimulant. In general the latter outweigh the former. At present there seems to be some promise of widespread recognition and use of coca preparations in North America, while in Europe doctors scarcely know them by name. The failure of coca to take hold in Europe, which in my opinion is unmerited, can perhaps be attributed to reports of unfavorable consequences attendant upon its use, which appeared shortly after its introduction into Europe; or to the doubtful quality of the preparations, their relative scarcity and consequent high price. Some of the evidence which can be found in favor of the use of coca has been proved valid beyond any doubt, whereas some warrants at least an unprejudiced investigation. Merk's [sic] cocaine and its salts are, as has been proved, preparations which have the full or at least the essential effects of coca leaves.

a) *Coca as a stimulant*. The main use of coca will undoubtedly remain that which the Indians have made of it for centuries: it is of value in all cases where the primary aim is to increase the physical capacity of the body for a given short period of time and to hold strength in reserve to meet further demands—especially when outward circumstances exclude the possibility of obtaining the rest and nourishment normally necessary for great exertion. Such situations arise in wartime, on journeys, during mountain climbing and other expeditions, etc.—indeed, they are situations in which the alcoholic stimulants are also generally recognized as being of value. Coca is a far more potent and far less harmful stimulant than alcohol, and its widespread utilization is hindered at present only by its high cost. Bearing in mind the effect of coca on the natives of South America, a medical authority as early as Pedro Crespo (Lima, 1793) recommended its use by European navies; Neudörfer (1870), Clemens (1867) and Surgeon-Major E. Charles[52] recommended that it should be adopted by the armies of Europe as well; and Aschenbrandt's experiences should not fail to draw the attention of army administrators to coca. If cocaine is given as a stimulant, it is better that it should be given in small effective doses (0.05–0.10g) and repeated so often that the effects of the doses overlap. Apparently cocaine is not stored in the body; I have already stressed the fact that there is no state of depression when the effects of coca have worn off.

At present it is impossible to assess with any certainty to what extent coca can be expected to increase human mental powers. I have the impression that protracted use of coca can lead to a lasting improvement if the inhibitions manifested before it is taken are due only to physical causes or to exhaustion. To be sure, the instantaneous effect of a dose of coca cannot be compared with that of a morphine injection; but, on the good side of the ledger, there is no danger of general damage to the body as is the case with the chronic use of morphine.

Many doctors felt that coca would play an important role by filling a gap in the medicine chest of the psychiatrists. It is a well-known fact that psychiatrists have an ample supply of drugs at their disposal for reducing the excitation of nerve centers, but none which could serve to increase the reduced functioning of the nerve centers. Coca has consequently been prescribed for the most diverse kinds of psychic debility—hysteria, hypochondria, melancholic inhibition, stupor, and similar maladies. Some successes have been reported: for instance, the Jesuit, Antonio Julian (Lima, 1787) tells of a learned missionary who was freed from severe hypochondria; Mantegazza praises coca as being almost universally effective in improving those functional disorders which we now group together under the name of neurasthenia; Fliessburg[53] reports excellent results from the use of coca in cases of "nervous prostration"; and according to Caldwell,[54] it is the best tonic for hysteria.

E. Morselli and G. Buccola[55] carried out experiments involving the systematic dispensation of cocaine, over a period of months, to melancholics. They gave a preparation of cocaine, as prescribed by Trommsdorf, in subcutaneous injections, in doses ranging from 0.0025–0.10g per dose. After one or two months they confirmed a slight improvement in the condition of their patients, who became happier, took nourishment, and enjoyed regular digestion.*

On the whole, the efficacy of coca in cases of nervous and psychic debility needs further investigation, which will probably lead to partially favorable conclusions. According to Mantegazza coca is of no use, and is sometimes even dangerous, in cases of organic change and inflammation of the nervous system.

b) *The use of coca for digestive disorders of the stomach.* This is the oldest and most firmly founded use of coca, and at the same time it is the most comprehensible to us. According to the unanimous assertions of the oldest as well as the most recent authorities (Julian, Martius, Unanuè, Mantegazza, Bingel,[56] Scrivener,† Frankl, and others) coca in its most various forms banishes dyspeptic complaints and the disorders and debility associated therewith, and after protracted use results in a permanent cure. I have myself made a series of such observations.

Like Mantegazza** and Frankl,[57] I have experienced personally how the painful symptoms attendant upon large meals—viz, a feeling

---

* Their assertions about the physiological effects of cocaine accord with those of Mantegazza. They observed, as an immediate effect of cocaine injections, dilation of the pupils, temperature heightened by up to 1.2 degrees, quickening of the pulse and respiration. There is never an attack of sickness.
† *Loc. cit.* "an excellent tonic in weakness of the stomach."
** Mantegazza's exhaustive medical case-histories impress me as being thoroughly credible.

of pressure and fullness in the stomach, discomfort and a disinclination to work—disappear with eructation following small doses of cocaine (0.025–0.05). Time and again I have brought such relief to my colleagues; and twice I observed how the nausea resulting from gastronomic excesses responded in a short time to the effects of cocaine, and gave way to a normal desire to eat and a feeling of bodily well-being. I have also learned to spare myself stomach troubles by adding a small amount of cocaine to salicylate of soda.

My colleague, Dr. Josef Pollak, has given me the following account of an astonishing effect of cocaine, which shows that it can be used to treat not merely local discomfort in the stomach but also serious reflex reactions; one must therefore assume that cocaine has a powerful effect on the mucous membrane and the muscular system of this organ.

"A forty-two-year-old, robust man, whom the doctor knew very well, was forced to adhere most strictly to a certain diet and to prescribed mealtimes; otherwise he could not avoid the attacks about to be described. When traveling or under the influence of any emotional strain he was particularly susceptible. The attacks followed a regular pattern: They began in the evening with a feeling of discomfort in the epigastrium, followed by flushing of the face, tears in the eyes, throbbing in the temples and violent pain in the forehead, accompanied by a feeling of great depression and apathy. He could not sleep during the night; toward morning there were long painful spasms of vomiting which lasted for hours. Round about midday he experienced some relief, and on drinking a few spoonfuls of soup had a feeling 'as though the stomach would at last eject a bullet which had lain in it for a long time.' This was followed by rancid eructation, until, toward evening, his condition returned to normal. The patient was incapable of work throughout the day and had to keep to his bed.

"At 8:00 PM on the tenth of June the usual symptoms of an attack began. At ten o'clock, after the violent headache had developed, the patient was given 0.075g *cocaïnum muriaticum*. Shortly thereafter he experienced a feeling of warmth and eructation, which seemed to him to be 'still too little.' At 10:30 a second dose of 0.075g of cocaine was given; the eructations increased; the patient felt some relief and was able to write a long letter. He alleged that he felt intensive movement in the stomach; at twelve o'clock, apart from a slight headache, he was normal, even cheerful, and walked for an hour. He could not sleep until 3:00 AM, but that did not distress him. He awoke the next morning healthy, ready for work, and with a good appetite."

The effect of cocaine on the stomach—Mantegazza assumes this as well—is two-fold: stimulation of movement and reduction of the organ's sensitivity. The latter would seem probable not only because of the local sensations in the stomach after cocaine has been taken but because of the analogous effect of cocaine on other mucous membranes. Mantegazza claims to have achieved the most brilliant successes in treatments of gastralgia and enteralgia, and all painful and cramping afflictions of the stomach and intestines, which he attributes to the anesthetizing properties of coca. On this point I cannot confirm Mantegazza's experiences; only once, in connection with a case of gastric catarrh, did I see the sensitivity of the stomach to pressure disappear after the administration of coca. On other occasions I have observed myself, and also heard from other doctors, that patients suspected of having ulcers or scars in the stomach complained of increased pain after using coca; this can be explained by the increased movement of the stomach.

Accordingly, I should say that the use of coca is definitely indicated in cases of atonic digestive weakness and the so-called nervous stomach disorders; in such cases it is possible to achieve not merely a relief of the symptoms but a lasting improvement.

c) *Coca in cachexia.* Long-term use of coca is further strongly recommended—and allegedly has been tried with success—in all diseases which involve degeneration of the tissues, such as severe anemia, phthisis, long-lasting febrile diseases, etc.; and also during recovery from such diseases. Thus McBean[58] noted a steady improvement in cases of typhoid fever treated with coca. In the case of phthisis, coca is said to have a limiting effect on the fever and sweating. Peckham[59] reports with regard to a case of definitely diagnosed phthisis that after fluid extract of coca had been used for seven months there was a marked improvement in the patient's condition. Hole[60] gives an account of another rather serious case in which chronic lack of appetite had led to an advanced condition of emaciation and exhaustion; here, too, the use of coca restored the patient to health. R. Bartholow[61] observed, in general, that coca proved useful in treating phthisis and other "consumptive processes." Mantegazza and a number of other authorities attribute to coca the same invaluable therapeutic quality: that of limiting degeneration of the body and increasing strength in the case of cachexia.

One might wish to attribute such successes partly to the undoubted favorable effect of coca on the digestion, but one must bear in mind that a good many of the authors who have written on coca regard it as a "source of savings"; i.e., they are of the opinion that a system which has absorbed even an extremely small amount of cocaine is capable, as a result of the reaction of the body to coca, of amassing a greater store of vital energy which can be converted into work than would have been possible without coca.[62] If we take the amount of work as being constant, the body which has absorbed cocaine should be able to manage with a lower metabolism, which in turn means a smaller intake of food.

This assumption was obviously made to account for the, according to von Voit,[63] unexplained effect of coca on the Indians. It does not even necessarily involve a contradiction of the law of conservation of energy. For labor which draws upon food or tissue components involves a certain loss, either in the utilization of assimilated food or in the conversion of energy into work; this loss could perhaps be reduced if certain appropriate steps were taken. It has not been proved that such a process takes place, however. Experiments designed to determine the amount of urine eliminated with and without the use of coca have not been altogether conclusive; indeed, these experiments have not always been conducted in such conditions that they could furnish conclusive results. Moreover, they seem to have been carried out on the assumption that the elimination of urine—which is known not to be effected by labor—would provide a measure of metabolism in general. Thus Christison noted a slight reduction in the solid components of his urine during the walks on which he took coca; Lippmann, Demarle, Marvaud, and more recently Mason[64] similarly concluded from their experiments that the consumption of coca reduces the amount of urine elimination. Gazeau,[65] on the other hand, established an *increase* of urine elimination of 11–24% under the influence of coca. A better availability of materials already stored in the body explains, in his opinion, the body's increased working power and ability to do without food when under the influence of coca. No experiments have been carried out with regard to the elimination of carbon dioxide.

Voit proved that coffee, which also rated as a "source of savings," had no influence on the breakdown of albumen in the body. We must regard the conception of coca as a "source of savings" as disproven after certain experiments in which animals were starved, both with and without cocaine, and the reduction of their body weight and the length of time they were able to withstand inanition were observed. Such experiments were carried out by Cl. Bernard,[66] Moréno y Maïz, Demarle, Gazeau, and von Anrep. The result was that the animals to which cocaine had been administered succumbed to inanition just as soon—perhaps even sooner—than those which had received no cocaine. The starvation of La Paz—an experiment carried out by history itself, and reported by Unanuè—seems to contradict this conclusion, however, for the inhabitants who had partaken of coca are said to have escaped death by starvation. In this connection one might recall the fact that the human nervous system has an undoubted, if somewhat obscure, influence on the nourishment of tissues; psychological factors can, after all, cause a healthy man to lose weight.

The therapeutic quality of coca which we took as our argument at the outset does not, therefore, deserve to be rejected out of hand. The excitation of nerve centers by cocaine can have a favorable influence on the nourishment of the body afflicted by a consumptive condition, even though that influence might well not take the form of a slowing down of metabolism.

I should add here that coca has been warmly praised in connection with the treatment of syphilis. R. W. Taylor[67] claims that a patient's tolerance of mercury is increased and the mercury cachexia kept in check when coca is administered at the same time. J. Collan[68] recommends it as the best remedy for *stomatitis mercurialis* and reports that Pagvalin always prescribes it in conjunction with preparations of mercury.

d) *Coca in the treatment of morphine and alcohol addiction.* In America the important discovery has recently been made that coca preparations possess the power to suppress the craving for morphine in habitual addicts, and also to reduce to negligible proportions the serious symptoms of collapse which appear while the patient is being weaned away from the morphine habit. According to my information (which is largely from the *Detroit Therapeutic Gazette*), it was W. H. Bentley[69] who announced, in May 1878, that he had substituted coca for the customary alkaloid in the case of a female morphine addict. Two years later, Palmer, in an article in the *Louisville Medical News,* seems to have aroused the greatest general interest in this treatment of morphine addiction; for the next two years "*Erythroxylon coca* in the opium habit" was a regular heading in the reports of the *Therapeutic Gazette*. From then on information regarding successful cures became rarer: whether because the treatment became established as a recognized cure, or because it was abandoned, I do not know. Judging by the advertisements of drug dealers in the most recent issues of American papers, I should rather conclude that the former was the case.

There are some sixteen reports of cases in which the patient has been successfully cured of addiction; in only one instance is there a report of failure of coca to alleviate morphine addiction, and in this case the doctor wondered why there had been so many warm recommendations for the use of coca in cases of morphine addiction.[70] The successful cases vary in their conclusiveness. Some of them involve large doses of opium or morphine and addictions of long standing. There is not much information on the subject of relapses, as most cases were reported within a very short time of the cure having been effected. Symptoms which appear during abstention are not always reported in detail. There is especial value in those reports which contain the observation that the patients were able to dispense with coca after a few weeks without experiencing any further desire for morphine.[71] Special attention is repeatedly called to the fact that morphine cachexia gave way to excellent health, so that the patients were scarcely recognizable after their cure.[72] Concerning the method of withdrawal, it should be made clear that in the majority of cases a gradual reduction of the habitual dose of the drug, accompanied by a gradual increase of the coca dose, was the method chosen; however, sudden discontinuation of the drug was also tried.[73] In the latter case

Palmer prescribes that a certain dose of coca should be repeated as often during the day as the desire for morphine recurs.* The daily dose of coca is lessened gradually until it is possible to dispense with the antidote altogether. From the very beginning the attacks experienced during abstinence were either slight or else became milder after a few days. In almost every case the cure was effected by the patient himself, whereas the cure of morphine addiction without the help of coca, as practiced in Europe, requires surveillance of the patient in a hospital.

I once had occasion to observe the case of a man who was subjected to the type of cure involving the sudden withdrawal of morphine, assisted by the use of coca; the same patient had suffered severe symptoms as a result of abstinence in the course of a previous cure. This time his condition was tolerable; in particular, there was no sign of depression or nausea as long as the effects of coca lasted; chills and diarrhea were now the only permanent symptoms of his abstinence. The patient was not bedridden, and could function normally. During the first days of the cure he consumed 3dg of *cocaïnum muriaticum* daily, and after ten days he was able to dispense with the coca treatment altogether.

The treatment of morphine addiction with coca does not, therefore, result merely in the exchange of one kind of addiction for another—it does not turn the morphine addict into a *coquero;* the use of coca is only temporary. Moreover, I do not think that it is the general toughening effect of coca which enables the system weakened by morphine to withstand, at the cost of only insignificant symptoms, the withdrawal of morphine. I am rather inclined to assume that coca has a directly antagonistic effect on morphine, and in support of my view I quote the following observations of Dr. Josef Pollak on a case in point:

"A thirty-three-year-old woman has been suffering for years from severe menstrual migraine which can be alleviated only by morphia injections. Although the lady in question never takes morphia or experiences any desire to do so when she is free of migraine, during the attacks she behaves like a morphine addict. A few hours after

---

* T[herapeutic] G[azette], July 1880. The preparation used was mostly the fluid extract, manufactured by Parke, Davis and Co.

the injection she suffers intense depression, biliousness, attacks of vomiting, which are stopped by a second morphine injection; thereupon, the symptoms of intolerance recur, with the result that an attack of migraine, along with all its consequences, keeps the patient in bed for three days in a most wretched condition. Cocaine was then tried to combat the migraine, but the treatment proved unsuccessful. It was necessary to resort to morphine injections. But as soon as the symptoms of morphine intolerance appeared, they were quickly relieved by 1dg of cocaine, with the result that the patient recovered from her attack in a far shorter time and consumed much less morphine in the process."

Coca was tried in America for the treatment of chronic alcoholism at about the same time as it was introduced in connection with morphine addiction, and most reports dealt with the two uses conjointly[74] In the treatment of alcoholism, too, there were cases of undoubted success, in which the irresistible compulsion to drink was either banished or alleviated, and the dyspeptic complaints of the drinkers were relieved. In general, however, the suppression of the alcohol craving through the use of coca proved to be more difficult than the suppression of morphomania; in one case reported by Bentley the drinker became a *coquero*. One need only suggest the immense economic significance which coca would acquire as a "source of savings" in another sense, if its effectiveness in combating alcoholism were confirmed.

e) *Coca and asthma.* Tschudi and Markham[75] report that by chewing coca leaves they were spared the usual symptoms of the so-called mountain sickness while climbing in the Andes; this complex of symptoms includes shortness of breath, pounding of the heart, dizziness, etc. Poizat[76] reports that the asthmatic attacks of a patient were arrested in every case by coca. I mention this property of coca because it appears to admit of a physiological explanation. Von Anrep's experiments on animals resulted in early paralysis of certain branches of the vagus; and altitude asthma, as well as the attacks characteristic of chronic bronchitis, may be interpreted in terms of a reflex excitation originating in the pulmonary branches of the vagus. The use of coca should be considered for the treatment of other vagus neuroses.

f) *Coca as an aphrodisiac.* The natives of South America, who represented their goddess of love with coca leaves in her hand, did not doubt the stimulative effect of coca on the genitalia. Mantegazza confirms that the *coqueros* sustain a high degree of potency right into old age; he even reports cases of the restoration of potency and the disappearance of functional weaknesses following the use of coca, although he does not believe that coca would produce such an effect in all individuals. Marvaud emphatically supports the view that coca has a stimulative effect; other writers strongly recommend coca as a remedy for occasional functional weaknesses and temporary exhaustion; and Bentley reports on a case of this type in which coca was responsible for the cure.[77]

Among the persons to whom I have given coca, three reported violent sexual excitement which they unhesitatingly attributed to the coca. A young writer, who was enabled by treatment with coca to resume his work after a longish illness, gave up using the drug because of the undesirable secondary effects which it had on him.

g) *Local application of coca.* Cocaine and its salts have a marked anesthetizing effect when brought in contact with the skin and mucous membrane in concentrated solution; this property suggests its occasional use as a local anesthetic, especially in connection with affections of the mucous membrane. According to Collin,[78] Ch. Fauvel strongly recommends cocaine for treating diseases of the pharynx, describing it as *"le tenseur par excellence des chordes vocales."* Indeed, the anesthetizing properties of cocaine should make it suitable for a good many further applications.

CHAPTER 6

Cocaine and Its Salts

OCTOBER 1884

"*Cocain und seine Salze*" von E. Merck, Klinische Monatsblätter für Augenheilkunde, Zeherder: Vol. 22, November 1884.
"Cocaine and its Salts" by E. Merck, *Chicago Medical Journal and Examiner* 50:157–163, February 1885.
Translated by Wm. M. Smith, M.D.

The European supplier of cocaine was E. Merck of Darmstadt, Germany. This firm, predecessor of the modern Merck, Sharpe and Dohme, produced the cocaine originally used by Freud. The present article by the founder, E. Merck, was translated and published in 1885 in the "translations" section of the Chicago Medical Journal and Examiner. *American doctors were thereby made aware of the most recent European developments in the study of cocaine. Ed.*

$C_{17} H_{24} NO_4$ (Lossen)*

Cocaine is an alkaloid of the coca leaves (Erythroxylon Coca Lam.), which was isolated by Niemann in 1860. In 1862 Lossen found a second, volatile, base, hygrin, which has been little investigated up to the present time; but it is apparently weak, and without the characteristic action of the cocaine. Other extracts of the leaves are: Ecgonin, coca tannic acid, and a peculiar wax. The cocaine crystals belong to the monoclinic system; they melt at 98° C., dissolve easily in alcohol, still more easily in ether, but only in 704 parts water at 12° C. The salts of cocaine, on the contrary, are readily soluble in water.

The first intelligence of the action of coca, taken internally, was furnished in the 16th century (Dr. Monardes, Sevilla, 1569). In 1749, the plant was brought to Europe, described by Jussie, and named *Erythroxylon coca,* by Lamarck. Tschudi, Markham, Poeppig, and other investigators who traveled in South America, observed the natives chewed the coca leaves when they wished to neutralize the effects of over–fatigue. The Indians macerate the leaves with ash of chenopodium quinoa, in order to eliminate the tannic acid by means of the alkali, and to free the alkaloid.

I produce the cocaine–alkaloid pure, as also its combinations, with muriatic acid, salicylic acid, hydrobromic acid, tartaric acid, and citric acid. Since the production of the cocaine has been accomplished, it is believed that in this substance the active principle of the coca leaves has been found.

At first it seemed probable that a similar action might be found as a quality of one of the analogous alkaloids, such as caffein, theine or theobromin. However, nothing has yet occurred to support this idea.

* This is the formula for cocaine. *Ed.*

Cocaine acts upon the nerve centers, but also upon other nerve regions—in small doses, as a stimulant; in large ones it causes paralysis. It kills warm–blooded animals, by arresting pulmonary action, though they are less affected by it than the cold–blooded animals. Although no doubt exists, therefore, that cocaine is a poison, still its toxic qualities are relatively small, and its action is not cumulative.

Schroff, who in 1862 made the first experiments with the remedy, saw, in puppies, after a dose of 0.05 grm. *per os.,* fluctuating respiration and transitory mydriasis. The same dose, administered subcutaneously, caused the death of the animal experimented upon, with epileptiform convulsions and very decided mydriasis, which immediately disappeared as soon as death occurred. With frogs, the application of 0.001 grm. is followed by complete loss of the power to move; *dosis lethalis* 0.002 grm.

According to Fronmüller, who, in 1863, examined the narcotic action of cocaine, 0.03 to 0.33 grm. administered to man internally produced no important effect; in one case, sleep intervened. Pulse and breathing were somewhat accelerated at first, later were subnormal. On one occasion, when taken with suicidal intent, 1.5 grm. cocaine was not followed by any serious effect upon the health. The fatal dose for man, therefore, must be very great if it cannot be established that the preparations of that date were not pure cocaine.

So far as the coca infusion have been experimented with, it may be considered that the leaves contain between 0.02 to 0.2 per cent. of cocaine. Of my cocaine mur. sol., 0.05 grm. appears to be an effective dose for man.

After subcutaneous injection of an attenuated solution of cocaine in man, a sensation of warmth is felt at first, then loss of sensation in the region about the injection; finally, a circumscribed redness of the skin, and after about thirty minutes, a return to the normal condition. Applied to the tongue, it benumbs the nerve sensibility of the same.

Quite lately, Dr. Th. Aschenbrandt, in the No. 50 (1883) of the *Deutsche Med. Wochenschrift,* has appeared as a champion of the cocaine, in that he accredits it with most remarkably beneficial qualities in great debility, particularly that produced by diarrhœa. During the last month, Prof. Dr. E. v. Fleischl, in Vienna, and Dr. Sigm. Freud, Physician in the General Hospital in Vienna, have diligently occupied themselves with this preparation. The former, particularly, has determined that the cocaine, by hypodermic injection, has proved itself to be an invaluable adjuvant against the continued use of morphia; also, against a single fatal dose. This fact alone should give the remedy an enduring place among the treasures of the physician.

Those above referred to have given the medicine in the form of its muriatic acid combination, in doses of 0.05 to 0.15 grm., and as much as 0.5 grm., in a watery solution, has been given per day. Dr. Freud has made a number of experiments upon himself and others, and besides a constant increase in physical strength, he has recognized a true coca–euphrasy. The feeling of hunger and the want of sleep disappear during the action of the coca.

With the attempt, in the following lines, to answer the question as to the therapeutic worth of the cocaine, I must likewise remark that up to the present time only the foundation can be given for future research. To this end, the remedy will be diligently experimented with in the various fields of medical science, so that it may be hoped that decided results as to its real worth may be obtained at an early date.

Cocaine is a stimulant which is peculiarly adapted to elevate the working ability of the body, without any dangerous result. Its action is stronger than that of alcohol. Its use for this purpose in marching or mountain climbing is self-evident. The dose in such cases may be from 0.05 to 0.01 grm., repeated as required.

It is still an open question as to whether mental labor may be carried on a greater length of time or made lighter by its use or not. Even so must it remain undetermined for the present as to whether the psychiater will be able to make use of cocaine for the purpose of inducing a continued elevation of the powers of the nerve centers. The subcutaneous use of cocaine in a daily dose of from 0.0025 to 0.1 grm. has been applied for months to patients suffering from melancholy, with some definite results.

Cocaine is a stomach remedy, in so far that after debauches in eating and drinking, it has produced rapid amelioration, and a normal longing for food, when used in doses of from 0.025 to 0.05 grm.

In atonic weakness of digestion and nervous disturbances of the stomach, a lasting return to the normal condition may be attained from time to time by the use of cocaine.

Also in cachexia is the continued use of cocaine recommended: in phthisis, great anaemia and wasting fevers. Further threatened mercurial cachexia from the continued use of quicksilver has been avoided by the incorporation of cocaine.

In any event, cocaine has its greatest future in morphia, and perhaps, also, in alcohol-abstinence. An American, W. H. Bentley, published in 1878 the observation that coca may paralyze the morphium hunger of the opium–eater. If all that has been recently published in this connection should be confirmed, the remedy is of incalculable worth. Relapses do not occur; on the contrary, the disuse of coca may take place promptly at the proper time without a return of the morphium hunger. Depression and nausea do not occur during the cure; diarrhœa and chills are the only symptoms observable.

In case of gradual or long–continued withdrawal of opium, decreasing doses of morphia and increasing doses of cocaine are given. In cases of absolute and sudden abstinence, doses of 0.1 grm. are injected as often as the morphium hunger is felt. Confinement in institutions becomes quite unnecessary with this method. Dr. Freud, who, with others, saw such a case, after ten days cocaine treatment (0.1 grm. subcutaneously three times per day), pass into positive convalescence, is of the opinion that a direct antagonism exists between morphium and cocaine.

The treatment for the alcohol habit is far more difficult. The first experiments date also from America, and seem to have turned out favorably.

The remedy has also been recommended as an aphrodisiac, and Dr. Freud has undoubtedly observed sexual excitation occur after the use of cocaine.

As already remarked, as soon as cocaine comes in contact with the mucous membrane it produces a transitory loss of sensation of the same. Therefore not only attempts to cure certain laryngeal and throat affections are made, but it is hoped that in operations in the larynx it may be employed as a local anaesthetic. An important and obviously frequent employment of cocaine seems to be assured in the field of ophthalmology.

On the 15th of September, at the meeting of the Ophthalmological Society in Heidelberg, the experiments of Dr. Koller, instituted in

Vienna, were discussed. Dr. Koller has experimented on the eyes of animals, also upon his own, a number of times, and has found that immediately after dropping in a 2 per cent. solution of cocaine mur., a brief burning occurs, continued for not more than a half minute, which is soon succeeded by an uncertain feeling of dryness. The opening of the lids of the experimented eye appears wider; reflex action, which otherwise occurs upon approaching the cornea, motion of the head, of the lids, and shrinking back of the eye–ball, disappears. In this condition a small scoop can be passed over the cornea without producing an unpleasant sensation; or the conjunctiva bulbi may be taken up with the forceps.

The anaesthesia of the eye lasts about ten minutes, though lack of sensation may persist some hours. Twenty to thirty minutes after the instillation the pupil dilates and returns to its normal state in a few (say twelve) hours. A slight, easily–overcome paralysis of the accommodation during this time is the only abnormality observed. As to the rest, the functions of the eye remain intact.

Dr. Koller has determined the anaesthetic action of the cocaine in animals in which he had produced a keratitis by irritation with a foreign body. He prognosticates a future for the cocaine in the removal of foreign bodies from the cornea, and in greater operations (cataract–extractions, iridectomy), or as a narcotic in corneal and conjunctival affections. Which salt of cocaine can be used to the greatest advantage in eye-practice will be very shortly determined.

It remains to be said that the experiments, the results of which I have here reported, have been made, without exception, with the preparations brought into commerce under the name of *"Cocaïn mur. solut. Merck;"* only for these are the doses and action, as above stated, to be relied upon.

E. Merck
October, 1884

CHAPTER 7

"Coca"

DECEMBER 1884

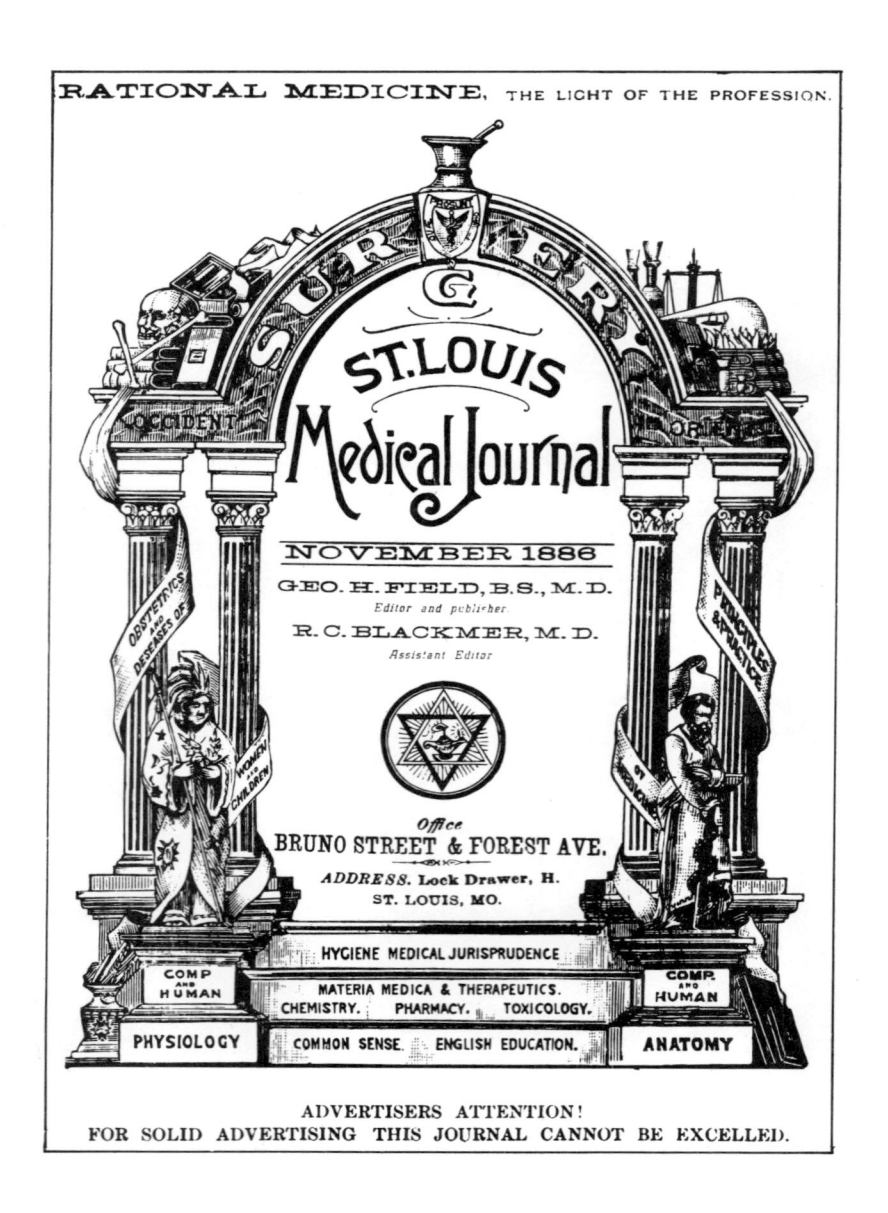

"Coca" by S. Freud (*centralblatt für die gesammte Therapie*) in *The Saint Louis Medical and Surgical Journal,* December 1884, Vol. XLVII, pp. 502–05.
Translated by S. Pollak, M.D.

Many American journals published regular columns of translations from the foreign literature. The following article which was the first appearance of Über Coca *in English is not a translation in the usual sense. It is both an abstract of the original and a compendium from several sources. In particular one should note that the opinion on the use of cocaine in the treatment of morphinism is from Fleischl not Freud, probably derived from the article by E. Merck. Ed.*

The shrub Erythroxylon coca is largely cultivated in South America especially in Peru and Bolivia. The shrub was known to and stood in high favor with the Spanish conquerors of Peru; it was intimately connected with religious ceremonies. The leaves were sacrificed to the gods, masticated during worship and thrust into the mouth of the dead, in order to secure a favorable welcome yonder. The council of Lima forbade the use of it as heathenish and sinful. But when the Spaniards saw that the Indians could not perform the heavy tasks imposed upon them in the mines without it, they repealed the interdiction. They dealt it out to their laborers three to four times a day, a custom still prevailing.

The Indians carry in their wanderings a bag of coca leaves, and also a flask of wood ashes. Of the leaves they make a bolus in their mouth, which they perforate with a thorn dipped in the ashes, then masticate it under a flow of saliva. Three to four ounces a day is a moderate allowance. They form the habit of chewing coca leaves in early youth, which is never relinquished. When they have a long journey before them, or when they take wives to themselves, or do any thing demanding great physical exertion, they increase the allowance of coca leaves. There are abundant proofs that the Indians are capable of performing the heaviest labor without feeling the necessity of food while chewing coca.

The immoderate use of coca will cause a cachexia, exhibiting indigestion, loss of flesh and strength, mental ethical depravity, apathy to any and everything, a condition resembling very much alcoholism and morphinism. This coca cachexia is always the result of an excessive use of it, but never from a disproportion of labor to the quantity used.

An effective substance of coca leaves is cocaine. This crystal tastes bitter, causes anesthesia of the mucosa, is difficult of solution in water, easier in alcohol and diluted acids, especially hydrochloric or muriatic acid.

The result of experiments is, that coca in small doses is stimulating, in large doses paralyzing to the nerves, the latter particularly so in small animals. Cocaine after a brief stimulation is paralyzing in frogs, first the ends of sensory nerves, later the sensory nerves themselves are impaired, breathing at first hurried, is later brought to a standstill, the action of the heart is gradually slowed to a diastolic rest. 2mg will cause toxic symptoms. Cocaine in warm-blooded animals is exciting of the psychic and cerebral centres. Dogs after 0.01g of cocaine per kilo, show maniacal perturbations, also pendulous movements of the head.

Cocaine will cause accelerated respiration, increased frequency of pulse from paralysis of the N. vagi, mydriasis, increased peristalsis, high blood pressure and diminished secretions.

The effect of cocaine on man does not differ much from that of coca leaves. The writer took 0.05g cocaine in a 1% solution while fatigued and ill at ease. This solution tasted at first bitter but soon became quite pleasant. After a few minutes he felt exhilarated and perfectly comfortable. Lips and tongue were furred and later unusually warm. Respiration was slower and deeper, he felt tired and sleepy, with yawning and mental confusion. After a few minutes began the true cocaine euphoria, with frequent cool eructations. Pulse at first slower, later of an increased frequency, great heat about the head.

Other experimentalists found evanescent erythema, increased micturition, dryness of conjunctiva and the mucosa of the nose, mouth and throat.

The physical effect of *cocaïn. mur.* in doses of 0.05–0.10g is exhilaration and constant euphoria. Exhilaration like that of alcohol is entirely wanting. One feels self reliant, vigorous and active, not the mental excitement of alcohol, **theine**, and caffein but simply normally strong, capable of doing work. Now came the most marvelous effects of coca. Long, persistent, intense mental or muscular work can be performed without fatigue. Food and sleep so imperatively demanded of all, are wholly disregarded. In cocainism one can eat and drink, but the conviction that it could be dispensed with prevails. One can forego sleep, though sleep will come if desired. In the early stage of cocainism, insomnia is the rule, but it is by no means annoying and painful.

The effect of an ordinary dose of cocaine subsides gradually, so that it is difficult to determine its relative duration. If while under the influence of cocaine intensely heavy work is performed for about four to five hours, a repetition of the dose will be required in order to guard against fatigue; the effect will last longer if the work is not too heavy. No lassitude will follow the coca euphoria, the effect of 0.05g dose will last twenty-four hours.

Therapeutically it is used as a stimulant wherever and whenever an increase of physical capacity is required to be maintained without food and without rest; thus in wars, in long journeys, in mountain ascents etc. where alcohol is so highly prized, coca is a far better force-giving stimulant than it and absolutely harmless in long use, the great cost of it is the objection.

Also in disturbed digestion is coca recommended; it is the oldest, best known and highest recommended corrective of digestion. The various preparations are given in all forms of dyspepsia, especially those arising from general debility. Pressure, fullness of the stomach, lassitude, inability to work disappear after small doses of cocaine (0.025–0.05g).

It has also been given with good results in cachexia and syphilis, also in morphinism and alcoholism, it is considered an absolute antidote against morphine, also in asthmatic trouble it has proven of great benefit.

Above all has recently the local anesthetic effect of muriate of cocaine in ophthalmic surgery been discovered and confirmed by oculists of the U.S.A. and Europe.

Professor Fleischl of Vienna confirms the fact that muriate of cocaine is invaluable, subcutaneously injected in *morphinism* (0.05–0.15g dissolved in water) a gradual withdrawal of morphine requires a gradual increase of cocaine, but a sudden abstinence from morphine, requires a subcutaneous injection of 0.1g of cocaine. *Inebriate asylums can be entirely dispensed with;* in ten days a radical cure can be effected by an injection of 0.1g of cocaine three times a day.* It is evident that there is a direct antagonism between morphine and cocaine.

It is the best stomachic after a debauch either in eating or drinking, 0.025–0.05g will promptly bring about a restoration to normal condition.

---

*The two preceding paragraphs are not in Freud's *Über Coca*. Cf. E. Merck pg. 80 *Ed.*

CHAPTER 8

Papers on Coca and other Prospects

JANUARY 1885

From *The Letters of Sigmund Freud*, edited by Ernst L. Freud.

Freud's continued use of cocaine is documented in his letters to Martha Bernays, his fiancée. It has been suggested by Vom Scheidt[1] that the development of psychoanalysis and ego psychology was partially the result of Freud's attempt to deal with the different state of consciousness produced by cocaine. In these letters his involvement with the use of the drug as a euphoriant is obvious. Ed.

To MARTHA BERNAYS
Vienna, Wednesday
January 7, 1885

My beloved darling

At last a letter from you again, which makes me laugh, for it informs me that you now possess three copies of the article* you wanted. Now you can send one on to Rosa.

On one point I cannot agree with you, Marty. You say how sensible we are now and how foolishly we treated one another in the past. I gladly agree that we are now sensible enough to believe in our love without any doubts, but we would never have reached this point had it not been for all that went before. It was the very intensity of my misery brought about by the many hours of suffering you caused me two years ago and since, that convinced me of my love for you. Today, what with all the work, chasing after money, position, and reputation, all of which hardly allows me time to drop you an affectionate line, I could never reach that conviction. Let us not despise the times when for me a day was made worth living merely by a letter from you, when a decision from you meant a decision between life and death. I really don't know what else I could have done at that time; it was a difficult period of struggle and finally of victory, and only after it was all over could I find the inner peace to work toward our future. In those days I was fighting for your love as I am now for your person, and you must admit that I had to work as hard for the one as I am now for the other.

During the past few days I have been feeling a bit seedy, engaged as I am in the twofold struggle which forms the content of *Auch Einer:*† struggle against a cold and against "the object." I have

---

* *Über Coca.*
† Novel by the German author Friedrich Theodor Vischer.

a combination of nose–throat–gums–ear catarrh and am correspondingly miserable. I suggest you read about it in Vischer.

My object has a specific name, it is called neuralgia—face–ache. The question is whether I shall succeed in curing it. I have already told you about one case which has very much improved; but now I am treating a second, a clear, much nicer case, at Prof. Weinlechner's. The result of the first day was very good. But what will the following days produce? I am so excited about it, for if it works I would be assured for some time to come of attracting the attention so essential for getting on in the world. Everything we hope for would be there and perhaps even Fleischl could benefit from it. And even if it isn't absolutely sensational, something is bound to come out of it.

I now have eleven subscribers for the lecture course, but wretchedly few cases, and I am continuously worried as to how I am to find the necessary material, but I will manage.

Yesterday evening I went to see Breuer, where I met Fleischl, who was very talkative but not in a particularly pleasant way. If only I could relieve him of the pain!

Goodnight, my little woman. You are quite right, it is sad that we cannot exchange kisses, only letters.

Your
Sigmund

Vienna, Friday
January 16, 1885
My sweet darling

A very affectionate greeting for the seventeenth; do you realize, by the way, that my lecture course also started on a seventeenth? And here, quickly, is my news, to make you happy at once. The die is cast. Today I had my wild beard trimmed and went to see Nothnagel.... I promised to be brief. "You once said you would be willing to assist me, and I believed it because it was you who said so. Now the opportunity has arrived. I would like to ask your opinion whether on the strength of my existing publications I should apply for the *Dozentur* or whether I should wait till I have more." "What are your papers on, Doctor? Coca—" (So coca is associated with my name.) I interrupted him to produce my collected writings, those from the pre–

Marty days and those of a later date. He just glanced at the number. "You seem to have eight or nine," he said. "Oh, by all means send in your application. When I think of the kind of people who get the *Dozentur*...! There won't be the slightest objection." "But I have several more things to be published, two of them in the immediate future." "You won't need them; these are more than enough." "But there isn't much about neuropathology among them." "That doesn't matter. Who knows anything about neuropathology unless he has studied anatomy and physiology? You do want the *Dozentur* for neuropathology, don't you? In that case three people will be chosen to report—Meynert, Bamberger,* and probably myself. There won't be any opposition, and if any objection is raised on the faculty, surely we are men enough to put it through?" "So I may assume that you will support my application for the *Dozentur?* I know Meynert will." "Certainly, and I don't think there will be any objections; if there are, we'll push it through just the same." I added: "It's a question of legalizing an unauthorized lecture course I'm giving. Actually, I'm only lecturing to some English people in their language, but there's quite a run on it." Then we shook hands warmly and off I went as the newest *Dozent*. I will send in my application next week. This time you won't miss your golden snake.

Let one fond kiss stand for many from
Your
Sigmund

---

* Dr. Heinrich von Bamberger, Professor of Pathology at the Universities of Würzburg and Vienna.

CHAPTER 9

Contribution to the Knowledge of the Effect of Cocaine by Sigmund Freud

JANUARY 1885

Beitrag zur Kenntniss der Cocawirkung. Von Dr. Sigm. Freud, Sekundararzt im k. k. Allgemeinen Krankenhause in Wien. Wiener Medizinische Wochenschrift. Sonnabend, den 31. Jänner 1885. Nr. 5. Fünfunddreissigster Jahrgang, pp. 130–133.
Contribution to the Knowledge of the Effect of Cocaine by Dr. Sigmund Freud, house officer of the General Hospital of Vienna.
Translated by Robert S. Potash, M.D.

In contrast to the former article, Freud concerns himself in this paper not with subjective reactions to the use of cocaine but with the drug's objective effects on measurable quantities of muscular energy and of reaction times. Experiments with the use of a dynamometer and a neuroamoebimeter are reported in detail.
It is interesting to note that increased functioning after the use of cocaine is not understood as a consequence of the drug's direct action on the musculature but as the result of a state of increased general well–being which secondarily improves motor action. Anna Freud.

TO BRING THE COCA PLANT and its alkaloid, cocaine, to the attention of physicians, I published in the July issue of Dr. Heitler's *Journal of Therapy*[1] a study on this subject based on a review of reports contained in the literature and on my own experiments with this long-neglected drug. I can report the unexpectedly rapid and complete success of that effort. While Dr. L. Königstein, at my suggestion, undertook to test the action of cocaine in alleviating pain and restricting secretions in pathological eye conditions, Dr. Carl Koller, quite independently, happened upon the felicitous idea of inducing complete anesthesia and analgesia of the cornea and conjunctiva by means of cocaine whose power to numb mucous membrane had been long known.* Dr. Koller demonstrated, moreover, the practical value of this local anesthetic by experiments on animals and by operations on humans. As a consequence of Koller's report at this year's Ophthalmological Congress at Heidelberg, cocaine has now won general acceptance as a local anesthetic.

In pursuing my researches on cocaine I attempted to investigate objectively and at the same time test and measure quantitatively an impressive general effect of this alkaloid consisting of the creation of a mood of elation and an increase in physical and mental capacity and endurance. I did so because I noticed that the subjective symptoms of the cocaine effect are different for different persons. While some report a euphoria even more intense than that observed by me

---

* The seventh of the uses of cocaine indicated by me deals with local application and closes: "Indeed the anesthetizing properties of cocaine should make it suitable for a good many further applications."

in my own subjective experiments, others, after taking cocaine, feel confused, uncomfortable, and definitely toxic. Schroff senior seems to have belonged to the latter. Schroff was the first (1862) to test the action of cocaine and his personal predisposition, which happened to be non-responsive to cocaine, must bear a share of the blame for the setback of this alkaloid at the time. I expected, too, that an objective method of measurements would reveal greater uniformity in the action of the coca.

As a means of designating the action of coca by changes in measurable quantities (possibly even in different directions), I decided to investigate the motor power of certain muscle groups and psychic reaction time. For the first test I made use of a dynamometer, a spring-metal clasp which upon being pressed together moves a pointer connected to it along a graduated scale. The pointer remains locked at peak pressure. I had at my disposal two instruments: One gave striking results because it was heavier and could be operated with both hands but had the disadvantage of demanding great effort, thereby producing rapid fatigue; the other, a light dynamometer, was designed by Dr. V. Burq for measuring the pressure of one hand only. I soon grew to trust the performance of the dynamometer for I found that the effects of pressure, especially the maximum effects, were free to the highest degree from any influence owing to arbitrary action of the person applying the pressure, and that the manner of applying pressure caused only slight and negligible changes. For testing psychic reaction time I used Exner's neuroamoebimeter. This instrument consists of a metal strip that vibrates 100 times per second. The subject stops the vibrations as soon as he hears the tone caused by the release of the set strip. The time elapsing between the perception of the tone and the completed action of stopping the spring is the reaction time. The number of vibrations is recorded directly in hundredths of a second by a pen. For more detailed uses of this small apparatus and the precautions necessary in handling it the reader is directed to Exner's *"Experimentelle Untersuchung der einfachsten psychischen Prozesse."*[2]

Dr. Herzig was kind enough to cooperate with me in these exacting experiments.

I repeatedly carried out on myself or had carried out these two series of experiments. I realize that such self-observations have the shortcoming, for the person engaged in conducting them, of claiming two sorts of objectivity for the same thing. I had to proceed in this manner for reasons beyond my control and because none of the subjects at my disposal had such a regular reaction to cocaine. The results, though, were also confirmed by my testing of others, mainly colleagues.

On testing with the dynamometer, 0.05–0.10g *cocaïn. mur.* produces a marked increase in the motor power of the arm; i.e., in my case the maximum action of the cocaine begins in about ten to fifteen minutes and remains in a somewhat lessened degree for a number of hours. I shall now discuss a few experiments in detail:

Experiment of November 9, 1884. Dynamometer for two hands;

Time	Pressures	Max.	Average	Remarks
8:00	66–65–60	66	63.6	fasting
10:00	67–55–50	67	57.3	after morning rounds
10:22	67–63–56	67	62	after breakfast
10:30	65–58–67	67	63.6	—
10:33	0.10 *cocaïnum muriaticum*[*]			
10:45	82–75–69	82	75.3	first ruptus
10:55	76–69–64	76	69.6	tired
11:20	78–71–77	78	75.3	euphoria
12:30	72–66–74	74	70.6	before lunch
12:55	77–73–67	77	72.6	—
1:35	75–66–74	75	71.6	after lunch
1:50	76–71–61	76	69.3	—
3:35	65–58–62	65	61.6	euphoria over

[*] Freud did not state the measurement here but it was almost certainly grams, as later specified in his experiment of November 26, 1884. *Ed.*

the pressure is given in pounds. In order to study the influence of fatigue each test consisted of applying pressure three times in quick succession.

As can be seen, cocaine caused a very marked increase in motor power regardless of whether average or maximum values are considered. This increase continued for approximately five hours. My general condition on the day of the experiment was very poor and my motor power was diminished.

Another experiment may demonstrate the action of cocaine in the case of higher starting figures for motor power:

Experiment of November 10, 1884. [Same apparatus.]

Time	Pressures	Max.	Average	Remarks
8:00	60	60	60	tired
10:00	73–63–67	73	67.6	after rounds
—	thereupon, a small indeterminate quantity of cocaine			
10:20	76–70–76	76	74	cheerful
10:30	73–70–68	73	70.3	—
11:35	72–72–74	74	72.6	—
12:50	74–73–63	74	70	—
2:20	70–68–69	70	69	—
4:00	76–74–75	76	75	normal condition
6:00	67–64–58	67	63	after strenuous work
8:30	74–64–67	74	68.3	somewhat tired
—	thereupon, 0.10 *cocaïnum muriaticum**			
8:43	80–73–74	80	75.6	ruptus
8:58	79–76–71	79	75.3	—
9:18	77–72–67	77	72	buoyant feeling

* Once again, Freud did not state the measurement here but it was almost certainly grams. *Ed.*

After continuing these experiments over a period of weeks, I was struck by two facts: Firstly, *the figures for the motor energy of a muscle group reveal a regular fluctuation in the course of a day;* secondly, *the same figures reach quite different absolute values on different days.* These results do not have much to do with the action of cocaine but are perhaps worth mentioning.

The report below may illustrate these daily fluctuations. Experiments of November 27 and 28, 1884. Pressure in kilograms; Burq's dynamometer; the figures refer to the maximum value of three pressures each with the right hand:

November 27			November 28		
Time	Max.	Remarks	Time	Max.	Remarks
7:20	32	on arising	7:20	32	on arising
9:30	35	after rounds fasting	7:50	34–5	fasting
12:00	37+	after many hour's work	10:00	37−	after rounds
2:45	37−	after coffee only	10:30	36–7	after breakfast
4:00	38	after lecture	1:40	36	after work
5:45	37+	after three hours' work	2:40	36	before lecture
6:45	38−	—	4:00	36	after lecture
7:15	35+	tired	5:30	36	after rounds
8:00	36.5	at rest	8:30	37	after coffee
9:15	34	after supper	10:30	35+	after supper

From these as well as from other observations it follows that motor power is at its lowest in the morning—so to say, it has not yet fully wakened—then it increases rapidly, reaches its peak before noon, where it remains constant for the rest of the day, then decreases at a slow and steady rate in the evening but never drops to the morning level. Strenuous work, as long as it does not lead to serious exhaustion, seems rather to increase motor efficiency. The taking of or omission of a meal produced no recognizable effect. Daily fluctuations of motor power seem to coincide with the daily temperature curve.

After these studies were completed, Dr. Max Buch's preliminary report in which he deals with daily fluctuations of motor energy was brought to my attention.[3] Buch's statements deviate from mine only in respect to the afternoon. He found that there is a drop from the afternoon peak to a lower peak in the evening from which point the nightly tapering off of strength then occurs. It may be left open whether or not the difference in our way of life or the fact that Buch used an apparatus marked into smaller units (¼ kg) was the cause for this slight difference in our results. Buch also cites an inaugural dissertation by Powarin,[4] where the essential fact that strength in the morning is at a minimum was already noted.

I have quoted as a second noteworthy fact that motor power attains to different values on different days with the result that the daily fluctuation drops down to a level which can be higher or lower. I have, therefore, listed some days which I began with a minimum force of 28kg and could not achieve any higher than 35kg. The greatest span between daily minimum and maximum values was in my case 6kg; on the other hand, the greatest span on different days was only 4kg.

It became clear to me that the above mentioned variation in motor power which does not depend on the time of day is an expression of the general state of well-being; after all, the subjective phenomenon of this state as bodily feeling [*Gemeingefühl* (coenesthesia)] and mood is to a great extent associated with motor efficiency. I do not consider the cocaine action itself to be a direct one—possibly on the motor-nerve substance or on the muscles—but indirect, effected by an improvement of the general state of well-being. Two facts support this view. Muscular energy increases most obviously after taking cocaine when cocaine euphoria has developed but before the total quantity can be absorbed into the circulation; and motor power in-

Experiment of November 26, 1884.

Time	Reaction times	Max.	Min.	Av.	Remarks
7:10	15½–21½–19–21–18½–24–24	24	15½	20.5	motor energy, 36—, tired

about 7:30, 0.10g cocaïn. mur.

Time	Reaction times	Max.	Min.	Av.	Remarks
7:38	17–21½–16–21–17–16	21½	16	18	motor energy, 39+
8:05	17–17–18–17	18	17	17.2	a little more cocaine
8:15	13½–11–16–15–16–12	16	11	13.9	euphoria
10:30	15½–14½–15–13½–17½	17½	14½	15.2	remaining good feeling motor energy, 37.5

Experiment of December 4, 1884. Well-being. No cocaine.

Time	Reaction times	Max.	Min.	Av.	Remarks
8:15	13½–13–14½–13½	14½	13	13.6	motor energy, 38–39k
8:30	15–14–14–19–15½–15½	19	14	15.5	during 4th reaction a disturbing sound
8:45	11½–13½–14½–12½–16½	16½	12½	13.7	—
9:00	12½–13–13–15½–14–18½	18½	12½	14.2	motor energy, 38

creases considerably if the cocaine takes effect when the general condition is poor and motor power diminished. In this case results achieved under the influence of cocaine even exceed the maximum under normal conditions.

In assessing the value of standard physical quantities to designate the condition of an individual, preference will be given to those magnitudes which, like temperature, show little individual variation. The motor power of a prominent muscle group should not be rejected to designate various conditions in an individual.

A similar, but vaguer, conclusion resulted from the experiments on the influence of cocaine on reaction time. I often noticed that under cocaine my reaction times were shorter and more uniform than before taking the drug; but sometimes, in a more cheerful and efficient mood, my psychic reactions were just as good. Change in reaction time is then a characteristic of cocaine euphoria to which I have also ascribed the increase in muscular strength.

CHAPTER 10

Addenda
to
Über Coca
by Sigmund Freud

FEBRUARY 1885

Nachträge Über Coca. Von Dr. Sigm. Freud, Secundararzt im k. k. Allgemeinen Krankenhause in Wien. Neu durchgesehener und vermehrter Separat-Abdruck aus dem Centralblatt für die gesammte Therapie." Wien, 1885. Verlag Von Moritz Perles.
Addenda to On Coca, by Dr. Sigmund Freud, house officer of the General Hospital of Vienna. A revised and added to reprint from the Centralblatt für die gesammte Therapie, Vienna 1885, Press of Von Moritz Perles.
Translated by Steven A. Edminster; additions to the translation by Frederick C. Redlich.

In early 1885, in response to the many requests for further information which he had received since the July 1884 publication of Üeber Coca, *Freud decided to reprint his essay in pamphlet form in an issue of five hundred copies. He took advantage of this opportunity to add an Addenda, and the title was amended to* Über Coca. *The pamphlet was published in February 1885 under the Moritz Perles imprint. The major differences between the Perles offprint and the July 1884* Centralblatt *article are:*

1) On page 294 of the Centralblatt *article, Freud gives the formula for cocaine as* $C_{17}H_{24}NO_4$. *The 1885 monograph reads* $C_{17}H_{24}N_4$, *an obvious misprint. Modern textbooks, however, cite* $C_{17}H_{21}NO_4$ *as the formula for cocaine.*

2) In the footnote on page 299 of the Centralblatt *article, the spelling of* Merk *has been corrected to* Merck, *and the following sentences have been deleted: "This preparation may be bought in Vienna in* Haubner's Engelapotheke am Hof *at a price which is not much higher than Merk's, but which must, nevertheless, be regarded as very high. The management of the pharmacy in question is trying, as they have been kind enough to inform me, to lower the price of the new drug by establishing new sources of supply."*

3) On page 304 of the Centralblatt *article, the spelling of the word* Merk'sche *has been corrected to* Merck'sche.

4) The word nach *is missing before the name Fliessburg both on page 306 of the* Centralblatt *article and the 1885 Perles offprint. It has been included in the translation by the translator.*

Steven A. Edminster

1. The Effect of Coca On Healthy Human Beings

SINCE THE PUBLICATION of this essay, which appears here as a reprint, I have had occasion to observe the effects of cocaine on quite a number of people; and as a result of my findings I must stress, even more emphatically than before, the diversity of individual reactions to cocaine. I have found some individuals who showed signs of a coca euphoria exactly like my own and others who experienced absolutely no effect from doses of 0.05–0.10 g. Yet others reacted to coca with symptoms of slight intoxication, marked by talkativeness and giddy behavior. On the other hand, an increased capacity for work seemed to me to be a constant symptom of the coca effect. Prompted by my experiences in this respect, I carried out an experiment which was designed to demonstrate the effect of coca by a comparison of the variations in certain measurable quantities in living beings. The successful results of this experiment were reported in the *Wiener medicinische Wochenschrift* of January 31, 1885; they relate to the investigation of muscular power of the arm by means of a dynamometer, and to the examination of mental reaction time with the aid of the neuroamoebimeter, an instrument devised by Professor Exner. I was able to determine, in experiments on myself after taking 0.10g of *cocaïnum muriaticum,* that the pressure which could be exerted by one hand was increased by 2–4kg, and that which could be exerted by both hands, by 4–6kg. In this connection it is interesting to note that the effect of coca is dependent on the condition of the subject at the time the experiment is carried out, and that the effect is more striking when the initial measurement of motor power is low rather than high. The increase in motor power induced by coca occurs suddenly after some fifteen minutes, and lasts, decreasing gradually, for a period of four to five hours. It runs parallel, therefore, to the coca euphoria, and it also seems to stem from an increase in the general preparedness for work, from an improvement in general well-being, rather than from any direct influence of the drug on the motor organs. A variation in mental reaction time was also observed. In my own case, after I had taken coca my mental reaction time was the same as it is when I am in the very best of health, even though beforehand it had been irregular and protracted as a consequence of a rather less perfect state of health.

The power of cocaine to increase muscular strength, which can be proved by the dynamometer, can be considered as conclusive confirmation of reports of the effect of coca on the Indians.

2. The Effect of Coca In Cases of Morphine Addiction

The usefulness of cocaine in cases of morphine collapse has recently been confirmed by Richter (Pankow), who also favors the view, expressed in the above text,* that there is an antagonistic relationship between the effect of cocaine and that of morphine.

3. The Internal Application of Cocaine

As, at present, many authorities seem to harbor unjustified fears with regard to the internal use of cocaine, it is not out of place to stress that even subcutaneous injections—such as I have used with success in cases of long standing sciatica—are quite harmless. For humans the toxic dose is very high, and there seems to be no lethal dose.

4. The Local Effect of Cocaine

The fact that cocaine can be indicated as a local anesthetic has received wide acceptance as a result of Koller's use of it to anesthetize the cornea, and thanks also to the work of Königstein, Jelinek, and countless others; cocaine is thus assured of a lasting value among our medicinal resources. It is to be expected that the internal use of cocaine will lead to just such gratifying results. However, the present still artificially high price of the drug is an obstacle to all further experiments.

---

* See Über Coca, Chapter 5.

CHAPTER 11

On the General Effect of Cocaine by Sigmund Freud

MARCH 1885

Ueber die Allgemeinwirkung des Cocaïns. Vortrag, gehalten im psychiatrischen Verein am 5. Marz 1885 von Dr. Sigm. Freud, Medicinisch-chirurgisches Centralblatt, Nr. 32, pp. 374–375, August 1885.
On the General Effect of Cocaine. A lecture given at the Psychiatric Union on March 5, 1885 by Dr. Sigmund Freud.
Translator unknown.

In this paper read before the Psychiatric Society, Freud attempts to interest his Viennese colleagues in the internal application of cocaine and its ability to raise the general feeling of well–being. After reporting on his own investigations, as described in Contributions to the Knowledge of the Effect of Cocaine, *he advocates experimentation with the drug in psychiatric states of functioning at a reduced level, as for example in nervous weakness, depression without organic lesions, etc. He stresses nevertheless that the usefulness of cocaine in psychiatric practice needs still to be proved.*

What he regards with greater optimism at this juncture is the use of cocaine in withdrawal cures from morphia and other addictions. This was discovered in America and observed by himself in one particular instance. Anna Freud.

LAST SUMMER I made a study of the physiologic action and therapeutic use of cocaine. I am now speaking to you because I believe that some points in this area may also be of interest to a psychiatric society. In this talk, I have excluded entirely the external use of cocaine, which has been introduced so successfully into ophthalmology and is also so valuable in other branches of practical medicine. We are interested only in the effects of cocaine when it is administered internally.

With the conquest of the lands of South America by the Spaniards, it became known that the leaves of the coca plant were used by the natives there as a source of enjoyment, and that the effects of coca, according to the most reliable informants, lay chiefly in a remarkable increase in efficiency. It is easy to understand, therefore, why great expectations were aroused in Europe when the Novara expedition brought a quantity of coca leaves to Europe, and Niemann, one of Wöhler's pupils in Göttingen, prepared a new alkaloid, cocaine, from them. Since then, numerous experiments have been performed with this substance, as well as with the leaves themselves, in order to obtain results similar to the effects of coca on the Indians, but the over-all results of these efforts have been a great disappointment and a tendency to question the credibility of the reports from the lands where coca grows. I do not wish to go into any details here about the probable reasons for these failures, but there are some findings even from those times (60 and 70 years ago) that indicate a heightening of efficiency by cocaine. In the winter of 1883, Dr. von Aschenbrandt reported that Bavarian soldiers who had become fatigued as a result of exposure to such exhausting factors as overexertion, heat, and so forth recovered after they had received very small amounts of cocaine hydrochloride. Perhaps my only merit lies in the fact that I gave credence to these reports. They prompted me to study the effects of coca on my own person and on others.

I can describe the effects of cocaine when taken internally as follows: If one takes a minimally active dose (0.05 to 0.10 g) while in excellent health and does not expect any special exertion thereafter, one can hardly perceive any surprising effect. It is different, however, if this dose of cocaine hydrochloride is taken by a subject whose general health is impaired by fatigue or hunger. After a short time (10–20 minutes), he feels as though he had been raised to the full height of intellectual and bodily vigor, in a state of euphoria, which is distinguished from the euphoria after consumption of alcohol by the absence of any feeling of alteration. However astonishing this effect of ingestion of coca may be, the absence of signs that could distinguish the state from the normal euphoria of good health makes it even more likely that we will underestimate it. As soon as the contrast between the present state and the state before the ingestion of cocaine is forgotten, it is difficult to believe that one is under the influence of a foreign agent, and yet one is very profoundly altered for four to five hours, since so long as the effects of the drug persist, one can perform mental and physical work with great endurance, and the otherwise urgent needs of rest, food, and sleep are thrust aside, as it were. During the first hours after cocaine, it is even impossible to fall asleep. This effect of the alkaloid gradually fades away after the aforesaid time, and is not followed by any depression.

In my paper "On Coca" (*Heitler's Centralblatt für die gesammte Therapie,* July 1884; printed separately by Moritz Perles, 1885), I have given several examples of the disappearance of legitimate fatigue and hunger, etc., which I observed largely among colleagues who had taken cocaine at my request. Since that time, I have made many similar observations, among them that of a writer who for weeks before had been incapable of any literary production and who was able to work for 14 hours without interruption after taking 0.1 g of cocaine hydrochloride. I could not fail to note, however, that the individual disposition plays a major role in the effects of cocaine, perhaps a more important role than with other alkaloids. The subjective phenomena after ingestion of coca differ from person to person, and only few persons experience, like myself, a pure euphoria without alteration. Others already experience slight intoxication, hyperkinesia, and talkativeness after the same amount of cocaine, while still others have no subjective symptoms of the effects of coca at all. On the other hand, heightened functional capacity appeared much more regularly as a symptom of the action of cocaine, and I directed my efforts toward an objective demonstration of the latter, perhaps through changes in values that are readily determined in the living subject and that relate to physical and mental functional capacity. For this purpose, I decided to test the force exerted in a given action by means of a dynamometer and to determine the mental reaction time with Exner's neuramoebimeter. As we know, a dynamometer is an elastic metal clasp whose drawing together moves a pointer along a graduated arc, on which one can read the force needed to move it back in pounds or kilograms. An instrument of this type is useful if it is graduated correctly and does not require too great exertion in handling and if the application of pressure to it involves only the kind of action that we are accustomed to performing in the daily use of our extremities, the form of motion of which thus lies ready, as it were, in our nervous system. The action that I performed was to press one hand or both hands while the arm was stretched out, and I soon convinced myself that it is very easy to obtain constant or constantly changing values with this instrument. The results of my experiments were very surprising. Ingestion of 0.4 g of cocaine hydrochloride increases the effective work of one hand by 2–3 kilograms and that of both hands by 3–4 kilograms, and this effect sets in after a few minutes, at about the same time as the coca euphoria, and gradually fades away in about the same time. In connection with these dynamometric measurements, I had an opportunity to confirm the fact found by M. Buch that muscle force, like temperature, shows regular daily fluctuation. The minimum motor performance is found in the morning after awakening. It rises rapidly in the morning, reaches a maximum in the afternoon, and drops slowly toward evening. I found the difference between maximum and minimum to be 4 kilograms.

I should like to point out a second fluctuation of the muscle force, which is independent of the time of the day and is reflected in the fact that on many days one starts from a lower minimum and reaches only a lower maximum, so that the daily fluctuation takes place on a lower level. I have never been able to find any connection between this lowering of the muscle force and a depressed general state, and for this reason I was compelled to conclude that the effect of cocaine results from an elevation of the central readiness for work rather than from any influence on the motor tract. It must also be remembered that the action of cocaine is more remarkable when the drug is taken by a subject whose motor forces are at their lowest level than when the subject's health is excellent and his motor efficiency at its maximum. The determination of the mental reaction time led to the same results as the dynamometric measurements. The mental reaction time, as we know, refers to the time that elapses between the reception of a sensory impression and the onset of a stipulated motor reaction in response to it. This time is given in hundredths of a second on the small Exner apparatus by the number of oscillations that a pen can make on a soot-covered plate until it is discovered by the reaction of the person under investigation. The tone that is produced when the swinging pen is released serves as the sensory stimulus that prompts the reaction. It was now found that my reaction times became short and more regular, if they had been uneven and longer before. On another occasion, however, I obtained an equally favorable reaction when I performed the experiments initially without cocaine but while in an excellent state of well-being. Here again, the relation between the effect of cocaine and the euphoria elicited by cocaine was evident.

I now come to the two points that are of direct psychiatric interest. Psychiatry is rich in drugs that can subdue over-stimulated nervous activity but deficient in agents that can heighten the performance of the depressed nervous system. It is natural, therefore, that we should think of making use of the effects of cocaine that we have described above in the forms of illness that we interpret as states of weakness and depression of the nervous system without organic lesions. As a matter of fact, cocaine has been used since its discovery against hysteria, hypochondria, etc., and there is no shortage of reports of individual cures obtained with it. Morselli and Buccola have used cocaine in a more extended and systematic fashion in the treatment of melancholiacs and indicate that they obtained slight improvement. On the whole, it must be said that the value of cocaine in psychiatric practice remains to be demonstrated, and it will probably be worthwhile to make a thorough trial as soon as the currently exorbitant price of the drug becomes more reasonable.

We can speak more definitely about another use of cocaine by the psychiatrist. It was first discovered in America that cocaine is capable of alleviating the serious withdrawal symptoms observed in subjects who are abstaining from morphine and of suppressing their craving for morphine. The *Detroit Therapeutic Gazette* has published in recent years a whole series of reports on morphine and opium withdrawals that were achieved with the aid of cocaine, from which it may be concluded, for example, that the patients did not require constant medical surveillance if they were directed to take an effective dose of cocaine whenever they felt a renewed craving for morphine. I myself have had occasion to observe a case of rapid withdrawal from morphine under cocaine treatment here, and I saw that a person who had presented the most severe manifestations of collapse at the time of an earlier withdrawal now remained able, with the aid of cocaine, to work and to stay out of bed, and was reminded of his abstinence only by his shivering, diarrhea, and occasionally recurring craving for morphine. He took about 0.40 g of cocaine per day, and by the end of 20 days the morphine abstinence was overcome. No cocaine habituation set in; on the contrary, an increasing antipathy to the use of cocaine was unmistakably evident. On the basis of my experiences with the effects of cocaine, I have no hesitation in recommending the administration of cocaine for such withdrawal cures in subcutaneous injections of 0.03–0.05 g per dose, without any fear of increasing the dose. On several occasions, I have even seen cocaine quickly eliminate the manifestations of intolerance that appeared after a rather large dose of morphine, as if it had a specific ability to counteract morphine.

Richter,[1] in Pankow, has recently confirmed my experiences with the value of cocaine in the treatment of morphine addicts. I know very well that cocaine appears to be of no value in certain cases of withdrawal treatment, and I am prepared to believe that there are differences in the individual reactions to the alkaloid. Finally, I believe that I should mention that the American physicians have seen fit to report on the cure or palliation of the craving for alcohol in alcoholics.

CHAPTER 12

Parke's Universal Panacea

AUGUST 1885

Gutt[macher, H.], "Neue Arzneimittel und Heilmethoden. Über die verschiedenen Cocäin-Präparate und deren Wirkung," Wiener Medizinische Presse. *August 9, 1885.*

Gutt[macher, H.] "New Medications and Therapeutic Techniques. Concerning the different Cocaine Preparations and Their Effect." *Vienna Medical Press.* August 9, 1885.

Translated by Stephen Fleck, Ferenc Gyorgyey and Robert Byck.

Parke Davis & Company, Detroit and New York, 1885. "Coca Erythroxylon and its Derivatives."

The following article has, in the past, been listed as one of Freud's "Cocaine Papers." It was published in the Wiener Medizinische Presse *and signed with the abbreviation "Gutt." Herman Guttmacher was a co-editor of* Wiener Klinische Wochenschrift *at about the time of the report. It was customary for editors to sign news articles with abbreviated names. Guttmacher's article quotes Freud on Parke's cocaine.* Ed.

The Different Cocaine Preparations and Their Effect

Less than a year ago Dr. Freud brought the attention of the medical world to the effects of the coca plant, that "divine plant" of the Indians, which nourishes the hungry, strengthens the weak, and makes all forget their misfortunes. Cocaine alkaloid from the coca leaves is now used in ophthalmology, and has achieved a status in therapy comparable to essential drugs such as morphine, and quinine. By fulfilling a real need, coca has already made a triumphant march through Europe. It is hard to believe that the plant, whose effects have been known for hundreds of years by the South Americans and to Europeans thru the reports of travellers such as Lossen and Niemann has been ignored for so long. Coca was disregarded until 1859 when our excellent consul, Dr Scherzer, brought leaves back from the expedition on the Austrian frigate Novara and sent the material to Professor Woehler for examination. To a certain extent, we can explain this neglect of coca by the fact that dry coca leaves, which are the only ones which arrive in Europe, have lost some of their effectiveness through both the drying and storage processes. E. Merck found that these old coca leaves did not seem useful for commercial purposes. While this may be a partial explanation for the neglect of cocaine, we must also consider that the majority of cocaine preparations which have been released for use have been almost ineffectual. The effective preparations of Merck and of Gehe are exceptions. Another problem is that cocaine decomposes rapidly in solution, and especially after heating, breaking up into methyl alcohol, benzoic acid and ecgonin. It has been reported that cocaine deteriorates in acid solution, and decomposition can be caused by potassium carbonate forming potassium benzoate. Since great care is required to produce medications of full effectiveness, many preparations containing no active cocaine have come into use.

All of these factors plus the high price of cocaine prevented an even more widespread introduction of the drug. Recently, even the preparations of Merck and Gehe, with which Drs. Freud, Koller, and Koenigstein obtained their excellent results, have become unavailable. The manufacturers suspended cocaine production because of the poor quality of the raw material which they could obtain.

We can, therefore, understand why attention has shifted to America, where the cocaine plant is native and where the raw material can be obtained in fresh condition. Parke Davis & Co., the most prominent pharmaceutical firm in America, already known for the introduction of many new drugs, has now produced a cocaine which is not equal to, but even seems preferable to the European preparations. This cocaine is more soluble, pure white (it has no yellow tinge like the Merck preparations), is free of hygrin, and has an aromatic odor. These properties suggest the greater purity of Parke product. Many clinicians in America and Europe can attest to the effectiveness of the Parke product. Here in Vienna, Professor Schnitzler and Dr. Beregszaszy at the Polyclinic have experimented with cocaine obtained from Parke Davis & Co. and found it to be satisfactory in every respect.

Dr. Beregszaszy has established that the cocaine hydrochloride produced by Parke Davis in Detroit is therapeutically equivalent to other preparations in the practice of rhinology and laryngology.

Dr. Beregszaszy tried solutions of 2%, 5%, 10%, 20% concentrations; he anesthetized the larynx with 10% and 20% solutions, whereas he used 2% and 5% solutions to produce vasoconstriction.

Dr. Freud, the rediscoverer of the coca plant, experimented with Parke's cocaine about which he made the following statement:

"I have examined cocaine muriaticum produced by Parke Davis for its physiological effects and can state that it is fully equal in effect to the Merck preparation of the same name. When taken internally it produces the characteristic coca euphoria. Increases in muscular strength were measured with the dynamometer after equal doses of Parke and Merck cocaine, and they were found to be the same. Parke's cocaine, when applied in 2% solution, anesthetizes the cornea and conjunctiva of the eye equally to the Merck product. Subcutaneously the Parke cocaine produces the same spasms and paralytic effects in animals. The only difference I can detect between the two preparations is that in their taste. The satisfactory results found with Parke cocaine are probably the result of the greater availability of coca leaves in America, and since the price is lower than European products because of lowered transportation expenses, this preparation should have a very great future."

Here, we would like to recapitulate the indications that Dr. Freud proposed for cocaine in July of last year; these are:

(a) *coca as a stimulant;*
(b) *coca in the treatment of gastric disorders;*
(c) *coca in cachexia;*
(d) *coca for the treatment of morphine and alcohol addicts;*
(e) *coca for the treatment of asthma;*
(f) *coca as an aphrodisiac; and*
(g) *the local application of coca.*

The last named use, which is to say, local anesthesia, has been decisive in the general acceptance of cocaine. As Freud said, "There will be a certain increase in [therapeutic] applications which are based on the anesthetic properties of cocaine." This is more than true; the drug has been used beyond our greatest expectations in local anesthesia. Most spectacular in this respect has been the use of the anesthetic and secretion-decreasing effects of cocaine in diseases of the eye. This usage, which Dr. Koenigstein and Dr. Koller independently developed at the suggestion of Dr. Freud, was first presented by Dr. Koller in a lecture at the Heidelberg Congress of Ophthalmologists where he recommended the general usage of cocaine as a local anesthetic.

It was not long before the anesthetic and analgesic properties of cocaine were proven in diseases of the nose, the larynx, and the pharynx; cocaine has even found some therapeutic uses in gynecology. Lastly, it has been useful wherever a local pain-relieving effect is desired—as for instance, with small ulcers. Furthermore, cocaine has been used with excellent result in minor operations on a great number of parts of the body when it has been used to obtain anes-

ADVERTISING DEPARTMENT.

TO PHYSICIANS!

Bromidia.

Formula.—Every *fluid drachm* contains 15 GRS., EACH of pure Brom. Potas. and *purified* Chloral and 1-8 gr. EACH of *gen. imp. ext* Cannabis Ind. and Hyoscyam.

Dose.—*One-half* to *one fluid drachm* in WATER or SYRUP every hour until sleep is produced.

BROMIDIA

is the Hypnotic *par excellence*

It produces refreshing sleep, and is *exceedingly* valuable in sleeplessness, nervousness, neuralgia, headache, convulsions, colics, etc., and will relieve when *opiates fail*. *Unlike* preparations of opium *it does not lock up the secretions*. In the restlessness and delirium of Fevers *it is absolutely invaluable*.

BATTLE & CO., Chemists,
ST. LOUIS.

TO PHYSICIANS!

≡Iodia.≡

Formula.—IODIA is a combination of Active Principles obtained from the green roots of Stillingia, Helonias, Saxifraga, Menispermum and Aromatics. Each *fluid* drachm also contains *five* grains IOD. POTAS. and *three* grains PHOS. IRON.

Dose.—One or two *fluid* drachms (more or less as indicated) *three* times a day before meals.

IODIA

is the *Ideal* Alterative.

☞It has been LARGELY PRESCRIBED in syphilitic, scrofulous, cutaneous and female diseases, and has an established reputation as being the best alterative ever introduced to the Profession.

BATTLE & CO., Chemists,
ST. LOUIS.

The Anodyne Principle of Opium.

≡Papine.≡

PAPINE is the *Anodyne* or *Pain-Relieving* Principle of Opium in a pleasant liquid form. Its advantages are: That it produces *the good effects* of Opium with less tendency to cause nausea, vomiting, constipation, etc. It is the *safest* and *most pleasant* of all the preparations of Opium, and is uniform in strength. It can be relied upon in all cases where Opium or Morphia *is indicated*.

ONE FLUID drachm represents one grain of Opium in Anodyne Power.

AVERAGE DOSE, one-half to one teaspoonful.

—o—

Prepared *EXCLUSIVELY* for *Physicians' Prescriptionc.*

—o—

BATTLE & CO., Chemists,
ST. LOUIS.

EXHILARATING! NOURISHING!

Cocalac.

COCALAC is a combination of Coca and the Cereal Lacto-Phosphoids.

DOSE.—*One tablespoonful three times a day, or oftener, as indicated.*

☞**Stimulation without Reaction.**

☞COCALAC is a scientific blending of Coca with the Lacto-Phosphoidal principle of wheat and oats; it is a fine TONIC and NUTRITIVE, *being capable of sustaining life without any other food or drink*, and therefore valuable for the convalescing, dyspeptic, or nervous patient. *It is also delicious to the taste and* ACCEPTABLE *to the stomach*.

—o—

BATTLE & CO., Chemists,
ST. LOUIS.

☞Send for pamphlet of Testimonials and Cases, and mention this JOURNAL.

thesia of mucuous membranes. The literature about cocaine has, in the last few months, become so voluminous that it would require a much longer and more extensive article than this to summarize all of the reports, even if we were to attempt to be brief. However, therapeutic experiments with cocaine have not ended and a whole new field has been opened up by the availability of Parke's cocaine, a reliable, effective, and purer cocaine. This is a beautiful white powder (available at a low price). In addition, 2% and 4% stable solutions of cocaine, citricum and cocaine salicylicum, as well as cocaine olienicum, are available here in Europe. The salicylate and citrate salts produced by Parke Davis are particularly stable and, therefore, can be used in aqueous solutions. Parke's cocaine olienicum can be used externally in both suppositories and ointments.

Because of the low price and stability of the Parke product, we hope to see more application of cocaine's wonderful, general therapeutic effects. These consist of mood elevation, increased physical and mental performance, as well as increased endurance. The experiments of Dr. Freud, which were done with the assistance of Dr. Herrig using the Burq dynamometer and the Exner neuroamoebimeter, demonstrate to us with mathematical certainty that doses from .05 to .10 grams improve the motor strength in the arms. It would be a pity if these outstanding properties of cocaine were left unexploited.

Gutt.

The following material has been abstracted from Parke, Davis and Company's 1885 promotional brochure, Coca Erythroxylon and Its Derivatives. *This has been edited with a view to presenting that material most pertinent to the present volume and to convey a representative sampling of the type of material contained therein. Ed.*

COCA ERYTHROXYLON

AND ITS DERIVATIVES

A *Résumé* of their History; Botanical Origin; Production and Cultivation; Chemical Composition; Therapeutic Application; Physiological Action; and Medicinal Preparations.

—EMBRACING—

REPORTS ON THEIR EMPLOYMENT

—IN—

General and Minor Surgery; Ophthalmology; Otology; Laryngology; Gynaecology; Genito–Urinary, Nasal and Dental Surgery; in the Treatment of the Alcohol and Opium Habits; in General Medicine; etc. etc.

Compiled by the
SCIENTIFIC DEPARTMENT OF PARKE, DAVIS & CO.,
Detroit and New York

1885

Introduction

A simple narrative of facts regarding the Coca shrub and its derivatives, and especially of its alkaloid—Cocaine—and the wonderful role its preparations now play in practice would, it is believed, form a chapter in the history of medicine and surgery full of interest not only to the practical physician and surgeon, and the progressive therapeutist, but to all who recognize the importance of a drug which, through its stimulant properties, can supply the place of food, make the coward brave, the silent eloquent, free the victims of the alcohol and opium habits from their bondage, and, as an anesthetic, render the sufferer insensitive to pain, and make attainable to the surgeon heights of what may be termed "aesthetic surgery," never reached before.

It is the purpose of this compilation to present these facts for the convenience of the medical profession, thus exhibiting the wide range of application of the drug and its derivatives, and point out some of the most eligible preparations for its internal use and appliances for its external application, which have been placed before the profession.

Application in Medicine and Surgery, and Eligible Preparations for Internal, Topical, and Hypodermic Use

An enumeration of the diseases in which coca and cocaine have been found of service would include a category of almost all the maladies that flesh is heir to. The medical press teems with reports of its efficacy in such a variety of affections that the sanguine might think it not too much to suppose that in coca and its derivatives the universal panacea for human ills had at last been discovered.

Allowing for the exaggeration of enthusiasm, it remains the fact that already cocaine claims a place in medicine and surgery equal to that of opium and quinine, and coca has been held to be better adapted for use as a popular restorative and stimulant than either tea or coffee.

A writer in the *Centralblatt für Klinische Medicine* [sic]* thus summarizes the therapeutic application of cocaine.

1. *As a stimulant if one wishes to do extra physical or mental work.*
2. *In gastric indigestion.*
3. *In the cachexiae.*
4. *In combating the effects of morphine and alcohol.*
5. *In asthma.*
6. *As an aphrodisiac.*
7. *As a local anesthetic.*

Its utility has thus far been more fully demonstrated as a local anesthetic than in any other role. It is certainly the best agent at the command of the physician or surgeon in facilitating minor surgical procedures, examinations, and operations of every variety. It has proved a boon not alone to the ophthalmologist, the otologist, the laryngologist, the gynecologist, the rhinoscopist, the dermatologist, the dental surgeon, and the genito–urinary surgeon, but also to the general practitioner.

Eligible Preparations of Coca and Cocaine, and Appliances for Their Convenient Administration and Application

Among these may be mentioned the following, which, it is believed, embrace all that will be needed by physicians and surgeons to meet the requirements of practice:†

Fluid extract coca.	Cocaine alkaloid.
Wine of coca.	Cocaine citrate solution, 4%.
Coca cordial.	Cocaine hydrobromate pure in crystals.
Coca cheroots.	Cocaine hydrobromate solution, 4%.
Coca cigarettes.	Cocaine muriate, pure in crystals.
Cocaine inhalant.	Cocaine muriate solution, 2%.
Cocaine oleate, 5%.	Cocaine muriate solution, 4%.
	Cocaine salicylate solution, 4%.

---

* This is probably referring to *Über Coca*. The reference should be *Centralblatt für gesammte therapie*. Ed.
† Manufactured by Parke, Davis & Co., Manufacturing Chemists. Descriptive circulars, etc., mailed on application.

COCA CORDIAL.

— A —

PALATABLE PREPARATION

OF

COCA ERYTHROX- YLON

CONTAINING

In an agreeable vehicle the active medicinal principle, free from the bitter astringent constituents of the drug.

THE SEDATIVE, tonic, and stimulants effects of coca erythroxylon and its preparations, and their wide application in medical practice are now too well known to the medical profession to need extended comment.

Coca has been extensively used with gratifying success for the relief of morbid conditions depending on nervous exhaustion, in the nervous irritability following excesses of any kind, in neurasthenia, to facilitate digestion in dyspepsia, to relieve the morbid depression of spirits resulting from exhausting mental labor, in nausea and vomiting of reflex origin, and in the treatment of the alcohol and opium habits.

In a great variety of affections it has proved itself to be a drug ranking in therapeutic importance with opium and quinine.

The Coca Cordial presents the drug in a palatable form, commending it especially to the larsge class of person of delicate nervous organization, for whom it is most often indicated.

In its preparation the astringent and bitter constituents of Coca which are not essential to its medicinal action have been eliminated, while care has been taken to retain unchanged the active principle cocaine. One fluid ounce of the cordial represents 60 gains of coca leaves of good quality, the vehicle employed being an agreeable cordial of a rich vinous flavor.

☞ We shall be pleased to send on application a circular more fully descriptive of Coca Cordial and its application, and we trust physicians will communicate to us the results of their experience in the use of this preparation, so far as it is likely to be of general interest to the profession.

PARKE, DAVIS & CO.,
Manufacturing Chemists,
DETROIT, MICH.

0 Maide Street. } New York,
1 Liberty

In addition to these preparations there has been presented a very complete cocaine case, containing every essential for the topical application of cocaine, including a hypodermic syringe, camel's hair pencil, a minim pipette, a vial to contain a solution of cocaine muriate, five capsules, each containing one grain of cocaine muriate in crystals, and a card containing directions for making a two–per–cent. and four–per–cent. solution of muriate of cocaine.

Although the applications of the various preparations of cocaine will no doubt be suggested to the intelligent physician, we venture, nevertheless, to mention in a general way a few facts regarding the special adaptability of some of them for use in particular classes of disease.

Thus it is evident that the *Fluid extract of coca, Wine of coca,* and *Coca cordial* are best adapted for oral administration; the solutions of the salts for topical and hypodermic use for anesthetic purposes; the *Cocaine oleate* for treatment of neuralgia of superficial nerves, or for anesthetizing a sensitive tooth for filling; the *Coca cheroots* and *cigarettes* and *Cocaine inhalent* for affections of the respiratory tract, spasmodic cough, bronchitis, etc.

Coca–Leaf Cigars and Cigarettes[1]

I have been experimenting for some time with the leaf of erythroxylon coca in the form of a cigar—first, for the purpose of ascertaining whether the drug would thus produce its physiological effects, and, secondly, in view of a new therapeutic application. It is too soon yet to express a positive opinion in regard to the latter, but I have had sufficient experience with them to say something about the former; and as I find that others are already commencing to enter this field, I may be excused for calling the attention of the profession at this early date, my excuse being that I wish to receive what credit may accrue from my share in their introduction.

Some time after I commenced my experiments, I found that Dr. Louis Lewis of this city, was employing coca in the form of a cigarette in the treatment of throat affections with success, and, as he says he has been using the drug in this way for nine years, he is entitled certainly to the credit of priority.

Dr. Lewis' cigarettes are composed partly of coca– and partly of tobacco–leaf. This has its advantages and disadvantages. Without discussing this point, however, I employ a cigar made of pure coca–leaf, with a wrapper of mild imported tobacco of fine quality, and a cigarette of pure coca–leaf containing no tobacco, wrapped with the best quality of rice–paper. Those who do not object to the tobacco can use the cigars, while those who have objections to it can employ the cigarette; while for those who object to the tobacco wrapper and the paper wrapper also I prepare a "smoking tobacco," of the pure coca–leaf, without admixture of any kind, which may be smoked in a pipe.

Coca is too well–known to the profession to make it necessary for anything more than the briefest description of the plant, its history, or its virtues.

The erythroxylon coca grows in moist and woody regions on the eastern slope of the Andes, from 2,000 to 10,000 feet above the level of the sea, and is highly valued and cultivated by the natives of Peru, Chili, and Bolivia, who make great use of it as a medicine and as an article of diet. It answers as a substitute for the tea, coffee, tobacco, hashish, opium, etc., of other nations. The natives masticate the dried leaves with finely–powdered chalk, or with a highly alkaline substance prepared from roasted potatoes and the ashes of various plants and which they call *llicta*. It is said that its use enables them to endure fatigue and exertion for many hours, and even for many days, with but little nourishment of any other kind, and while under its influence they are said to perform prodigies of labor.

Let me compare, therefore, the action of these cigars with that said to be produced by the drug, not only by the natives, but by Bartholow, Wood, the United States Dispensatory, the National Dispensatory, and other authorities equally well known, who are investigating the properties of this remarkable drug.

First, all authorities agree that the use of coca, either in the leaf, fluid extract, or wine, is followed by a feeling of contentment and of well–being, the sense of fatigue is removed, drowsiness is experienced for a brief period, but is soon followed by wakefulness and increased mental activity. The celebrated pedestrian Weston, having learned their powers, was detected in the use of coca–leaves during one of his extraordinary feats in London. The question then, is, does coca, smoked, produce these effects?

I have testimony as to the feeling of contentment and well–being:

Dr. M., of Wilmington, Delaware, one of the leading physicians of that State, made some experiments in this direction for me. Being thoroughly acquainted with the effect of the drug, having frequently used it in connection with his extensive practice, and often experienced its effects on himself, what he has to say must be received as of weight. At the time of the experiment which was tried upon himself he was feeling somewhat depressed—had the blues, in other words—owing to the absence of his family and the loneliness of his house without them. After dinner he smoked a couple of the cigars, with the effect that the "blues" were expelled and he felt the exhilarating effect of the drug in the same manner as after a dose of the wine. It is his opinion that the effect of the cigars is milder than that of the wine, but he is satisfied that he experienced the peculiar power of the coca by smoking it. He will continue his experiments in other cases.

Mr. S., of the same city, who was suffering from dyspepsia and its attending depression, smoked the cigars after meals at my suggestion, the result being to dispel the depressed feeling and remove the fullness experienced after eating a meal. Repeated experiments confirm this. As coca is said to stimulate the gastric nerves and greatly facilitate digestion, the above experience seems to prove that the cigar has a similar effect.

Mr. C., a clerk in a cigar–manufactory, Philadelphia, smoked several of the cigars. He says that the first one was used during the hot weather of summer, when he was nervous and depressed by the heat. The effect was to stimulate him, remove the depression, and steady his nerves, and he felt well afterwards for the rest of the day. Repeated experiment confirms him in the belief as to the correctness of his view that coca–leaf smoked is a stimulant and tonic. He inhaled the smoke.

Dr. K., Philadelphia, has smoked a number of the cigars at my request. He is familiar with the effect of coca, having used it while a student as a stimulant during his researches on the heart at the physiological laboratory of the Jefferson Medical College. He recognizes the stimulating effect of the drug in the cigar.

Mr. M., Philadelphia, a chemist of much reputation and a very careful observer finds a stimulating effect from the cigar the same as his experience in the use of coca. He will continue to experiment with it.

Prof. S., for many years a teacher of pharmacy in Philadelphia, a gentleman of excellent powers of observation, says that he experiences the peculiar effect of coca on smoking the cigar.

Chief Engineer N., U.S.N., a member of a recent Arctic exploring expedition, says that he did not experience any exhilaration from the smoke of the coca–leaf. He will, however, continue his experiments still further, and report to me after doing so.

Personally, I have found the effect of smoking coca–leaves to bear out the statement that the drug produces a general excitation of the circulatory and nervous systems. Smoking and inhaling the smoke of one or two cigars will increase my own pulse–rate some eight or ten beats to the minute. It certainly relieves the sense of fatigue. Smoked at night, in my own case and in the cases of several of my patients, it produces wakefulness similar to strong coffee.

The exaltation produced by it does not seem to be followed by any feeling of languor or depression. I find it a relief after a full meal, like a good tobacco cigar. It seems to impart increased vigor to the muscular system as well as to the intellect, with an indescribable feeling of satisfaction. I have never experienced any intoxicating effect from smoking it. Dr. Bartholow says that coca, as is the case with tea and coffee, acts as an indirect nutrient by checking waste, and hence a less amount of food is found necessary to maintain the bodily functions; and it is probable that some of the constituents of coca are utilized in the economy as food, and that the retardation of tissue–waste is not the sole reason why work may be done by the same person better with than without it: and I have just learned, in a letter from Messrs. Parke, Davis & Co., that "a Mr. Stevens, a citizen of Abilene, Kansas, who was afflicted with hay–fever, and was about to go to the mountains, had concluded to remain at home, having obtained relief from the use of cigarettes of coca. Every morning he uses a cigarette, and finds perfect relief. He uses three per day, and also has used an application of a two–per–cent. solution of muriate, but finds that the cigarettes relieve him quicker and the effects last longer."

To sum up, therefore, coca smoked seems to produce the same effect on the system as coca taken internally in the form of fluid extract, wine, or elixir, but not in such a marked degree. Coca itself is known to be stimulant, tonic, and restorative to the system in the treatment of various diseases marked by debility and exhaustion. Nervous debility and exhaustion in all its forms, whether caused by disease or excesses, are said to be relieved by it. Fatigue disappears, to be followed by a feeling of indescribable calm and satisfaction, increased strength of brain and muscle, and desire for mental and muscular occupation.

Coca has been used with great success in the treatment of the opium habit. It is also an excellent substitute for tobacco. It has been successfully used in dyspepsia, flatulency, colic, gastralgia, enteralgia, hysteria, hypochondria, spinal irritation, idiopathic convulsions, nervous erethism, and in the debility following severe acute affections. As it is a valuable restorative agent, checking tissue–waste, it is a useful remedy in consumption and wasting diseases generally. It is also of value in the nervous forms of sick–headache, *migraine*. It is said to be an aphrodisiac.

Now, my object in publishing this article is to introduce coca–leaf cigars to the profession. I have furnished what information I have to prove the cigars are capable of producing the action of the drug. In my own mind I have no doubts on the subject, though the effects are milder than those resulting from the employment of the fluid preparations of coca internally. I have also summed up the properties said to be possessed by coca as a therapeutic agent. I have produced evidence, in addition to that furnished by Dr. Lewis, that it is of value in the treatment of hay–fever; and, as it is important that the true value of this form of using coca–leaf should be known, I have had some made, and I will send samples to members of the profession, free of charge, who may desire to test them, and will publish the results, favorable or otherwise, in the medical press. I have no proprietary interest in them, nor have I copyrighted this article concerning them. The idea of coca in this form, and all information concerning it, is free to the use of the profession.

Hypodermic Use of Cocaine

The hypodermic use of cocaine has been ably discussed by J. M. DaCosta, M.D., in the following paper, entitled "Some Observations on the Use of the Hydrochlorate of Cocaine, Especially its Hypodermic Use," read before the College of Physicians of Philadelphia, and published in the *Medical News,* December 13, 1884:

Hydrochlorate of cocaine is a drug evidently of such power that, on reading the effects produced on the eye, I determined to investigate its properties in other respects, with a view of ascertaining whether it might be of use to the physician as well as to the ophthalmologist. I shall first detail some conclusions I have arrived at with reference to its *local* action.

On the *throat* it undoubtedly diminishes the sensibility, and is serviceable in causing the laryngoscope to be better borne. Moreover, it is of use in irritable relaxed throats, and in instances in which there is spasmodic difficulty in swallowing associated with this irritability, or from other causes. In ulcers at the back of the throat, connected with dysphagia, painting the parts two or three times daily affords considerable relief. Only, for this to last, the solutions employed must be stronger than those which have been used—not from two to four, but from eight to twelve per cent. In tubercular laryngitis the action is excellent. Even a four–per–cent. solution gives hours of relief, in some cases as many as six hours freedom from the sense of irritation and the difficulty of swallowing; and stronger solutions relieve for a longer time. The result obtained is far more certain and decided than from the local use of morphia. Compared with iodoform, it is probably less permanent, but as good, or better, at the time.

Dr. Jurist, whom I asked to employ the hydrochlorate of cocaine at the throat clinic of the Jefferson Medical College, has favored me with a note in which he speaks of the remedy being "brilliantly successful" in relieving pain and making deglutition easy in painful diseases of the pharynx and larynx, preeminently in tuberculosis and in syphilis.

Using chromic acid and the galvanic-cautery frequently, he found that, by first painting the parts with a four per cent. solution, the employment of these agents could be made comparatively painless, and that the efficacy of these, or, indeed, of all caustic and destructive means, is not interfered with.

In syphilitic ulcerations especially this was tested, and much suffering prevented. Where only four–per–cent. solutions are employed, the patient may not feel the caustic application to the abraded surface for about twenty or thirty minutes, but after this it becomes painful. All trials should be preceded by careful cleansing of the parts. The local action of the cocaine is also astringent and hemostatic, as well as one destroying sensibility. This local action may also be perceived on the tongue and gums. "Although facilitating intralaryngeal medication, it does not prevent spasms," Dr. Jurist writes me, "and consequently is valuable in intralaryngeal operations only on account of its anesthetic effects."

As regards the local use of cocaine on other portions of the human body I am able to record some observations made in my ward at the Philadelphia Hospital. In one instance, pain in a hollow molar tooth was speedily relieved by inserting a piece of cotton saturated with a four–per–cent. solution. It may, in passing, be remarked that cocaine used hypodermically in the same patient failed to mitigate an attack of intestinal pain of colicky kind which had lasted for two days. A case of earache which seemed to be neuralgia was at once relieved by instilling a few drops of a four–per–cent. solution into the meatus; and a similar observation was made by the resident physician in the ward of my colleague, Dr. Hutchinson. As regards facial neuralgias, the results were less decisive than anticipated. Perhaps they would become more so if we were to rub in an oleate of cocaine over the aching nerves, or larger nerve trunks, or to use a hypodermic for its local use where the disordered nerves are superficial and easily reached. In one instance of neuralgia of the face, in which the pain shot into the jaws, painting the gums of the upper jaw with a four–per–cent. solution gave very speedy relief. For the amelioration of painful and irritable affections of the nasal mucous membrane, hydrochlorate of cocaine, in not less than a four–per–cent. solution, is of use; and I have known applications with caustics made without pain when the membrane, after being well cleansed, had been painted with the solution. Since becoming acquainted with the action of the remedy, I have had no case of rose cold or hay fever; but it ought to be of service, and I would suggest its employ in these most troublesome affections.

While discussing its local use, it may not be inappropriate to refer to the fact that the solutions of the hydrochlorate of cocaine we all employ—Merck's hydrochlorate—contain less of the alkaloid than supposed; a four–per–cent. solution, for instance, is only of about three–per–cent. strength. My attention was called to this by Dr. Jurist, whose remarks, speaking of his observations, I append; and while writing these lines I find that Dr. Squibb has just published the same conclusion:

"The difficulty experienced in obtaining the cocaine hydrochlorate in bulk, while the solutions were always at command, made it seem desirable to study the latter more closely. In conjunction with my friend, Mr. Stedem, a number of examinations were made. Our later investigations included Merck's manufacture in bulk.

"*Experiment I.*—On adding a dilute solution of ammonia to a solution of the cocaine salt, and then agitating with chloroform, the ammonium hydrochlorate could readily be drawn off with a pipette, leaving the cocaine in solution in the chloroform. By carefully evaporating both solutions, the ammonium salt was readily obtained in pure crystalline form. On the watch–crystal into which the chloroform solution was poured, there were formed a number of *white acicular crystals surrounded by an aureola of sticky, resinous material,* light yellow in color, and altogether amorphous in character. The crystals were soluble in hot and cold water; the resinous product in dilute *hydrochloric acid,* but not in water.

"*Experiment II.*—Another portion of the solution was carefully evaporated over a water-bath. The resulting mass was similar in appearance to the first, but was readily soluble in water. The difference in solubility is accounted for by the acid state of the residue. When it is remembered that cocaine and its salts have heretofore been described as colorless and crystallizable, and that Merck's product is amorphous granular, and of a light straw color, and further, that chemical manipulations separate a resinous mass from the commercial article, the proposition that our present solutions do not contain the full proportion of the active principle, appears to be well grounded."

But what has interested me much about the drug, and what, so far as I know, has not been as yet investigated, is its hypodermic employ, elucidating its general action. In the observations I am about to detail, I have been greatly aided by Dr. Ecroyd, the resident physician in my ward at the Pennsylvania Hospital, and by Dr. Woodbury. We have tried the remedy both on the well and the sick, especially in cases of neuralgia and other painful affections, and have arrived at certain definite conclusions. But first let me speak of the dose. We began with one minim of a two, then of a four–per–cent. solution, only to find them inert. No influence could be detected on pulse, respiration or temperature; nor was any local anesthesia produced at the point of injection. Indeed, no decided effects are produced with less than eight minims of a four–per–cent. solution, or one–third of a grain of the hydrochlorate of cocaine; and half a grain will show these effects even more strikingly. In some instances two thirds of a grain were used.

As regards the local influence at the point of injection, there is considerable difference whether a superficial or a deep hypodermic be used. A hypodermic thrown into the superficial layers occasions local anesthesia, so that the part may be pricked with needles without these being felt. In one case in which we tried one of these superficial injections in a boy of nineteen, a wheal was produced which was quite insensitive, while all around it sensation was preserved, though perhaps slightly reduced. It is evident, therefore, that if it be desirable to use the hypodermic means of producing local insensibility for the removal of small tumors and the like, a superficial injection immediately into or very close to the parts to be removed will have to be practiced. These superficial injections do not occasion subsequent inflammation or abscesses. This is equally true of deeper injection into the tissue below the skin in the manner in which hypodermics are generally given. But the deeper injections do not produce local anesthesia of the surface.

Now, as regards the *general* effect of hydrochlorate of cocaine hypodermically employed, it has a little, but not very much, influence on *sensation*. Most patients speak of a sense of warmth all over the body, which, beginning at the point of injection, becomes general in from five to ten minutes; it is, however, not of long duration, the arm in which the injection was practiced feeling numb or heavy, or, as one expressed it, "funny." In him, half a grain having been thrown into the left forearm, the sensibility of the skin was diminished from the elbow down to the fingers on that side, and two sharp points were not as distinctly as previously distinguished at the tips of the fingers. There was no change of general sensibility in the legs. The mucous membrane of the lips, tongue, and fauces, was slightly less sensitive to sharp points; the conjunctiva was less sensitive, the pupils were dilated.

On the whole, then, there is some general reduction of sensibility, though it is not marked, and is transitory. And this observation accords with others in which one-third of a grain was used, where the alteration of sensibility showed even less; and with a few in which two-thirds of a grain were employed. The general sensibility is therefore only slightly altered.

On the *temperature*, the effect is to heighten it somewhat. This is the record taken by Dr. Ecroyd in the case of a well-nourished man suffering from pains in back and gluteal region, seemingly due to muscular rheumatism:

One-third of a grain of hydrochlorate of cocaine was used; no local anesthesia was produced at the point of injection, and there was no influence on the pain.

At 11.00 A.M. (before injection), pulse 76; resp. 17; temp. 97.5°.
At 11.25 A.M. (after injection), pulse 70; resp. 16; temp. 98.5°.
At 11.40 A.M. (after injection), pulse 66; resp. 16; temp. 98.5°.
At 11.55 A.M. (after injection), pulse 64; resp. 16; temp. 98.4°.
At 12.10 P.M. (after injection), pulse 68; resp. 16; temp. 99°.

Similar observations were made in other cases; and it may, in general terms, be stated that the temperature rises from half a degree to a degree and a half; that it does not do so abruptly; but that the rise is maintained for several hours. Within ten minutes after the injection has been given, an increased heat is registered. In one case it was four–tenths of a degree above the figure of starting, and it never reached more than half a degree, which it did one hour and five minutes after the hypodermic injection of one-third of a grain.

The most striking effect of the hypodermic injection of cocaine is on the *circulation*. The pulse may be somewhat accelerated or slower; but it always becomes fuller and stronger. The frequency of beat was noted to fall from sixty-six to fifty-four, twenty minutes after the injection. In other instances there was but little variation; in a few a slight quickening was detected. But not in a single instance was there not a fuller and a stronger pulse. We made many observations on these points at intervals of fifteen minutes, the sphygmograph being kept in place to insure uniformity of pressure, and always with the same result.

On the *pupils* the influence is very marked. They become speedily dilated; and with the change, uncertainty of vision is complained of. The dilation of the pupils, following the hypodermic injection, does not last more than a couple of hours, and during this period ophthalmoscopic examination is of course very easy.

On the *secretions,* I have not as yet fully studied the drug. On the bowels it had no influence; the urine appeared increased in quantity, and the specific gravity decidedly lowered, while the phosphates were found to be increased. But our observations were not very numerous or definite on these points.

Summing up now some of the general effects observed, the drug, used hypodermically in the doses mentioned, failed to relieve attacks of intestinal pain, and was useless in cases of obstinate neuralgias, especially in sciatica. This was especially shown in a case at the Pennsylvania Hospital, in which about ten hypodermic injections were given, varying between one–third and a half grain, but in which no decided effect on the pain or the disease was produced. It is, however, fair to state that the case was of a year's standing, and had

NEW REMEDIES.

☞ **Your Special Attention is Called to the Note Below.**

QUININE FLOWER.—Used in the South during the late war, to some extent, as a substitute for quinine, and now introduced to the profession by us.

YERBA REUMA.—From the Pacific slope, now introduced by us. Used in diseases of the mucous passages, especially in catarrh, acute and chronic, leucorrhœa, gonorrhœa and dysentery.

KAVA KAVA.—From the Sandwich Islands. First introduced by us. An efficient and agreeable remedy in gonorrhœa, gleet, gout and rheumatism.

CASCARA SAGRADO.—Introduced by us. It has long been regarded by the residents of the Pacific coast as a sovereign remedy for habitual constipation and dyspepsia.

COTO BARK.—From Bolivia. First introduced by us. It is said to be almost a specific against diarrhœa in its various modifications.

COCA LEAVES.—A powerful nervous excitant, giving great vigor to the muscular system and sustaining the human frame under extreme physical exertion and fatigue.

PARAGUAY TEA.—Largely used in South America as a stimulant to sustain the system when undergoing hunger or great fatigue during the summer heats.

GUACO LEAVES.—This valuable remedy was also first introduced by us. Its use is indicated in cholera, diarrhœa, chronic rheumatism, etc.

BERBERIS AQUIFOLIUM.—A new California drug, now introduced by us, possessing extraordinary powers as a combined alterative and tonic, and valuable in syphilitic and scrofulous diseases, salt rheum, etc.

BOLDO LEAVES.—First introduced by us. The new South American tonic. In France it has been employed in cases where quinine could not be tolerated.

ARECA NUTS.—First introduced by us. From India. Strongly astringent. Used by Dr. Morris, of England, in the removal of tape worm.

GRINDELIA SQUARROSA.—From California. First introduced by us. An excellent and efficient remedy in malarial diseases, enlarged spleen, etc.

YERBA SANTA.—From northern California. First introduced by us. This drug is a standard remedy in the Western States in bronchial and laryngeal disorders.

FUCUS VESICULOSUS.—First introduced by us. An anti-fat remedy of great merit. No derangement of the stomach or general system seems to result from its use.

GRINDELIA ROBUSTA.—From the Pacific Slope. Since this drug was first introduced by us, it has earned for itself a reputation for almost specific curative action in ast ma. NOTE.—There are several false varieties of this plant, which are offered as genuine. Physicians will readily perceive the difference in the taste of the fluid extract, as compared with our preparation of the TRUE plant.

KOOSO, GUARANA, BAEL FRUIT, BUCKEYE BARK, URTICA DIOICA SOAP TREE BARK SANDAL WOOD, PULSATILLA, SUNDEW.	USTILAGO MADIS, MAGNOLIA FLOWERS AILANTHUS GLANDULOSA, FIVE-FLOWERED GENTIAN, NIGHT-BLOOMING CEREUS GRINDELIA COMPOUND, XANTHIUM SPINOSUM, WATER FENNEL SEED, POMEGRANATE BARK, EVENING PRIMROSE.	DAMIANA, BEARSFOOT, BROOMTOP, COUGHGRASS, CASTOR LEAVES PARSLEY SEED, ARBOR VITÆ, CHIRETTA, KAMALA.

NOTE.—For a detailed description of the botanical history and medicinal application of each drug, send stamp for our descriptive circular. We will also furnish our price list if desired. Any inquiry regarding these New Remedies will be promptly answered.

PARKE, DAVIS & CO.,
Manufacturing Chemists,
DETROIT.
FOR SALE BY

Richardson & Co., St. Louis.   Meyer Bros. & Co. St., Louis.
Morrisson, Plummer & Co., Chicago.

☞ In corresponding with advertisers please mention **The Medical Journal.** ☜

resisted blisters and chloroform injections. The cocaine influenced somewhat the dull pain; but did no permanent good. Neither in this case nor in others did it induce sleep. In certain very superficial neuralgias, its local action, not its constitutional influence, does temporary good. As an anesthetic, its local action is the one which will give it its great value; and in diseases of the eye, ear, throat, tongue, and nose, the insensibility to which it gives rise suggests a wide range of application. But this insensibility cannot be produced to a sufficient degree through the constitutional effect of a hypodermic.

Yet thus resorted to, the remedy has other and valuable uses. The effects on the pulse and temperature recorded in these observations, suggest its application in many a condition of collapse, of weak heart, or heart failure; and its employ in low fevers, too, as a cardiac stimulant is a self–evident proposition. How permanent the benefit, how often the doses must be repeated, are matters which experience alone can determine.

Cocaine in the Treatment of the Alcohol and Opium Habits, and as an Antidote in Cases of Opium Poisoning.

The extensive study of the effects of cocaine and its salts, which has resulted from the discovery of the anesthetic power of cocaine hydrochlorate, has brought into prominence the therapeutic value of this drug in the treatment of the opium and alcohol habits.

While the stimulant and tonic effects of coca and its derivatives have long been recognized as being of value in counteracting the depressant effects of opium and alcohol, it has remained for recent experimenters to claim that in cocaine we have a remedy, whose physiological action and therapeutic effects, as recorded by competent observers, leave no doubt as to its great efficacy in the treatment of the alcoholic habit, its almost specific action in affording relief to the victims of the opium habit, and its antidotal effect in cases of poisoning by opium and its preparations.

In an article by E. Merck, published in the *Klinische Monatsblätter für Augenheilkunde Zeherden* for October, 1884, a translation of which subsequently appeared in the *Chicago Medical Journal and*

Examiner, February, 1885, it is stated that Professor E. Fleischl and Dr. Sigm. Freud, of Vienna, have carefully studied the action of cocaine, and as a result of their observations, have determined that this drug has proved itself to be an invaluable aid against the continued use of morphia and also *against a single fatal dose.*

These experimenters have given the medicine in the form of its muriatic acid combination, in doses of 0.05 to 0.15 g, and as much as 0.5 g in a watery solution has been given per day.

Merck further remarks that cocaine has its greatest future in morphia and alcohol abstinence, that it apparently paralyzes the morphine hunger of the opium eater, relapses do not occur, and depression and nausea do not take place during the cure.

In case of gradual or long continued withdrawal of opium, decreasing doses of morphia and increasing doses of cocaine are given. In cases of absolute and sudden abstinence, doses of 0.01g are injected subcutaneously as often as the morphine hunger is felt. Confinement in institutions becomes quite unnecessary with this method.

Dr. Freud, who, with others saw such a case after 10 days of cocaine treatment (0.01 gramme subcutaneously three times a day) pass into positive convalescence, is of the opinion that a direct antagonism exists between morphine and cocaine.

Professor Fleischl confirms Dr. Freud's statement, recommending the gradual withdrawal of morphine and a gradual increase of cocaine, and that in case of sudden abstinence from morphine, a radical cure can be effected in ten days, by an injection of 0.01 of a gramme of cocaine three times a day, and further adds with reference to the value of cocaine in treating the alcohol habit, *that inebriate asylums can now be entirely dispensed with.*

If these claims are substantiated by more mature observation, and cocaine should prove to be, as the facts recorded would now indicate, the long sought for specific for the opium habit; the reliable antidote in poisoning by opium preparations; and the invaluable stomachic and tonic in alcoholism, it will indeed be the most important therapeutic discovery of the age, the benefit of which to humanity will be simply incalculable.

The Use of Cocaine in Nervous Affections.

At the recent meeting of the American Neurological Association, Dr. J. K. Bauduy, of St. Louis, read a paper in which he recounted his experience with the use of cocaine in the treatment of certain forms of psychical disturbance. We expect to publish Dr. Bauduy's paper shortly. In the meantime, we would call attention to a letter which has been shown us, written by Dr. L. Bremer, of St. Louis, from which we make the following extracts: "Dr. Bauduy, of this city, has been using the cocaine in cases of melancholia with the happiest results. During a recent visit at St. Vincent's Hospital I was, by the kindness of the doctor, afforded an opportunity of witnessing the rapid and wonderful effect which the hypodermic injection of one grain of the drug produced in the affection named. W. H., aged seventeen, who was under my treatment before his admission to the hospital, for hebephrenia, and whose mental state I am thoroughly familiar with, was, on our visit, found in a condition of great depression. Although he knew me well, he refused to speak to or recognize me. The expression of his face was that of utter dejection, despair, and disgust. All efforts to elicit an answer to my questions failed; he remained wrapped up in a sullen silence. The injection of one grain of cocaine changed the scene as by magic. Four minutes after the introduction of the drug the patient began to talk; the spell was broken, and he conversed freely and intelligently on the nature of his trouble. The almost mathematical precision of the effect of the remedy could only be compared to that of morphine in certain nervous affections.

"The second case in which the cocaine was tried in my presence, and yielded a like brilliant result, was that of a young man suffering from a severe form of melancholia combined with a refusal to take nourishment. Five minutes after the administration of the drug he became quiet and partook readily of the nourishment offered him. This patient would never eat except when under the influence of the drug; it was applied for the first time when he was approaching inanition, to avert which the feeding–tube was thought of as a last resort. . . . To my knowledge, Dr. Bauduy has been the first to try cocaine in melancholia."

Dr. Bauduy seems to have been the first to suggest the use of cocaine for the morning sickness of pregnancy. An interesting account of Dr. Scenck's experience with the remedy for that distressing condition will be found in the report of the proceedings of the St. Louis Medico–Chirurgical Society, published in the St. Louis Courier of Medicine for May, where it is expressly stated that the cocaine was used at the suggestion of Dr. Bauduy.—*New York Medical Journal*.

Failures with Cocaine.

Dr. F. C. Riley, of New York, makes a report of two cases in ophthalmic practice which demonstrate that the much lauded new remedy is not always as reliable as might be wished:

Case 1.—Granular lids with intense pannus occurring in a girl of ten years. The photophobia in this case was so marked that, upon facing the patient toward the window in an ordinarily well–lighted room, the eye–ball rolled upward and inward to such a degree as to completely hide the whole corneal expanse from view, unless the superior palpebral covering was lifted.

Two drops of a four–per–cent. solution of cocaine was instilled, at intervals of ten minutes, for a period of half an hour, or three instillations in all, with no perceptable effect either as regarded diminution of sensibility to light or touch. Neither was there any appreciable effect produced upon the size of the pupil, nor did the drug affect the circulation so far as it was possible to observe it.

Three days subsequent to the preceding trial, I determined upon operating to relieve the pannus, and again tried the same solution, instilling four drops every five minutes for a period of three–quarters of an hour, or in all, nine instillations. Careful efforts to touch the conjunctiva or cornea at any part thereof, between each instillation, failed to elicit the slightest evidence of anything even approximating a condition of anesthesia. Feeling that a fair trial had been given the drug in this case, I proceeded to the use of ether and performed syndectomy.

Case 2.—A lad about twelve years of age, who had a perforating ulcer of the cornea about six months since, with prolapsus of iris into the perforation, etc. Cornea almost completely cloudy or pearly. To the outer and upper segment yet remained a small spot of transparent tissue, at which point I deemed it advisable to perform an iridectomy in order to free the entrapped iris, which seemed to produce a constant irritability of the eye. Vision–perception of light only. Using the same solution of cocaine as in the former case, four drops every ten minutes for forty minutes, with absolutely no effect of any kind, either to cornea or conjunctiva, led me to the opinion that the solution was not what it should be. Subsequent results with the same solution have, however, dispelled my suspicion as to the sample used, as I have since obtained all the physiological effects so far noted by other observers. The two cases recorded, however, seem to me to prove beyond the suspicion of a doubt that there are certain conditions, pathological, may be, or individual idiosyncrasies, possibly both, that tend to militate against the verdict so generally expressed thus far in favor of the anesthetic effects of the drug. It seems to me that in the use of this substance, the cases of failure to obtain the desired end should be placed before your readers as well as the brilliant results obtained by so many of us. That it has been a great blessing to many during its short career there is no doubt, and that it will continue to prevent the attendant pain of many operations in the future I am confident. Even if it gives as universal satisfaction in time to come as it has in my hands thus far, it is indeed a friend to the suffering and distressed.—*Medical Record.*

Caution in the Use of Cocaine.[2]

Dr. Knapp, in the *New York Medical Record* for December 13, 1884, first called attention to the precaution which should be observed in the use of the new anesthetic. His reasons are based upon the symptoms presented by the two following cases:

Case 1.—Six minims of a four–per–cent. solution of cocaine were injected close to the posterior segment of the globe. Anesthesia was complete, and the operation successful, there being no disturbing element in the recovery. During the operation, however, it was noticed that the patient became pale.

Case 2.—Five minims of a three–per–cent. solution of cocaine were injected beneath a sebaceous tumor of the lid. Anesthesia was complete, and the somewhat laborious operation was satisfactorily completed; but, during the operation, the patient became as pale as a corpse, felt faint, asked repeatedly for drinks, and was covered with cold perspiration. All of these disagreeable features passed off in fifteen minutes.

Dr. Knapp, while recognizing the safety of injecting larger quantities of cocaine in other parts of the body, suggests that the vascularity of the orbit may allow quicker entrance of fluids injected here into the general circulation than elsewhere, and will hereafter be more cautious in the use of cocaine about the eye—will use one or two minims and feel his way.

The *New York Medical Record,* for January 17, 1885, under the head of "Disagreeable Experiences with Cocaine," refers to numerous communications from correspondents, relating more or less disagreeable or alarming experiences with this drug—some of which appear in its columns. Dr. E. S. Peck, of New York, has had the same experience as Dr. Knapp in operating for squint, under cocaine, in the person of a young lad. A four–per–cent. solution was used, and during the operation, was noted "increasing pallor of the face, together with a profuse, beady perspiration." This was at first attributed to apprehension or pain, but as no pain was experienced, it is thought to have been due to the drug.

Dr. George T. Stevens, of New York, injected four minims of a three–and–a–half–per–cent. solution of cocaine over the course of the rectus internus, preparatory to advancement of this muscle, in the person of a very nervous man. The operation was performed without pain, and ten minutes later the patient had convulsions, difficult breathing, loss of consciousness, and a livid face. All of these symptoms passed off in half an hour, and nothing out of the way could be discovered by a careful examination of the man, further than dilatation of the pupil ad maximum on the operated side. He refers to Dr. Knapp's observations, and suggests that the proximity of the orbit to the large nervous centres may, in part, account for the disagreeable symptoms.

Dr. E. C. River, of Denver, Col., reports the case of a man operated upon for strabismus under cocaine, where six drops of a four–per–cent. solution had been instilled into each eye. After completion of the operation the patient complained of nausea and a feeling of faintness, the face became pale, the hands cold, and the skin covered with cold perspiration; pulse 48. All of these symptoms passed off in a few minutes. The next day cocaine was used as before, without unpleasant effects. The patient said the distress previously experienced was due to the knowledge he had that he was being cut, though he had no pain. He had fainted on a former occasion while witnessing an operation.

The enthusiasm of success on the one hand, and the suspicion of novelty on the other, are two factors which greatly influence us in our estimates as to the value of all new remedies. Should the former outweigh the latter, prominence is quickly gained. A preponderance of the latter delays proper appreciation and recognition. Occasionally, however, they counterbalance, and correct opinions are then quickly gained; but usually this process of vacillation continues to make belief uncertain long after the question should have been definitely settled.

The unusual success which has been accorded to cocaine has given it impetus enough to override much that has been said against it—and I would fain call attention to such effects as the above, which have been ascribed to cocaine, and ask if the suspicions pointing to this agent as the cause have not been as premature as they are unjust.

Few operators in minor surgery have failed to observe the train of symptoms narrated above during operations without an anesthetic. Nay, more, the sight of instruments or of blood, or the mere description of an operation, will at times bring on the various stages of fainting, which may culminate in the patient's falling senseless to the floor in a state of syncope. And in another class of individuals—nervous and excitable—such surroundings will bring on hysterical phenomena, simulating as strongly serious disorders, as they are in themselves harmless. Having shown that it is not necessary to go so far as cocaine for an explanation of phenomena which have been observed during its use, it will be superfluous to state that physiological research has failed to reveal such properties as have been attributed to it upon the operating table. That cocaine can be used about the orbit with comparative impunity, it will suffice to say that three cases of enucleation which I am familiar with have been performed at the New York Eye and Ear Infirmary under its influence, the amount of the drug used being about 3 jss of a four–per–cent. solution in each instance. Two of these cases occurred in the practice of Dr. D. C. Cocks, the other two in my own, where the house surgeon, Dr. L. P. Walker, operated, and Dr. Walker informs me that he has a second case. No untoward symptom was noted in either of these four cases.

The importance of cocaine can hardly be over–estimated, yet it has its limitation; and not an unimportant one is the mental impressions which grow from a knowledge of what is going on during an operation performed under its influence. Local anesthesia does not necessarily bring mental quietude and self–control, and if these two latter conditions are absent, the imagination is apt to play an important role in any operation undertaken. Whether a prominent feature or not, the imagination must always be considered in operations performed without a general anesthetic.—*Medical Record,* February 7, 1885.

CHAPTER 13

"The Cocaine Episode,"
PART THREE

From *The Life and Work of Sigmund Freud* by Ernest Jones, M.D.

Freud had throughout been puzzled by the irregular action of cocaine in different subjects, one which greatly impeded its clinical employment. In order to have a means of testing its action objectively and, if possible, ascertaining on what these variations depended, he decided to make observations on muscular capacity and on swiftness of reactions under cocaine. For the former purpose he used a dynamometer, a not very accurate instrument, and in November 1884 he resumed with various colleagues the observations he had started with it in July with Koller. Incidentally, it seemed to have been an instrument with a special interest for him, since he bought one when he was in Paris so as to observe his own "nervous states."* For the second purpose he worked with Herzig, using Exner's neuro-amoebimeter. The results were published in the *Wiener medizinische Wochenschrift,* January 31, 1885. The paper is of interest as being the only experimental study Freud ever published, and its rather dilettante presentation shows that this was not his real field. The ideas are all good, but the facts are recorded in a somewhat irregular and uncontrolled fashion that would make them hard to correlate with anyone else's observations.

A few definite conclusions emerged from the work. One was that muscular strength, as thus tested, has considerable intrinsic variations, e.g., at different times of the day and on different days even in the same person. The increase produced by cocaine is very slight in perfect health and is pronounced only when the subject is fatigued or depressed. Freud concluded that cocaine has no direct action on the neuromuscular system, but only through improving, in certain circumstances, the general state of well-being.

At the turn of the year a popular article on Freud's monograph appeared in the *Neue Freie Presse,* which was copied in the American press.† It was his old school friend, Franceschini, who wrote it. For some time afterwards Freud was plagued by having to answer letters demanding further information or help. He decided to reprint his essay in pamphlet form in an issue of 500 copies, and to take the

---

* Letter from Freud to Martha Bernays dated January 27, 1886.
† Unpublished letters from Freud to Martha Bernays dated January 9 and February 13, 1885.

opportunity to make various additions to it. This was published in the middle of February 1885 under the same title of "On Coca."

In March he reported that after giving two more lectures on the subject he hoped to have done with it. It was probably the same lecture and was delivered on March 3 at the Physiological Club and on March 5 at the *Psychiatrische Verein* (Psychiatric Society); it was published in the *Medico-Chirurgische Centralblatt,* August 7, 1885. It seems to have met with considerable success. Freud was gratified at *The Lancet* abstracting it.

The lecture was a general review of the topic. He pointed out that, while psychopathology is rich in methods that reduce overstimulated nervous action (bromides, etc.), it was poor in those that can raise any lowered activity, e.g., with weakness or depression of the nervous system. What the use of cocaine in certain cases proved was that an interfering agent of an unknown nature acting centrally could sometimes be removed by chemical means. He admitted that in some cases of morphia addiction it was not helpful, whereas in others it was of great value. He had seen no cases of cocaine addiction. (This was before Fleischl had suffered from cocaine intoxication.) So he could say that in such cases: "I should unhesitatingly advise cocaine being administered in subcutaneous injections of 0.03–0.05 grams per dose and without minding an accumulation of the drug."

But Freud was far from having done with the episode. Too much general interest, both pro and contra, had been aroused for that. In April an American firm offered him 60 gulden ($24) to test their cocaine in comparison with Merck's, and it proved to be as good. In the same month he was conducting "coca experiments" with Königstein, but he did not say what they were. In the next month we hear that there were always new uses being found for cocaine; the latest was that patients with hydrophobia could swallow after their throats had been painted with it.*

On April 5, 1885, Freud's father called on him with the news that there was something wrong with the sight of one of his eyes. Freud was inclined to make light of it and regard it as something temporary,

---

* Unpublished letter from Freud to Martha Bernays dated May 19, 1885.

but Koller, who happened to be there, examined it and made the diagnosis of glaucoma.* They called in their senior, Königstein, who operated, and very successfully, the next day, Koller, who administered the local anesthetic with Freud's assistance, gracefully remarked that the three people concerned with the introduction of cocaine were all present together. Freud must have been proud to have helped his father and to prove to him that he had after all amounted to something.

Freud remained on the friendliest terms with Koller. He was one of the most enthusiastic of the friends who congratulated him on the successful outcome of his duel with an anti-Semitic colleague, and he was greatly concerned about his serious illness later in the year. The last mention of him is of Freud's writing to congratulate him on an appointment in Utrecht, with the hope of visiting him there for Pan's.

To return to the story of Fleischl, which was of immense importance to Freud, not only in connection with cocaine. Something has been said of his personality in an earlier chapter. Freud first admired him from a distance, but after leaving the Brücke Institute he had come to know him more personally. In February 1884, for instance, he speaks of his "intimate friendship" with Fleischl. Earlier than this, in the month of his engagement, he wrote of him as follows:

Yesterday I was with my friend Ernst v. Fleischl, whom I have hitherto, before I knew Martha, envied in all respects. Now I have the advantage over him. He has been engaged for ten or twelve years to someone of his own age, who was willing to wait for him indefinitely and from whom he has now for some unknown reason parted. He is a most distinguished man, for whom both nature and upbringing have done their best. Rich, trained in all physical exercises, with the stamp of genius in his energetic features, handsome, with fine feelings, gifted with all the talents, and able to form an original judgment on most matters; he has always been my ideal and I could not rest till we became friends and I could experience a pure joy in his ability and reputation.†

---

* Unpublished letter from Freud to Martha Bernays dated April 6, 1885.
† An alternative translation of this excerpt from Freud's letter to Martha Bernays of June 27, 1882 is published in *The Letters of Sigmund Freud.* Ed.

He had promised Fleischl not to betray his "secret" that he was learning Sanskrit. Then followed a long fantasy how happy such a man with all these advantages could make Martha, but he broke off to assert his own claim to her. "Why shouldn't I for once have more than I deserve? Martha remains my own!"

On another occasion he wrote:

I admire and love him with an intellectual passion, if you will allow such a phrase. His destruction* will move me as the destruction of a sacred and famous temple would have affected an ancient Greek. I love him not so much as a human being, but as one of Creation's precious achievements. And you needn't be at all jealous.

But this wonderful man suffered on a grand scale. The quite unbearable nerve pain which had already tormented him for ten years gradually wore him down. His mind became periodically affected. He took large doses of morphia, with the usual consequences. Freud got his first insight into his condition on a short visit in October 1883.

I asked him quite disconsolately where all this was going to lead to. He said that his parents regarded him as a great *savant* and he would try to keep at his work as long as they lived. Once they were dead he would shoot himself, for he thought it was quite impossible to hold out for long. It would be senseless to try to console a man who sees his situation so clearly.

A fortnight later he had another affecting interview.

He is not the sort of man you can approach with empty words of consolation. His state is precisely as desperate as he says, and one cannot contradict him. . . . 'I can't bear,' he said, 'to have to do everything with three times the effort others use, when I was so accustomed to doing things more easily than they. No one else would endure what I do,' he added, and I know him well enough to believe him.

As was mentioned above, it was early in May 1884 that Freud first administered cocaine in the hope that thereby Fleischl would be able to dispense with the morphia, and for a short time this was very

---

* Referring to his terrible disease and approaching death.

successful. From then on Freud visited him regularly, helped him to arrange his library, and so on. But only a week later, in spite of the cocaine weaning him from morphia, Fleischl's condition was pitiable. After several vain attempts to get an answer to his knockings Freud procured help and he, Obersteiner, and Exner burst into the room to find Fleischl lying almost senseless with pain. Breuer, his doctor, then arranged that Obersteiner should get into his room every day with a master key. A couple of days later, Billroth, having had no success with several operations on the stump of the hand, tried the effect of electrical stimulation under narcosis; as one might expect, the result was disastrous and Fleischl's state worse than ever.

Fleischl shared Freud's optimistic view about the value of cocaine, and when a shortened translation of the monograph was published in the *St. Louis Medical and Surgical Journal,* in December 1884, he added a note describing his own good experiences with it in connection with the withdrawal of morphia. He considered the two drugs were antithetical.

In January 1885 Freud, who had now been trying to relieve the pain of trigeminal neuralgia by injecting cocaine into the nerve, hoped to do the same for Fleischl's neuromata, but no good seems to have come of it. On an occasion in April Freud had sat up all night with him, Fleischl spending the whole time in a warm bath by his side. He wrote that it was quite impossible to describe this, since he had never experienced anything like it; "every note of the profoundest despair was sounded." It was the first of many such nights he passed in the following couple of months. By this time Fleischl was taking enormous doses of cocaine; Freud noted that he had spent no less than 1,800 marks ($428) on it in the past three months, which meant a full gram a day—a hundred times the quantity Freud was accustomed to take, and then only on occasion. On June 8 Freud wrote that the frightful doses had harmed Fleischl greatly and, although he kept sending Martha cocaine, he warned her against acquiring the habit. He noted Brücke's endless kindness to Fleischl, who was, it will be remembered, his Assistant at the Institute.

Even before this, however, Freud had lived through a good deal.

Every time I ask myself if I shall ever in my life experience anything so agitating or exciting as these nights.... His talk, his explanations of all possible obscure things, his judgments on the persons in our circle, his manifold activity interrupted by states of the completest exhaustion relieved by morphia and cocaine: all that makes an *ensemble* that cannot be described.

But the stimulation emanating from Fleischl was such that it even compensated for the horrors.

Among Fleischl's symptoms were attacks of fainting (often with convulsions), severe insomnia, and lack of control over a variety of eccentric behavior. The cocaine had for some time helped in all these respects, but the huge doses needed led to a chronic intoxication, and finally to a delirium tremens with white snakes creeping over his skin. This came to a crisis on June 4. On calling in the evening Freud found him in such a state—Brücke and Schenk were also there—that he went to fetch Breuer and then spent the night there. It was the most frightful night he had ever spent.

Towards the end of June Breuer told him that Fleischl's relatives wanted Freud to spend the month of August in St. Gilgen looking after him. It would have meant leaving the hospital prematurely, missing some courses, and also breaking off the anatomical researches in the middle, but Freud for personal reasons was inclined to consent. In the end Fleischl insisted on being alone. Freud thought he could not go on for more than another six months, but Fleischl lived six painful years longer.*

---

* This biographical summary is continued in Chapter Seventeen.

CHAPTER 14

Cocaine as a Means to an End

PARIS 1886

From *The Letters of Sigmund Freud*, edited by Ernst L. Freud.

In these letters to his fiancée, Freud casually describes his own use of cocaine. Ed.

To MARTHA BERNAYS
Paris,
Monday, 11 P.M.
January 18, 1886
My sweet Princess

...Today your sweet letter arrived at last, and I must now send off my answer in this mutilated form, otherwise you will have to wait even longer. I have so exhausted myself writing that I can barely hold the pen.... Yesterday I spent more than an hour with Charcot.... I would love to give you a description of his home; but this must wait for another day. What's more, he invited me (as well as Ricchetti) to come to his house tomorrow evening after dinner: "Il y aura du monde." You can probably imagine my apprehension mixed with curiosity and satisfaction. White tie and white gloves, even a fresh shirt, a careful brushing of my last remaining hair, and so on. A little cocaine, to untie my tongue. It is quite all right of course for this news to be widely distributed in Hamburg and Vienna, even with exaggerations such as that he kissed me on the forehead (à la Liszt). As you see, I am not doing at all badly and I am far from laughing at you and your plans.

My fondest greetings and I would love to be your dentist, who I am sure doesn't know how to value it, only how to charge.

Your
Sigmund

Wednesday
January 20, 1886
My beloved little woman

....I had meant to write to you at midnight, but couldn't find the matches, and so had to take off my elegant clothes and go to bed by the light of the moon. So let us begin at the beginning. On Saturday Charcot came up to Ricchetti and invited him to dine at his house on Tuesday before leaving. Startled, R. declined, and finally accepted to go after dinner. Then Charcot turned to me and repeated the latter form of invitation, which I accepted with a bow, feeling delighted. . . .

After Charcot had reminded us once more of our appointment on Tuesday morning, we spent all the afternoon preparing for the evening. Ricchetti, who hitherto had been going about in the most incredibly shabby clothes, had been persuaded by his wife to buy a new pair of trousers and a hat; his tailor is said to have told him that for a party it is quite unnecessary to wear a tail coat and that he could go in a redingote, with the result that he was the only guest not in full evening dress. My appearance was immaculate except that I had replaced the unfortunate ready–made white tie with one of the beautiful black ones from Hamburg. This was my tail coat's first appearance; I had bought myself a new shirt and white gloves, as the washable pair are no longer very nice; I had my hair set and my rather wild beard trimmed in the French style; altogether I spent fourteen francs on the evening. As a result I looked very fine and made a favorable impression on myself. We drove there in a carriage the expenses of which we shared. R. was terribly nervous, I quite calm with the help of a small dose of cocaine, although his success was assured and I had reasons to fear making a blunder. We were the first after–dinner guests and as we had to wait for the others to come from the dining room, we spent the time admiring the wonderful salons. But then they came and we were under fire: M. and Madame Charcot; Mlle Charcot; M. Léon Charcot; a young M. Daudet, an unattractive youth, son of Alphonse Daudet; Prof. Brouardel,* doctor of forensic medicine, a manly, intelligent head; M. Strauss, an assistant of Pasteur and well known for his work on cholera; Prof. Lépine† of Lyons, one of France's most distinguished clinicians, a small sickly man; M. Giles de la Tourette, former assistant to Charcot, now to Brouardel, a true Provençal; a Prof. Brock, *membre de l'Institut,* mathematician and astronomer who at once started talking German and turned out to be a Norwegian; then came Charcot's brother, a gentleman who looked like Prof. Vulpian but wasn't, and several others whose names I never learned; also an Italian painter,

---

* Paul Camille Hyppolite Brouardel, Professor of Forensic Medicine, later for many years doyen of the Faculty of Medicine in Paris.
† Professor Raphaël Lépine, member of the French Academy of Science.

Toffano.* And now you will be anxious to know how I fared in this distinguished company. Very well. I approached Lépine, whose work I knew, and had a long conversation with him; then I talked to Strauss and Giles de la Tourette, and accepted a cup of coffee from Mme Charcot; later on I drank beer, smoked like a chimney, and felt very much at ease without the slightest mishap occurring. Indeed, one couldn't help feeling at ease, for the whole atmosphere was so informal and a great deal of attention was paid to us foreigners. Lépine suggested I should join him in Lyons, which I wouldn't mind doing; he asked me a great many questions about the Vienna hospital staff and at one moment I became the center of attention. R. had been paying court to Mademoiselle and Madame and the latter suddenly became full of enthusiasm and announced: "qu'il parle toutes les langues. Et vous, Monsieur?" asked Madame Charcot, turning to me. "German, English, a little Spanish," I replied. "And French only very badly." She found this sufficient, and Charcot added: "Il est trop modeste, il ne lui manque que d'habituer l'oreille." I then admitted that I often don't understand what has been said until half a minute later, and compared this failing to the symptoms of tabes, which went very well.

These were my achievements (or rather the achievements of cocaine), which left me very satisfied. I also received permission to attend Prof. Brouardel's course in the Morgue, where I have been today. The lecture was fascinating, the subject matter not very suitable for delicate nerves. It is described as the latest murder in every Paris newspaper. . . .

I very much wonder, by the way, whether this invitation will be the last. I believe it may, for in fact I owe it to Ricchetti. . . .

With a fond kiss
Your
Sigmund

Paris, Tuesday
February 2, 1886
My beloved sweet darling

You write so charmingly and sensibly and every time you speak your mind about something I feel soothed. I don't know how to

---

* Emile Toffano, whose picture "Enfin Seuls" (exhibited at the Paris Salon in 1880), was reproduced and sold all over the world.

thank you; I have recently decided to show you a special kind of consideration (you will laugh): by making up my mind not to be ill. For my tiredness is a sort of minor illness; neurasthenia, it is called; produced by the toils, the worries and excitements of these last years, and whenever I have been with you it has always left me as though touched by a magic wand. So I must aim at being with you very soon and for a long time, and since this is hardly possible except by marrying I must try soon to earn the famous 3000 florins a year; and as I am not unindustrious and the prospects aren't bad, I am not unhappy either and am not concerned about my nervousness....

The news of the day is that I received a very friendly letter from Obersteiner, in whose good will I place, as you know, a certain—though still rather vague—hope. Among other things, he tells me of the scientific scandals going on at the moment in Vienna. To think of the Viennese circle of highly respectable people does me good, even from a distance. One really must try not to become as wicked as people make one out, but one should learn to be careful....

The bit of cocaine I have just taken is making me talkative, my little woman. I will go on writing and comment on your criticism of my wretched self. Do you realize how strangely a human being is constructed, that his virtues are often the seed of his downfall and his faults the source of his happiness? What you write about the character of the family Bernays is of course quite correct. But I have no reason to grumble about it. It is to this exaggeration (to which you yourself so charmingly admit) that I owe my luck, for otherwise I would never have found the courage to court you. Whether it was luck for you too, we won't go into. But if today were to be my last on earth and someone asked me how I had fared, he would be told by me that in spite of everything—poverty, long struggle for success, little favor among men, oversensitiveness, nervousness, and worries—I have nevertheless been happy simply because of the anticipation of one day having you to myself and of the certainty that you love me. I have always been frank with you, haven't I? I haven't even made use of the license usually granted to a person of the other sex—of showing you my best side. For a long, long time I have criticized you and picked you to pieces, and the result of it all is that I want nothing but to have you, and have you just as you are.

Do you really find my appearance so attractive? Well, this I very much doubt. I believe people see something alien in me and the real reason for this is that in my youth I was never young and now that I am entering the age of maturity I cannot mature properly. There was a time when I was all ambition and eager to learn, when day after day I felt aggrieved that nature had not, in one of her benevolent moods, stamped my face with that mark of genius which now and again she bestows on men. Now for a long time I have known that I am not a genius and cannot understand how I ever could have wanted to be one. I am not even very gifted; my whole capacity for work probably springs from my character and from the absence of outstanding intellectual weaknesses. But I know that this combination is very conducive to slow success, and that given favorable conditions I could achieve more than Nothnagel, to whom I consider myself superior, and might possibly reach the level of Charcot. By which I don't mean to say that I will get as far as that, for these favorable conditions no longer come my way, and I don't possess the genius, the power, to bring them about. Oh, how I run on! I really wanted to say something quite different.... You know what Breuer told me one evening? I was so moved by what he said that in return I disclosed to him the secret of our engagement. He told me he had discovered that hidden under the surface of timidity there lay in me an extremely daring and fearless human being. I had always thought so, but never dared tell anyone. I have often felt as though I had inherited all the defiance and all the passions with which our ancestors defended their Temple and could gladly sacrifice my life for one great moment in history. And at the same time I always felt so helpless and incapable of expressing these ardent passions even by a word or a poem. So I have always restrained myself, and it is this, I think, which people must see in me.

Here I am, making silly confessions to you, my sweet darling, and really without any reason whatever unless it is the cocaine that makes me talk so much. But now I must go out to supper and then dress myself up and do some more writing. Tomorrow I will report to you quite truthfully on how the evening at Charcot's turned out. You of course must tell everyone that I had a wonderful time, and I shall write the same to Vienna. The truth is for us alone.

12:30 A.M.

Thank God it's over and I can tell you at once how right I was. It was so boring I nearly burst; only the bit of cocaine prevented me from doing so. Just think: this time forty to fifty people, of whom I knew three or four. No one was introduced to anyone, everyone was left to do what he liked. Needless to say, I had nothing to do; I don't think the others enjoyed themselves any better, but at least they could talk. My French was even worse than usual. No one paid any attention to me, or could pay attention to me, which was quite all right and I was prepared for it.... Only toward the end I embarked on a political conversation with Giles de la Tourette, during which he of course predicted the most ferocious war with Germany. I promptly explained that I am a Jew, adhering neither to Germany nor Austria. But such conversations are always very embarrassing to me, for I feel stirring within me something German which I long ago decided to suppress.—At about 11:30 we were ushered into the dining room, where there was a lot of drink and something to eat. I took a cup of chocolate.—You mustn't think that I was disappointed; one cannot expect anything more from a *jour fixe,* and all I know is that we will never have such a thing. But please don't tell anyone how boring it was. We shall always talk about the first evening only. And now goodnight, my sweet darling, fondest greetings from

Your
Sigmund

Paris, Wednesday
February 10, 1886
My lovable darling

What a magic city this Paris is!... I couldn't help thinking what an ass I am to be leaving Paris now that spring is coming, Nôtre Dame looking so beautiful in the sunlight,... But I feel neither courageous nor reckless enough to stay any longer....

For a week now there has been a foreigner in the Salpêtrière, a definitely Germanic type and yet somehow different; I can't quite make him out. Wednesday is the day we go to the ophthalmological room, and there this foreigner suddenly began behaving with some authority; when he exchanged cards with Charcot's ophthalmologist, the latter became very polite and expressed the hope that Monsieur would often return so that he could learn something from him. Whereupon we all began wondering who he might be. Before leaving he came over to us Viennese and said: "I heard you speaking German. I'd like to introduce myself." My *bête noire* exchanged cards with him first and I was still trying to find mine when the foreigner said: "I am a German, but I emigrated to America long ago." At last I gave him my card, but it happened to be one without an address. He glanced at it and said: "Could you be Dr. F. from Vienna? I've known your name for a long time, from your publications, especially the one on cocaine." I was a little surprised and inquired after his name, which turned out to be Knapp.* Now, Knapp is the foremost ophthalmologist in New York, who has also written a lot about cocaine and to whom I once wrote a letter in Koller's name. I greeted him accordingly and my *bête noire* stood there looking rather sheepish, first of all because he had failed to recognize the man, and second because he had again managed to make a fool of himself. When he heard the word *cocaine* mentioned he asked: "Have you also written about cocaine?" Whereupon Knapp replied: "Of course he has, it was he who started it all." This morning my Viennese was much more malleable and talked exclusively of the great practice that awaited me in Vienna. . . .

Fondest greetings and kisses, my little woman. . . .

Your
Sigmund

---

* Dr. Hermann Knapp.

CHAPTER 15

Craving for and
Fear of Cocaine
by Sigmund Freud

JULY 1887

Beiträge über die Anwendung des Cocaïn. Zweite Serie. I. Bemerkungen über Cocaïnsucht und Cocaïnfurcht mit Beziehung auf einem Vortrag W.A. Hammond's. Von Dr. Sigm. Freud, Dozent für Nervenkrankheiten in Wein. 1887. Weiner Medizinische Wochenschrift Nr. 28, p. 929–932, 9 Juli 1887.
Contributions about the Applications of Cocaine. Second Series. I. Remarks on Craving for and Fear of Cocaine with reference to a lecture by W. A. Hammond by Dr. Sigmund Freud, Lecturer in Neurology in Vienna.
Translated by Leona A. Freisinger.

In this paper, Freud defends cocaine against the accusation of being dangerous and habit-forming, in the words of a German psychiatrist "the third scourge of mankind," next to alcohol and morphia. Quoting his own and other authors' experiences, he maintains that cocaine addiction occurs only with morphia addicts who, during withdrawal attempts, misuse the cure, retain their drug dependency and merely change from one substance to another, in this instance from morphia to cocaine. In all other cases, cocaine is found to be not habit-forming, can be given up at will and, after longer use, may cause aversion to rather than a craving for it.

On the other hand, Freud finds the general usefulness of cocaine limited by an element of unreliability. Apart from its anesthetic effect which is invariable, reaction to it fluctuates according to the individual state of excitability and the individual state of the vasomotor nerves on which the cocaine acts. Anna Freud.

CARL KOLLER's brilliant use of the anesthetic properties of cocaine for the benefit of the ill and the advancement of medical science had for a time obscured the right of the new drug to be considered in the treatment of internal and nervous disorders. Later, however, one of these uses of cocaine, which I may attribute to my study "On Coca," published in the July 1884 issue of the *Centralblatt für Therapie*, came to the notice of physicians. I refer to the use of cocaine to combat morphine addiction and the alarming withdrawal symptoms that occur in effecting a cure. I had drawn attention to this property of cocaine based on American reports (in the *Detroit Therapeutic Gazette*) and at the same time reported the surprisingly favorable results of the first morphine withdrawal by means of cocaine carried out on the Continent. (It is perhaps well to mention at this point that I do not speak of experiments carried out on myself, but of another whom I advised on the matter.)

Observations similar to the above led Prof. H. Obersteiner to report on the effectiveness of cocaine in treating morphine addiction to the Medical Congress of Copenhagen. He made little impression, however. The new use of cocaine was first brought to the general attention of physicians—and also, unfortunately, of morphine addicts —through the pamphlets of E. Merck Co., Darmstadt, and an extravagant article by Wallé in the *Deutsche Medizinalzeitung* (No. 3, 1885).

Erlenmeyer (in his *Centralblatt,* 1885), on the basis of an impressive series of tests, very forcefully disputed any effective use of cocaine in morphine withdrawal and represented it as a highly dangerous drug owing to its effect on the vascular innervation. Erlenmeyer's conclusions, however, rested on a serious experimental error, which was immediately detected by Obersteiner, Smidt, Rank, et al. Instead of administering the drug according to my recommended effective dose (several decigrams) *per os,* Erlenmeyer had given minimal amounts injected subcutaneously and thus obtained, from a dosage, ineffective over a long period, a transient toxic effect. In the opinion of the authors refuting him, my original statements had in no way been invalidated.

The value of cocaine for morphine addicts is lost, however, for other reasons. The patients began to get hold of the drug themselves and to become addicted to it as they had been to morphine. Cocaine became for them a substitute for morphine, and an unsatisfactory substitute at that, since most morphine addicts rapidly attained a tolerance to the enormous dose of 1g *pro die* injected subcutaneously. As it has turned out, cocaine used in this way is a far more dangerous enemy to health than morphine. Instead of a slow marasmus, we have rapid physical and moral deterioration, hallucinatory states of agitation similar to delirium tremens, a chronic persecution mania, characterized in my experience by the hallucination of small animals moving in the skin, and cocaine addiction in place of morphine addiction —these were the sad results of trying to cast out the devil by Beelzebub. Many morphine addicts who until that time had held their own in life now succumbed to cocaine. Erlenmeyer, in a position to carry on his agitation against the new alkaloid more successfully owing to his first publication on "cocaine addiction," spoke of a "third scourge" of the human race, worse than the first two (alcohol and morphine).

Inasmuch as the first reports of the toxic effects of cocaine were received at about the same time from eye and throat specialists, cocaine began to get the reputation of a highly dangerous drug whose use over a long period of time produces a "habit" or "condition similar to morphinism." I find this warning in the most recent publication on cocaine (by O. Chiari, this *Wochenschrift,* No. 8).

I believe that this has gone much too far. I cannot resist making a comment which comes to mind and will do away with the horror of the so-called "third scourge of the human race," as Erlenmeyer so pathetically labels cocaine. *All reports of addiction to cocaine and deterioration resulting from it refer to morphine addicts,* persons who, already in the grip of one demon are so weak in will power, so susceptible, that they would misuse, and indeed have misused, any stimulant held out to them. *Cocaine has claimed no other, no victim on its own.* I have had broad experience with the regular use of cocaine over long periods of time by persons who were not morphine addicts, and have taken the drug myself for some months without perceiving or experiencing any condition similar to morphinism or any desire for continued use of cocaine. On the contrary, there occurred more frequently than I should have liked, an aversion to the drug, which was sufficient cause for curtailing its use. My own experience with the usefulness of cocaine in certain nervous conditions and the absence of any subsequent addiction to cocaine, coincides so completely with that reported recently by W. Hammond, a well-known foreign authority, that I prefer to translate his remarks rather than reiterate statements I have already made in my paper "On Coca" (*Centralblatt für Therapie,* 1884) and a later essay ("Beitrag zur Kenntnis der Cocawirkung," *Wr. med. Wochenschrift,* No. 5, 1885). I shall only make a few remarks beforehand on the acute cocaine poisoning which has been observed by eye and throat specialists.

The condition is to some extent merely a manifestation of postoperative collapse, such as occurs after any surgery, particularly on sensitive parts of the body, and can hardly be attributed to the alkaloid, which is often used in minimal doses. Another set of observations must, however, be characterized unequivocally as cocaine poisoning because of their similarity to symptoms which can be produced experimentally by an overdose of cocaine: stupor, dizziness, increase of pulse rate, irregular respiration, anorexia, insomnia, and eventually delirium and muscular weakness. These conditions, undoubtedly caused by cocaine, have been the result sometimes of resorption of the drug by the mucous membranes of the head and, more frequently, of subcutaneous injections of the drug. Compared with the frequency of the use of cocaine in the last two years, they are of rare occurrence, and in no case have they endangered life. Thus it is with good reason that most physicians are left with the impression that the possibility of toxic effects need not preclude the application of cocaine to attain a desirable end. It is important to note that some toxicity also occurs with small doses of cocaine. So the sensitivity of certain individuals to cocaine, together with the absence of any reaction to larger doses in other cases, has aptly been labeled an idiosyncrasy. I believe this one unreliability of cocaine—that one does not know when a toxic effect will appear—is very intimately connected with another, which must be attributed to the drug itself—that one does not know when and with whom a general reaction is to be expected. (I disregard, of course, the anesthetic effect.) The connection, which may facilitate the understanding of this peculiarity, would seem to be as follows: Cocaine has a very obvious effect on the vascular innervation. Applied locally, as can easily be observed in a cocainized eye, etc., it induces vasoconstriction, that is, ischemia of the tissue. According to B. Fränkel (discussion in the *Berlin Medical Society* of November 4, 1885) cocaine produces vasodilation on the tongues of curarized frogs, vasoconstriction beginning only with a dilution of 1:20,000. According to Erlenmeyer, cocaine begins to act in doses as low as 0.005g by injection, paralyzing the vasomotor centers and reducing the arterial tension; according to Litten (discussion, etc.) it has an exquisitely tonic effect, elevating the blood pressure. I could cite a whole series of resounding, contradictory statements from various investigators, in all of which one thing stands out—that cocaine acts on the blood vessels, specifically, according to concentration, method of application, and disposition of the subject to various effects. I would like to add that the descriptions of acute cocaine poisoning all point to a state of vasoconstriction or vascular paralysis. The variable factor on which the diversity of the action of cocaine depends seems to me, therefore, to lie in the conditions prevailing and in the lability of the vascular innervation. There can be no doubt that the irritability of the vasomotor nerves (or vasonervous centers) is very different in different individuals and varies even within the same individual. It is likely that one of the main symptoms of the nervous state occurs in the lability of the cerebral vascular innervation. One need only recall the various effects of galvanization on the back according as it is carried out on a healthy person or on a neurotic of this or that disposition. In like manner, cocaine, if its general effect is created by influencing cerebral circulation, will in the case of a stable vascular *tonus,* sometimes be ineffective, and at other times, through a rapidly occurring change, induce a toxic effect. In between lie other cases in which a favorable tonic or hyperemic action is manifested. I suspect that *the reason for the irregularity of the cocaine effect lies in the individual variations in excitability and in the variation of the condition of the vasomotor nerves on which cocaine acts.* Since little attention has been paid to this factor of individual predisposition, and the degree of excitability generally cannot be known, I consider it advisable to abandon so far as possible subcutaneous injection of cocaine in the treatment of internal and nervous disorders.

The following is a summary of the report on cocaine by W. Hammond at a meeting of the New York Neurological Society on November 2, 1886:

According to his statement, he used a prepared coca wine, containing 2 grains of the muriatic salt to a pint of wine, and with it performed numerous experiments on himself and others. This coca preparation produced excellent effects in cases of so-called spinal irritation, effects which he could not attribute to the wine alone. He used it also as a tonic and stimulant. He himself was for a long time in the habit of taking a wineglassful after the day's work and found himself refreshed each time, without any subsequent depression.

He goes on to say that he also used the preparation in some cases of dyspepsia with great sensitivity of the stomach and noted a very striking soothing action. He gave doses of 2–3 teaspoonfuls every fifteen to twenty minutes to a total of about six doses. The first spoonfuls were mostly vomited. The one following, however, were retained for longer periods of time until finally the vomiting stopped. Cases of stomach sensitivity which were probably related to spinal irritation (neurasthenia) were found to be alleviated after a few hours of this treatment.

Dr. Hammond then touched briefly on the physiological aspect of the action of coca and remarked that the first authors who reported on the use of coca among South American natives had greatly exaggerated its noxiousness. Their reports were repeatedly warmed over and served anew, without reference as to source, and thus inspired the currently prevailing bias. To test the truth of reports appearing recently in the journals that have aroused a great deal of fear, he injected himself repeatedly with cocaine, the mild toxic effect of which he described in detail. He did not, however, become addicted to cocaine, and could give up the drug whenever he wished. As far as the so-called cocaine habit is concerned, so he asserted, he gave the drug to a woman suffering from Graves's disease in doses of 1–5 grains for a period of three months. Nevertheless, she was able to discontinue its use without any difficulty. He also treated a morphine addict with the drug, administering it by subcutaneous injection of up to 5 grains daily for some months. In all of these patients, as with himself, cocaine induced an extraordinary increase in heart activity, elevation of blood pressure and temperature, breaking out into sweat and insomnia.

In three cases of female melancholia with mutism, he succeeded in bringing the patients round to speech by injections of cocaine, sometimes to decided advantage.

Dr. Hammond placed the habituation to cocaine on a par with that of coffee or tea, an entirely different sort of habit from morphia addiction. He did not believe that there is a single verified case of cocaine addiction on record (except among morphine addicts), that is to say, of the sort in which the patient would be incapable of discontinuing use of the drug at will. In long continued use of cocaine, however, damage to the heart and other organs may be expected.

CHAPTER 16

"Coca:
Its Preparations and their
Therapeutical Qualities, with
some Remarks on the
So–called 'Cocaine Habit.' "

NOVEMBER 1887

From a "Volunteer Paper" by William A. Hammond, M.D., Surgeon General, U.S. Army (Retired List) of New York, N.Y. Transactions of the *Medical Society of Virginia,* November, 1887, pp. 212–26.

This is one of the few reports in the medical literature of the determination of a dose-effect curve for cocaine. The fact that the experiments were done by a former Surgeon General on himself makes the report even more remarkable. It is worthwhile to compare the effects in chronic users described by Hammond with those seen by Lewin. Such candid reporting by a major medical figure may seem astounding to today's readers but attitudes and laws about drug taking were different in the nineteenth century. Ed.

Dr. William A. Hammond, in attendance upon the Session by invitation, under call for a paper or remarks, read a paper having the above title, which he had prepared as a contribution for the *November, 1887,* number of the *Virginia Medical Monthly.* As the paper is published in full in that journal, the Publishing Committee present simply a full synopsis of it, followed by the Secretary's report of the remarks made by Fellows, etc., in the discussion of the subject.—*Note by Recording Secretary.*

Dr. Hammond confined his remarks almost entirely to an account of his personal experience with the preparations of Erythroxylon coca. The three preparations he has employed are the fluid extract, the wine, and the hydrochlorate of cocaine.

(1) The *fluid extract* in one or two fluid dram doses, three times daily, sometimes acts well; but is so disagreeable to the taste as to be apt to excite nausea. Besides, being the extract of the leaves, as a whole, it contains substances that materially interfere with the action of the active principle of the drug. These are chiefly tannin and a resinous substance, to which the nauseous taste is mainly due. The fluid extract is rarely admissible with children, as the irritant ingredients named often cause vomiting shortly after taking it. It seems to act better in persons of advanced age, as the tonic and astringent qualities of these very ingredients are often beneficial for them. But these matters are antagonistic to the action of cocaine, and present insuperable objections to the employment of the fluid extract when we desire to obtain solely the action of the alkaloid.

(2) *The wines of coca* as usually prepared, present like objections. Experience has taught the Indians of Peru and Bolivia how to get the best results from the employment of the leaves of coca. They make

the leaves into a mass with lime, and then chew them. The action of the saliva on this mass measurably separates the alkaloid, which is absorbed into the system, while the woody fiber, tannin and extractive matters are ejected from the mouth. But all the wines of coca are preferable, so far as taste and effect are concerned, to the fluid extract. But as now found in the market, they are generally uncertain, and often absolutely inert, except in so far as regards the wine entering into their composition. They vary greatly in the amount of cocaine they contain, and some of them are almost entirely free from this essential constituent. Dr. Hammond, therefore, got Messrs. Thurber, Whyland & Co., of New York City, who have an exceedingly competent chemist in their employ, to prepare a wine of coca with full bodied and absolutely pure wine, that should contain a fixed proportion of cocaine, and at the same time be free from tannin, resin, and other inert or resinous substances present in the leaves. The result was a wine of coca containing two grains of cocaine to the pint, absolutely free from tannin and resinous matter, and pleasant to the taste, and giving about a sixth of a grain of cocaine to each ordinary wineglassful.

This wine of coca is beneficial in *spinal irritation,* especially in that very common yet distressing stomach irritability, marked by vomiting, with or without nausea, the moment any kind of food enters the stomach. In such instances, give the wine in teaspoonful doses every five minutes until eight or ten doses are taken. The first dose may be rejected almost as soon as swallowed, but the second will be retained longer, and the third longer still, and the fourth will probably not be thrown up at all. After tolerance is thus established, the wine may be given in larger quantities—say a wineglassful just before eating—with the effect, in most cases, of producing entire relief of gastric irritation. It may then be continued, so long as may be necessary, as an agent of great value in curing spinal irritation, and as a tonic to the system. Indeed, this wine is beneficial in all instances in which it is desirable to increase the vital powers. Coca appears to be the one agent that can be thus employed without fear of the depression that so generally follows the use of other stimulants.

As a *tonic to the vocal apparatus,* it is of great value where fatigue follows the excessive use of the voice, or where the voice breaks down in the midst of some supreme effort. Where such fatigue or failure is feared, a full claret–glass of the wine, taken just before beginning to speak or sing, will almost invariably accomplish the object.

Cerebral hyperemia is generally the result of excessive mental exertion, or of intense emotional disturbance. Nothing can be more beneficial in this condition than is this remedy. Dispensing with all other stimulants, Dr. Hammond advises a claret–glassful of the wine of coca with each meal. The influence is felt almost immediately, the vital powers seem to be at once restored, and the mind soon regains its former vigor. If sleep has been disturbed or absent, it becomes regular and in sufficient quantity, after the remedy has been taken for a few days. Such are the cases, passing under the names of nervous prostration and neurasthenia, general debility, etc., in which the influence of the wine of coca is most distinctly shown.

In another form of mental depression, often accompanying hysteria in the female, or a like condition in the male, attended usually with some disorder of the generative system, this wine of coca is invaluable—often curing it without any other medicine. Under its continuous use for several months, the emotions become more and more expansive, the disposition to brood over imaginary or slight troubles disappears, tears are no longer shed over mere nothings, and the countenance becomes hopeful. He has never had any trouble in causing the patient to stop the use of the wine of coca.

But he could not in a single paper mention all of the many morbid conditions of the nervous system in which he has found the wine of coca beneficial. In general, his own experience, coupled with that of other practitioners, establishes the fact that the wine of coca is very valuable as a tonic and stimulant to the weakened or exhausted nervous system. Physicians of eminence likewise speak of it in the highest terms in many such diseases as fevers, dysentery, heart and lung troubles, and especially in malarious disorders. It is very remarkable that its use is not followed by the depression of mind and body that so generally ensue upon the use of other excitants.

(3) *Cocaine Muriate or Hydrochlorate.* What is true of the wine is more emphatically true of the active principle, cocaine hydrochlorate, and should often be preferred even for internal administra-

tion. While best known as a local anesthetic in operations about the eye, nasal cavities, etc., it is a speedy and decided remedy in certain affections of the nervous system.

About two years ago, Dr. Hammond undertook a series of experiments with this agent on himself, with the object of obtaining more satisfactory information relative to its action than it seemed possible for him to get otherwise. To quote the record of these observations:

> I began by injecting a grain of the substance under the skin of the forearm, the operation being performed at 8 P.M. The first effect ensued in about five minutes, and consisted of a pleasant thrill which seemed to pass through the whole body. This lasted about ten minutes, and shortly after its appearance was accompanied by a sensation of fullness in the head and heat of the face. There was also noticed a decided acceleration of the pulse, with increase of force. This latter symptom was probably, judging from subsequent experiments, the very first to ensue, but my attention being otherwise engaged it was overlooked. On feeling the pulse five minutes after making the injection, it was found to be 94, while immediately before the operation it was only 82. With these physical phenomena there was a sense of exhilaration and an increase of mental activity that were well marked, and not unlike in character those that ordinarily follow a glass or two of champagne. I was writing at the time, and I found that my thoughts flowed with increased freedom and were unusually well expressed. The influence was felt for two hours, when it gradually began to fade. At 12 o'clock (four hours after the injection) I went to bed, feeling, however, no disposition to sleep. I lay awake till daylight, my mind actively going over all the events of the previous day. When I at last fell asleep it was only for two or three hours, and then I awoke with a severe frontal headache. This passed off after breakfast.
> On the second night following, at 7 o'clock, I injected *two grains* of the hydrochlorate of cocaine into the skin of the forearm. At that time the pulse was 84, full and soft. In four minutes and a half it had increased to 92, was decidedly stronger than before, and somewhat irregular in rhythm. The peculiar thrill previously mentioned was again experienced. All the phenomena attendant on the first experiment were present in this, and to an increased degree. In addition there were twitching of the muscles on the face, and a slight tremor of the hands noticed especially in writing. In regard to the mental manifestations there was a similar exhilaration as in the last experiment, but much more intense in character. I felt a great desire to write, and did so with a freedom and apparent clearness that astonished me. I was quite sure, however, at the time, that on the following morning, when I came to read it over, I would find my lucubrations to be

of no value. I was therefore agreeably disappointed when I came to peruse it, after the effects of the drug had passed off, that it was entirely coherent, logical, and as good if not better in general character as anything I had previously written. The effects of this dose did not disappear till the middle of the next day, nor until I had drunk two or three cups of strong coffee. I slept little or none at all, the night being passed in tossing from side to side of the bed, and in thinking of the most preposterous subjects. I was, however, at no time unconscious, but it seemed as though my mind was to some extent perverted from its usual course of action. The heat of the head was greatest at about 12 o'clock, and at that time my pulse was 112—the highest point reached. I had no headache until after arising, and the pain disappeared in the course of the morning.

Four nights subsequently I injected *four grains* of the hydrochlorate of cocaine into the skin of the left forearm. The effects were similar in almost every respect with those of the other experiments except that they were much more intense. The mental activity was exceedingly great, and in writing, my thoughts as before appeared to be lucidly and logically expressed. I wrote page after page, throwing the sheets on the floor without stopping to gather them together. When, however, I came to look them over on the following morning, I found that I had written a series of high-flown sentences altogether different from my usual style, and bearing upon matters in which I was not in the least interested. The result was very striking as showing the difference between a large and excessive dose of the drug; and yet it appeared to me at the time that what I was writing consisted of ideas of very superior character, and expressed with a beauty of diction of which I was in my normal condition altogether incapable.

The disturbance of the action of the heart was also exceedingly well marked, and may be described best by the word "tumultuous." At times, beginning within three minutes after the injection, and continuing with more or less intensity all through the night, the heart beat so rapidly that its pulsations could not be counted, and then its action would suddenly fall to a rate not exceeding 60 in a minute, every now and then dropping a beat. This irregularity was accompanied by a disturbance of respiration of a similar character, and by a sense of oppression in the chest that added greatly to my discomfort.

On subsequent nights I took *six, eight, ten and twelve grains* of the cocaine at a dose.... The effects ... were similar in general characteristics though of gradually increasing intensity in accordance with the dose taken to that in which four grains were injected.... In one, that in which *twelve grains* were taken, I was conscious of a tendency to talk, and as far as my recollection extends, I believe I did make a long speech on some subject of which I had no remembrance the next day. In all, the action of the heart was increased, was irregular in rhythm and force to such an extent that I was apprehensive of serious results. Insomnia was a marked characteristic, and there was invariably a headache the following morning. In all cases, however, the effects passed off about midday, and by evening I was as well as ever.

My experience had satisfied me that a much larger dose than any I had up to that time injected might, in my case at least, be taken with impunity. A consideration of the phenomena observed appeared to show that the effects produced by twelve grains were not very much more pronounced than those following six grains. I determined, therefore, to make one more experiment, and to inject *eighteen grains*. I knew that in a case of attempted suicide twenty-three grains had been taken into the stomach without seemingly injurious effect, and that in another case thirty-two grains were taken within the space of three hours without symptoms following of greater intensity than those I had experienced.

I had taken the doses of eight, ten and twelve grains in divided quantities, and this dose of eighteen grains I took in four portions within five minutes of each other. At once an effect was produced upon the heart, and before I had taken the last injection the pulsations were 140 to the minute, and characteristically irregular. In all the former experiments, although there was great mental exaltation, amounting at times almost to delirium, it was nevertheless distinctly under my control, and I am sure that at any time under the influence of a sufficiently powerful incentive I could have obtained entire mastery over myself, and have acted after my normal manner. But in this instance, within five minutes after taking the last injection, I felt that my mind was passing beyond my control, and that I was becoming an irresponsible agent. I did not feel exactly in a reckless mood, but I was in such a frame of mind as to be utterly regardless of any calamity or danger that might be impending over me. I do not think I was in a particularly combative condition, but I was elated and possessed of a feeling as though exempt from the operation of deleterious influences. I do not know how long this state of mind continued, for I lost consciousness of all my acts within, I think, half an hour after finishing the administration of the dose. Probably, however, other moods supervened, for the next day when I came downstairs, three hours after my usual time, I found the floor of my library strewn with encyclopedias, dictionaries and other books of reference, and one or two chairs overturned. I certainly was possessed of the power of mental and physical action in accordance with the ideas by which I was governed, for I had turned out the gas in the room and gone upstairs to my bedchamber and lighted the gas, and put the match used in a safe place, and undressed, laying my clothes in their usual place, had cleaned my teeth and gone to bed. Doubtless these acts were all automatic, for I had done them all in pretty much the same way for a number of years. During the night the condition which existed was, judging from the previous experiments, certainly not sleep; and yet I remained entirely unconscious until 9 o'clock the following morning, when I found myself in bed with a splitting headache and a good deal of cardiac and respiratory disturbance. For several days afterward I felt the effects of this extreme dose in a certain degree of languor and indisposition to mental or physical exertion; there was also a difficulty in concentrating the attention, but I slept soundly every night without any notable disturbance from dreams.

[Dr. Hammond remarked as follows:]

Certainly in this instance I came very near taking a fatal dose and I would not advise anybody to repeat the experiment. I suppose that if I had taken the whole quantity in one single injection instead of in four, over a period of twenty minutes, the result might have been disastrous. Eighteen grains of cocaine are equivalent to about 3,600 grains of coca leaves, and of course, owing to its concentration, capable of acting with very much greater intensity.

I am not aware that a fatal dose of cocaine has yet been indicated by actual fact. Probably eighteen grains would kill some people, and perhaps even smaller quantities might, with certain individuals, be fatal. But these are inferences and not facts; but so far as I know there is not an instance on record of a person dying from the administration of cocaine.

So far as my experiments extend (and I think it will be admitted that they have gone as far as is safe) I am inclined to think that a dose sufficient to produce death would do so *by its action on the heart*. Certainly it was there that in my case the most dangerous symptoms were perceived. The rapidity, force, and marked irregularity of the pulse all showed that the innervation of the heart was seriously affected.

It is surprising that no marked influence appeared to be exercised upon the spinal cord or upon the ganglia at the base of the brain. Thus there were no disturbances of sensibility (no anesthesia) and no interference with motility, except that some of the muscles, especially those of the face, were subjected to slight twitchings. In regard to sight and hearing, I noticed that both were affected, but that while the sharpness of vision was decidedly lessened, the hearing was increased in acuteness. At no time were there any hallucinations.

Acting upon these data, Dr. Hammond has always used hydrochlorate of cocaine, when employing it in its pure state, by hypodermic injections. For internal administration, he prefers the wine of coca. But as the substance applied to mucous membranes diminishes the caliber of the blood vessels and produces anesthesia of the part, he would give cocaine muriate by the mouth in certain stomach affections on the same principle as it is at present applied to mucous membranes of the nose, pharynx, larynx, etc.

In cases of *melancholia* and in *hysteria with great depression of spirits,* he has derived benefit from its hypodermic use, beginning with half grain and gradually increasing to two grains if required. One injection daily for three or four days will often make the most dismal melancholic cheerful, and act permanently.

He has used it entirely satisfactorily in two cases of *neuritis of the radial nerve,* attended with great pain, partial paralysis of the muscles supplied by the nerve, and numbness of the thumb, index and outer half of the middle finger. He injected half grain every two hours—eight times in one case, and ten times in the other—at the point, and deep enough to come as near as possible to the nerve, where the pain was greatest. The symptoms began to subside from the first injection, and there was no return after the last.

He has not had an opportunity to use it in *sciatica;* but in such a case he would inject at the upper part of the sciatic nerve, and try to throw the cocaine solution into the substance of the nerve itself.

In *neuralgia,* the cocaine should be injected very near the inflamed nerve, for it is only by its local action that it can have the desired effect.

Dr. Hammond purposely omitted reference to its established uses in ophthalmology, rhinology and laryngology so as to save time to speak about the *So-called Cocaine Habit.*

He is sure this has no existence *as such.* Morphia eaters, having heard that it is an antidote to their habit, undoubtedly have tried to cure themselves with it; but without stopping the morphine have simply engrafted the cocaine habit on the morphia habit—an exceedingly bad combination. But he emphatically denies that there is such a thing as a cocaine habit, pure and simple, which the individual cannot, of his own effort, altogether arrest. The pleasurable mental exhilaration induced by injections of half a grain or grain produces no weakening of the will–power, nor craving for the drug, such as is produced by morphia, etc. He has repeatedly given it for weeks, and has never had a single one, male or female, object to its being stopped—not even as much as to giving up tea or coffee, and nothing like as much as stopping alcohol or tobacco. Dr. Bosworth, of New York, took within the space of a few months, he thinks, between 500 and 600 grains, and stopped its use, without suffering the least inconvenience. Dr. Frank W. Ring (*Medical Record,* September 3, 1887) applied with an atomizer nightly for ten months two grains of a four-per-cent solution to the nasal mucous membrane—taking more than 600 grains during the ten months; and then he calmly decided to stop it, which he did. The inclination for it often seized him, but he crushed it with the perfect confidence that he shall never again indulge in its enchantments.

As a matter of personal experience, Dr. Hammond related that last March he was attacked by a *violent rhinitis* of a form not laid down in the books, and different in character, and of far greater intensity than any that any rhinologist he consulted had ever witnessed. There was great swelling of the nose and face; the discharge during the first stage was of an exceedingly acrid and thin fluid, followed by the formation of a very loosely attached membraniform substance not very unlike that of diphtheria, but with no disposition to extend beyond the nasal cavities. From March 1 to July 16, he applied by atomizers, camel's hair pencils, etc., an average of twenty grains a day of different percentage solutions, with great relief. He was always careful to make the applications far enough back until he tasted the cocaine. He used, therefore, about 600 grains a month, but nothing like this, of course, entered the system. Besides its local influence, its effects upon the system were a slight mental exhilaration, and sometimes an indisposition to sleep when he took more than his usual quantity. On July 16 he stopped the use of the remedy without the slightest difficulty, nor did he resume it again for six weeks, when his disease returned. From August 26 to October 1, he used nearly 800 grains, and then again ceased using it without the slightest difficulty. On neither occasion of stopping its use was there the slightest craving for it, or inconvenience.

Dr. W. L. Robinson, of Danville, Va., had seen prompt and permanent relief from sciatica by hypodermic injections of cocaine, deep down on the nerve, but had utterly failed with the same agent in facial neuralgia (*tic douleureux*). He did not believe it would do any good on a granular surface, and in his own case of hay fever, he had failed to receive any relief even with a twenty–per–cent solution, until the granular surface was cauterized. He could not think any remedy of such power could be used *ad libitum* without danger.

Dr. B. L. Winston, of Hanover, C. H., stated that he had used cocaine in the case of a virgin eighteen years old, who was suffering with vaginismus, hoping that with the aid of the drug, he would be able to forcibly distend the ostium vagina. So far as he could detect, however, it had no effect whatever on either the hyperesthesia or the spasmodic contraction of the sphincter vagina muscle. It was only after his patient was completely anesthetized with chloroform that he was able to distend the ostium vagina effectually. He did not use the cocaine stronger than a four–per–cent solution, which, perhaps, accounted for his failure.

Dr. Landon B. Edwards, of Richmond, thought Dr. Winston's case scarcely a fair test of the value of the agent, because of the small dose. In a case under his care, where the pain of intercourse with her husband was so painful as to make her dread the act, he directed that a sixteen-per-cent solution be applied with a small piece of absorbent cotton to the mouth of the vagina, or an ointment of like strength made with cosmoline, some fifteen minutes or so before she anticipated the intercourse. She afterwards said that the cocaine had relieved her to such a degree as to make the marital relationship enjoyable. He was rather surprised at the statement by Dr. Hammond that he did not believe that there was a cocaine habit, in the usual sense of the term, established by the too frequent and immoderate use of cocaine. He had heard of a case in this city.

Dr. Hugh M. Taylor of Richmond, Va., was surprised to hear Dr. Hammond express his disbelief in the existence of the cocaine habit, as he (Dr. Taylor) had seen a case ending in delirium or mania, which had lasted for several weeks, and which had deeply impressed him with the danger of habit, incident to the continuous use of cocaine. The unfortunate victim of the habit was a young physician, who had had the drug prescribed for him for the relief of some supposed kidney disease. He had been using cocaine hypodermically for eighteen months or two years, and gradually the size of the dose and its frequency had to be increased as his system became habituated to its effects, or as his depraved nervous system demanded a larger supply. From a small to a large dose, from longer to shorter intervals, and from a minor to a marked effect, the growth of the habit was easily traced until the victim's will-power was all gone, and he had not the will to will its discontinuance. Without known reason, he had left his practice in the country and had come to Richmond, where he had been for several weeks. His conduct was so strange that his friends were telegraphed to come and look after him. He had mixed himself up in all sorts of business transactions, and talked and behaved in such a suspicious way that his friends recognized the necessity of placing him under some restraint. When seen by Dr. Taylor, he had been quarantined in his room in the hotel for twenty-four hours. His hypodermic syringe with which he gave himself the cocaine, had been taken away from him and no form of substitute was allowed. He was about as rational as a man who had been taking whisky or opium freely, and about as nervous as one from whom these agents had been suddenly taken. Almost his first utterance was an appeal for the return of his syringe and permission to continue the use of cocaine. He did not want whisky nor opium— no substitute would do. He could not live without cocaine, and wanted it that moment. He pled for it on the ground of its being necessary for his health, insisted that he could not live without it, and did not hesitate to threaten his own and other lives if his request was not granted. His legs and arms were thick with needle punctures, and the blood specks on his underclothes showed the frequency of the dose.

With Dr. Taylor's consent he was placed in an institution for treatment, but in a few days he made his escape and returned to his country home. His brothers there took charge of him, shut him up in his room, put a guard over him, and kept him in confinement for a month or six weeks. At the end of that time his nervous system had recovered its tone, and he had lost his cravings for the drug, and was supposed to be well.

The history of this case, together with his own observations, left no doubt on Dr. Taylor's mind that cocaine should be classed with opium, chloral and chloroform, as one of the dangerous remedies to trust unreservedly in the hands of the uninitiated. While he appreciated the boon cocaine conferred upon suffering humanity, he felt called upon to insist upon the danger of continuing its use for a great length of time. He was unalterably of the opinion that the case he reported was one of cocaine habit, and as far as he knew, no other agents, such as opium, chloral, whisky, chloroform etc. were factors in the case.

Dr. L. Ashton, of Falmouth, Va., said that he had successfully treated one case of opium habit by the substitution of cocaine and then dropping the cocaine. In such a case as Dr. Edwards had reported, he would suggest its use as an ointment made with lanolin.

Dr. John N. Upshur, of Richmond, Va., said he thought that cocaine was a remedy that should be used with caution, not being at all times uniform in its action. He related the case of a lady recently under his care, who was suffering from uterine disease, subsequent to a miscarriage. There was intense hyperesthesia of the cervix and vagina. He used three–grain suppositories of cocaine twice daily for its relief, and with no unpleasant symptoms. She suffered however, some week or two later with intense pain of inflamed hemorrhoids, for which he used a suppository of cocaine grs. ij. opium and extract of belladonna āā gr. ¼. In an hour after the introduction of the first suppository, she was seized with the most intense hysterical excitement, face flushed, and developed symptoms of intoxication, which lasted for six or eight hours. He was satisfied that this condition was caused by the cocaine, and that neither the opium nor belladonna had anything to do with it, as she had repeatedly taken these agents, both by the mouth and hypodermically, without any unpleasant effects, nor were the symptoms in any way analogous to the physiological effects of opium or belladonna.

Dr. R. M. Slaughter, of Theological Seminary, Va., had used cocaine in a case of vaginismus without success: but he had not used the application in anything like the strength that has been referred to today.

Dr. E. W. Rowe, of Orange, C. H., thought it too hasty for Dr.

Hammond to draw the conclusion that there was no such thing as the cocaine habit, simply because he had not seen a case.

Dr. Rohé, of Baltimore, Md., said he was familiar with the use of cocaine in rectal diseases. He uses suppositories of three grains of cocaine with half–grain of extract of belladonna. It is certainly useful as an anesthetic in operating on hemorrhoids.

Dr. Thomas J. Moore, of Richmond, Va., cited two cases—one of operating for fissure as a result of piles, and the other to relieve pain while removing some stitches. In neither case did the cocaine application do any good.

Dr. Alex. Harris, of Jeffersonton, Va., has used it with great satisfaction in cases of conjunctivitis. It acts both as an astringent and anesthetic.

Dr. Samuel B. Morrison, of Rockbridge Baths, Va., has used it to irrigate the bowels, but had derived no effect. He agrees with Dr. Moore.

Dr. Hugh M. Taylor has used it preparatory for operation for vesico–vagina fistula, and also for lacerated perineum, etc., and was pleased with the effect.

Dr. J. F. Winn, of Richmond, Va., had used cocaine as a satisfactory anesthetic in removing piles.

Dr. Hammond said that the drug is something new, and we have not yet learned all of its uses nor its abuses. Even the early history of Peruvian bark showed that its uses were not properly understood; even deaths were then attributed to it, which we now know were not due to cinchona. He does not wish to be understood as saying that there is no such thing as the cocaine habit, but he does say that the habit is very much like that of the coffee habit. All of us feel that we have power left us of discontinuing its use if we choose to will to discontinue its use. This is not the feeling of a whisky–drinker or an opium–eater. When such a one wishes to discontinue the whisky or the opium, he finds himself almost powerless to put forth the necessary will force. In the case reported by Dr. Taylor, it should be taken into consideration that his doctor had advised him to take the cocaine, that the cocaine gave relief, and it may have been a determination to have the cocaine rather than to suffer the pain he was having. It was a case of preference, and not a case of irresistible habit. Cocaine is undoubtedly an antidote or a good substitute for morphine habit: for the former can be broken, while the latter cannot be easily broken except by medical treatment. It seems to be established that cocaine does not act satisfactorily when *applied* to inflamed tissues, but it does act when injected near the inflamed part so as to be absorbed. But there are exceptions even to the statement that it does not act when applied to inflamed surfaces; for it does act well when applied to inflamed surfaces of the eye and nose. Gen. Grant's case is too fresh in memory to have to repeat it here in illustration of its value when applied to inflamed tissues. In any of such surgical cases as have been referred to today, good would probably have resulted had a twenty–per–cent solution been used instead of a weaker preparation. He had recently given great relief to a lady while traveling on the cars, and who had gotten a cinder in her eye, which was causing inflammation, by pencilling the eye with the preparation he usually carried about with him. In three minutes her eye was painless, and no inflammation resulted. In the rare cases of injurious or threatening effects, to which allusions have been made, he would remind the gentlemen that other things act as peculiarly. For instance, Dr. J. B. St. John Roosa, the distinguished ophthalmologist of New York, had had a case in which an unusually small quantity of atropia solution applied to the eye produced severe symptoms of belladonna poisoning. He had not tried in his paper to state anything like the full list of diseases for which cocaine is useful. Hence he had not dwelt upon the value of the drug in mucous inflammations. In vaginismus, he had used something like a twenty–per–cent solution with invariable success. Among the odd uses to which he had satisfactorily put cocaine was one of masturbation in the female—the habit being established in her by rubbing or scratching an itching vulva. He simply kept the parts wet with a solution of cocaine, and she was relieved of both the pudendal irritation and the masturbatory habit. In the same way, keeping the prepuce wet with cocaine solution, will often cure masturbation in the male. As to rectal diseases, he has no experience with cocaine. He said that Dr. Milton Josiah Roberts was in the habit of using a twenty-four-per-cent solution, and thinks very highly of it. He is surprised at Dr. Wm. L. Robinson's statement that he had derived so little benefit from cocaine in his case of hay asthma. So far as he knows, it is about the only case on record in which it did not do great good in that disease. So generally valuable is it in that disease that the Hay Fever Association has adopted it as their remedy.

Dr. Charles M. Shields, of Richmond, Va., said that he uses a strong solution of cocaine in cauterizing and in like operations upon the mucous membrane of the nose, and yet has had no disagreeable effect from his daily use of it. He combines it almost invariably with atropia, and this combination acts well.

CHAPTER 17

"The Cocaine Episode,"
PART FOUR

From *The Life and Work of Sigmund Freud* by Ernest Jones, M.D.

The tide however, was beginning to turn. In July 1885, appeared the first of Erlenmeyer's pointed criticisms in the *Centralblatt für Nervenheilunkde,* which he edited. Freud's comment was:

It has the advantage of mentioning that it was I who recommended the use of cocaine in cases of morphium addiction, which the people who have confirmed its value there never do. Thus one can always be grateful to one's enemies.[1]

It contrasted with an overextravagant praise which Wallé had expressed earlier in the year.[2] At a medical congress held in Copenhagen in the summer, Obersteiner, in a paper entitled "On the Employment of Cocaine in Neuroses and Psychoses," had warmly defended Freud, as did some others; he sent a reprint of it to Freud in Paris together with a friendly letter. He confirmed the value of cocaine during the withdrawal of morphia, which he had tested in a number of cases in his private sanatorium at Oberdöbling. But in January of the following year, in a paper on intoxication psychoses, he had to admit that the continued use of cocaine could lead to a delirium tremens very similar to that produced by alcohol.

Early in 1886 Freud had the experience of meeting in Paris Dr. Knapp, then America's leading ophthalmologist. In a company of acquaintances Knapp greeted him as the man who had introduced cocaine to the world, and congratulated him on the achievement. It was a welcome balm.

In the same year, 1886, however, cases of cocaine addiction and intoxication were being reported from all over the world, and in Germany there was a general alarm. Erlenmeyer, in a second attack in May, doubtless written as a protest against Wallé's enthusiasm, voiced it in no uncertain terms: This was the occasion when he coined the phrase "the third scourge of humanity."[3] Erlenmeyer had written a book entitled *Über Morphiumsucht (On Morphia Addiction)* in 1884, and in its third edition, 1887, he incorporated what he had written about cocaine addiction in his first article.[4] At the end of the book he has a sentence praising the literary qualities of Freud's essay on coca, but adding without comment, "He recommends unreservedly the employment of cocaine in the treatment of morphinism." The third edition was reviewed by no less a person than Arthur Schnitzler, who broke a lance for Freud in the course of it.[5]

The man who had tried to benefit humanity or, at all events, to create a reputation by curing "neurasthenia" was now accused of unleashing evil on the world. Many must at least have regarded him as a man of reckless judgment. And if his sensitive conscience passed the same sentence, it could only have been confirmed by a sad experience a little later when, assuming it was a harmless drug, he ordered a large dose of it to a patient who succumbed as the result.[6] How much the whole episode affected Freud's reputation in Vienna is hard to say: all he said himself about it later was that it had led to "grave reproaches." It could not have improved matters when a little later in the year he enthusiastically supported Charcot's strange ideas on hysteria and hypnotism. It was a poor background from which to shock Viennese medical circles a few years later with his theories on the sexual etiology of the neuroses.

In a paper published in the *Wiener medizinische Wochenschrift* of July 9, 1887, Freud made a rather belated reply to all the criticisms.[7] It was occasioned by an article written by W. A. Hammond, which Freud quotes extensively in his support. He had two lines of defense. One was that no case of cocaine addiction was (then) known except in cases of morphia addictions, suggesting that no one else could fall a victim to it. Any habit formation was not, as was so commonly believed, the direct result of imbibing a noxious drug, but was due to some peculiarity in the patient. In this he was, of course, perfectly right, but the argument carried no conviction at the time.

The second line was more equivocal. The variable factor accounting for the uncertain effect of cocaine in different people he attributed to the lability of the cerebral blood vessels: if the pressure in them is stable, cocaine has no effect; in other cases it produces a favorable hyperemia, but in still others a toxic effect. Since this could not be determined beforehand, it was essential to refrain from giving subcutaneous injections of cocaine in any internal or nervous maladies. By the mouth cocaine was harmless, under the skin sometimes dangerous. He again claimed the Fleischl case (without naming him) as the first one of morphia addiction to have been cured by the use of cocaine.

In this second line of defense, which could only have been unconsciously determined, Freud had made a particularly bad shot. In January 1885 he had, very logically, tried to relieve trigeminal neuralgia by injections of cocaine into the nerve.[8] It was not successful, perhaps from lack of surgical skill. But in the same year W. H. Halsted, America's greatest surgeon and one of the founders of modern surgery, injected it into nerves with success, and thus laid the basis of nerve blocking for surgical purposes. He paid dearly, however, for his success, for he acquired a severe addiction to cocaine, and it took a long course of hospital treatment to free him from it. He was thus one of the first new drug addicts.

In seeking to avert from his magic substance the stigma of being a dangerous drug Freud could appeal to general prejudice in implicating hypodermic injections as the real peril. This prejudice against the hypodermic needle existed for many years, and indeed is only now dying away; analysis of patients who have an unwonted dread of it leaves no doubt about its symbolic meaning to the unconscious mind.

When Fleischl was offered cocaine he immediately administered it to himself in the form of subcutaneous injections. Years afterwards Freud asserted he had never intended this, but only oral administration.[9] There is, however, no evidence of any protest on his part at the time, and some months later he was himself advocating subcutaneous *injections* of large doses for just such cases as Fleischl's, i.e., withdrawal of morphine, and he presumably used them. It was his then chief, Professor Scholz, who had recently perfected the technique of the hypodermic needle, and doubtless Freud acquired it from him. He employed it a good deal in the next ten years for various purposes,[10,]* and at one place in his writings he mentions his pride at never having caused an infection thereby. On the other hand, in his dreams† the theme of injections occurs more than once in association with that of guilt.

In the references to his previous writings Freud gave in his apologia in 1887, in which he implicated the hypodermic needle as the

---

* He mentions having cured a case of sciatica in this way.
† See the Dream of Irma's Injection, Chapter Eighteen. *Ed.*

source of the danger in the employment of cocaine, he omitted any reference to the 1885 paper in which he had strongly advocated the evil injections. Nor is the latter paper included in the 1897 list of his writings he had to prepare when applying for the title of Professor. No copy of it is to be found in the collection he kept of his reprints. It seems to have been completely suppressed. If that were due to an unconscious repression, one would not be surprised to come across a similarly unconscious self-betrayal, since the two things so often go together. It was Wittels who first noticed that in *The Interpretation of Dreams* Freud referred to his recommendation of cocaine in 1885,[11] actually this mistake occurs in all the eight editions (including the *Collected Papers* and the *Collected Works*). Freud was so completely unaware of the trick his unconscious had played on him that he asked Wittels where he had written 1885 and added, "I suspect a mistake on your part."[12] Wittels did not himself perceive any significance in the slip, but the more alert Bernfeld did.[13] It was of course in 1884 when he recommended the use of cocaine, but it was in 1885 that he recommended the use of the (dangerous) injections.[14] That was the little scar remaining.

Koller later emigrated to New York, where, as Freud had predicted, he had a successful career. But even at the beginning of his achievement he committed a "symptomatic error" which indicated some disturbance in his personality that came to open expression in later years. When publishing the paper he had read in Vienna in October 1884, he quoted Freud's monograph as dating from August instead of July, giving thus the impression that his work was simultaneous with Freud's and not after it. Both Freud and Obersteiner noticed the "slip" and corrected it in subsequent publications. As time went on Koller presented the discrepancy in still grosser terms, even asserting that Freud's monograph appeared a whole year *after* his own discovery, which was therefore made quite independently of anything Freud had ever done.

Perhaps we may correlate this curious behavior with the fact that in hospital days Freud had treated him privately for a neurotic affection;* "negative transferences," as they are called, often endure.

---

* Unpublished letter from Freud to Martha Bernays dated April 4, 1885.

What is instructive in the cocaine episode is the light it throws on Freud's characteristic way of working. His great strength, though sometimes also his weakness, was the quite extraordinary respect he had for the *singular fact*. This is surely a very rare quality. In scientific work people continually dismiss a single observation when it does not appear to have any connection with other data or general knowledge. Not so Freud. The single fact would fascinate him, and he could not dismiss it from his mind until he had found some explanation of it. The practical value of this mental quality depends on another one: judgment. The fact in question may be really insignificant and the explanation of it of no interest; that way lies crankiness. But it may be a previously hidden jewel or a speck of gold that indicates a vein of ore. Psychology cannot yet explain on what the flair or intuition depends that guides the observer to follow up something his feelings tell him is important, not as a thing in itself, but as an example of some wide law of nature.

When, for example, Freud found in himself previously unknown attitudes towards his parents, he felt immediately that they were not peculiar to himself and that he had discovered something about human nature in general: Oedipus, Hamlet, and the rest soon flashed across his mind.

That is the way Freud's mind worked. When he got hold of a simple but significant fact he would feel, and know, that it was an example of something general or universal, and the idea of collecting statistics on the matter was quite alien to him. It is one of the things for which other, more humdrum, workers have reproached him, but nevertheless that is the way the mind of genius works.

I said that this quality could also be a weakness. That happens when the critical faculty fails in its duty of deciding whether the singular fact is really important or not. Such a failure is most often caused by some interference from another idea or emotion that has got associated with the theme. In the cocaine episode we have examples of both success and failure; hence its interest. Freud observed on his own person that cocaine could paralyze some disturbing element and thus release his full normal vitality. He generalized from this single observation and was puzzled why in other people it led to addiction, and ultimately to intoxication. His conclusion was right that they had within them some morbid element of which he was free, although it was many years before he was able to determine what precisely that was.

On the other hand, when he made the single observation of Fleischl's addiction to cocaine, he wrongly connected this with the unimportant fact that he used injections. He did not do so at first, when he was himself recommending the use of them. When, however, his later misfortunes concerning the use of cocaine came about, his reaction of self-reproach and sense of guilt had to be focused. It was focused on the heinous needle, his recommendation of which had then to be obliterated. That the choice accords well with the explanation given earlier of his self-reproach few would deny.

CHAPTER 18

Freud's Cocaine Dreams

From *The Interpretation of Dreams* by Sigmund Freud.
Translated by James Strachey.

It is widely thought that Freud's experimentation with and use of cocaine stopped in 1887, but a careful reading of the two dreams that follow reveal clearly that Freud was using the drug at least as late as 1895. Many of the personae who have appeared earlier in this book surface again, here, in Freud's dreams which also reveal some of the ways in which Freud's recollections at that time were linked to his cocaine experiences. One passage from the 1895 "Dream of Irma's Injection" is particularly interesting: "I was making frequent use of cocaine at that time to reduce some troublesome nasal swellings, and I had heard a few days earlier that one of my women patients who had followed my example had developed an extensive necrosis of the nasal mucous membrane. I had been the first to recommend the use of cocaine, in 1885, and this recommendation had brought serious reproaches down on me. The misuse of that drug had hastened the death of a dear friend of mine."

In view of recent reports that cocaine tends to suppress Rapid Eye Movement sleep (the phase associated with dreaming), it is noteworthy that the first dream Freud "submitted to a detailed interpretation" occurred during a time when Freud was taking cocaine. Ed.

The Dream of Irma's Injection   by Sigmund Freud, July 1895

I. Preamble

During the summer of 1895 I had been giving psycho–analytic treatment to a young lady who was on very friendly terms with me and my family. It will be readily understood that a mixed relationship such as this may be a source of many disturbed feelings in a physician and particularly in a psychotherapist. While the physician's personal interest is greater, his authority is less; any failure would bring a threat to the old–established friendship with the patient's family. This treatment had ended in a partial success; the patient was relieved of her hysterical anxiety but did not lose all her somatic symptoms. At that time I was not yet quite clear in my mind as to the criteria indicating that a hysterical case history was finally closed, and I proposed a solution to the patient which she seemed unwilling to accept. While we were thus at variance, we had broken off the treatment for the summer vacation.—One day I had a visit from a junior colleague, one of my oldest friends, who had been staying with my patient, Irma, and her family at their country resort. I asked him how he had found her and he answered: 'She's better, but not quite well.' I was conscious that my friend Otto's words, or the tone in which he spoke them, annoyed me. I fancied I detected a reproof in them, such as to the effect that I had promised the patient too much; and, whether rightly or wrongly, I attributed the supposed fact of Otto's siding against me to the influence of my patient's relatives, who, as it seemed to me, had never looked with favour on the treatment. However, my disagreeable impression was not clear to me and I gave no outward sign of it. The same evening I wrote out Irma's case history, with the idea of giving it to Dr. M. (a common friend who was at that time the leading figure in our circle) in order to justify myself. That night (or more probably the next morning) I had the following dream, which I noted down immediately after waking.*

DREAM OF JULY 23RD–24TH, 1895 *A large hall—numerous guests, whom we were receiving.—Among them was Irma. I at once took her on one side, as though to answer her letter and to reproach her for not having accepted my 'solution' yet. I said to her: 'If you still get pains, it's really only your fault.' She replied: 'If you only knew what pains I've got now in my throat and stomach and abdomen—it's choking me'—I was alarmed and looked at her. She looked pale and puffy. I thought to myself that after all I must be missing some organic trouble. I took her to the window and looked down her throat, and she showed signs of recalcitrance, like women with artificial dentures. I thought to myself that there was really no need for her to do that.—She then opened her mouth properly and on the*

---

* [Footnote added 1914:] This is the first dream which I submitted to a detailed interpretation.

right I found a big white* patch; at another place I saw extensive whitish grey scabs upon some remarkable curly structures which were evidently modelled on the turbinal bones of the nose.—I at once called in Dr. M., and he repeated the examination and confirmed it. . . . Dr. M. looked quite different from usual; he was very pale, he walked with a limp and his chin was clean-shaven. . . . My friend Otto was now standing beside her as well, and my friend Leopold was percussing her through her bodice and saying: 'She has a dull area low down on the left.' He also indicated that a portion of the skin on the left shoulder was infiltrated. (I noticed this, just as he did, in spite of her dress.) . . . M. said: 'There's no doubt it's an infection, but no matter; dysentery will supervene and the toxin will be eliminated.' . . . We were directly aware, too, of the origin of the infection. Not long before, when she was feeling unwell, my friend Otto had given her an injection of a preparation of propyl, propyls . . . propionic acid . . . trimethylamin (and I saw before me the formula for this printed in heavy type). . . . Injections of that sort ought not to be made so thoughtlessly. . . . And probably the syringe had not been clean.†

This dream has one advantage over many others. It was immediately clear what events of the previous day provided its starting-point. My preamble makes that plain. The news which Otto had given me of Irma's condition and the case history which I had been engaged in writing till far into the night continued to occupy my mental activity even after I was asleep. Nevertheless, no one who had only read the preamble and the content of the dream itself could have the slightest notion of what the dream meant. I myself had no notion. I was astonished at the symptoms of which Irma complained to me in the dream, since they were not the same as those for which I had treated her. I smiled at the senseless idea of an injection of propionic acid

---

* The word 'white' is omitted, no doubt accidentally, in the 1942 edition only. STRACHEY
† All ellipses appear in the original. *Ed.*

and at Dr. M.'s consoling reflections. Towards its end the dream seemed to me to be more obscure and compressed than it was at the beginning. In order to discover the meaning of all this it was necessary to undertake a detailed analysis.

ANALYSIS *The hall—numerous guests, whom we were receiving.* We were spending that summer at Bellevue, a house standing by itself on one of the hills adjoining the Kahlenberg.*: The house had formerly been designed as a place of entertainment and its reception–rooms were in consequence unusually lofty and hall–like. It was at Bellevue that I had the dream, a few days before my wife's birthday. On the previous day my wife had told me that she expected that a number of friends, including Irma, would be coming out to visit us on her birthday. My dream was thus anticipating this occasion: it was my wife's birthday and a number of guests, including Irma, were being received by us in the large hall at Bellevue.

I reproached Irma for not having accepted my solution; I said: 'If you still get pains, it's your own fault.' I might have said this to her in waking life, and I may actually have done so. It was my view at that time (though I have since recognized it as a wrong one) that my task was fulfilled when I had informed a patient of the hidden meaning of his symptoms: I considered that I was not responsible for whether he accepted the solution or not—though this was what success depended on. I owe it to this mistake, which I have now fortunately corrected, that my life was made easier at a time when, in spite of all my inevitable ignorance, I was expected to produce therapeutic successes.—I noticed, however, that the words which I spoke to Irma in the dream showed that I was specially anxious not to be responsible for the pains which she still had. If they were her fault they could not be mine. Could it be that the purpose of the dream lay in this direction?

Irma's complaint: pains in her throat and abdomen and stomach; it was choking her. Pains in the stomach were among my patient's symptoms but were not very prominent; she complained more of

---

* A hill which is a favourite resort in the immediate neighbourhood of Vienna.
STRACHEY

feelings of nausea and disgust. Pains in the throat and abdomen and constriction of the throat played scarcely any part in her illness. I wondered why I decided upon this choice of symptoms in the dream but could not think of an explanation at the moment.

She looked pale and puffy. My patient always had a rosy complexion. I began to suspect that someone else was being substituted for her.

I was alarmed at the idea that I had missed an organic illness. This, as may well be believed, is a perpetual source of anxiety to a specialist whose practice is almost limited to neurotic patients and who is in the habit of attributing to hysteria a great number of symptoms which other physicians treat as organic. On the other hand, a faint doubt crept into my mind—from where, I could not tell—that my alarm was not entirely genuine. If Irma's pains had an organic basis, once again I could not be held responsible for curing them; my treatment only set out to get rid of *hysterical* pains. It occurred to me, in fact, that I was actually *wishing* that there had been a wrong diagnosis; for, if so, the blame for my lack of success would also have been got rid of.

I took her to the window to look down her throat. She showed some recalcitrance, like women with false teeth. I thought to myself that really there was no need for her to do that. I had never had any occasion to examine Irma's oral cavity. What happened in the dream reminded me of an examination I had carried out some time before of a governess: at a first glance she had seemed a picture of youthful beauty, but when it came to opening her mouth she had taken measures to conceal her plates. This led to recollections of other medical examinations and of little secrets revealed in the course of them—to the satisfaction of neither party. *'There was really no need for her to do that'* was no doubt intended in the first place as a compliment to Irma; but I suspected that it had another meaning besides. (If one carries out an analysis attentively, one gets a feeling of whether or not one has exhausted all the background thoughts that are to be expected.) The way in which Irma stood by the window suddenly reminded me of another experience. Irma had an intimate woman friend of whom I had a very high opinion. When I visited this lady one evening I had found her by a window in the situation reproduced in the dream, and her physician, the same Dr. M., had pronounced that she had a diphtheritic membrane. The figure of Dr. M. and the membrane reappear later in the dream. It now occurred to me that for the last few months I had had every reason to suppose that this other lady was also a hysteric. Indeed, Irma herself had betrayed the fact to me. What did I know of her condition? One thing precisely: that, like my Irma of the dream, she suffered from hysterical choking. So in the dream I had replaced my patient by her friend. I now recollected that I had often played with the idea that she too might ask me to relieve her of her symptoms. I myself, however, had thought this unlikely, since she was of a very reserved nature. She was *recalcitrant,* as was shown in the dream. Another reason was that *there was no need for her to do it:* she had so far shown herself strong enough to master her condition without outside help. There still remained a few features that I could not attach either to Irma or to her friend: *pale; puffy; false teeth.* The false teeth took me to the governess whom I have already mentioned; I now felt inclined to be satisfied with *bad* teeth. I then thought of someone else to whom these features might be alluding. She again was not one of my patients, nor should I have liked to have her as a patient, since I had noticed that she was bashful in my presence and I could not think she would make an amenable patient. She was usually pale, and once, while she had been in specially good health, she had looked puffy.* Thus I had been comparing my patient Irma with two other people who would also have been recalcitrant to treatment. What could the reason have been for my having exchanged her in the dream for her friend? Perhaps it was that I should have *liked* to exchange her: either I felt more sympathetic towards her friend or had a higher opinion of her intelligence. For Irma seemed to me foolish because she had not accepted my

---

* The still unexplained complaint about *pains in the abdomen* could also be traced back to this third figure. The person in question was, of course, my own wife; the pains in the abdomen reminded me of one of the occasions on which I had noticed her bashfulness. I was forced to admit to myself that I was not treating either Irma or my wife very kindly in this dream; but it should be observed by way of excuse that I was measuring them both by the standard of the good and amenable patient.

solution. Her friend would have been wiser, that is to say she would have yielded sooner. She would then have *opened her mouth properly,* and have told me more than Irma.*

What I saw in her throat: a white patch and turbinal bones with scabs on them. The white patch reminded me of diphtheritis and so of Irma's friend, but also of a serious illness of my eldest daughter's almost two years earlier and of the fright I had had in those anxious days. The scabs on the turbinal bones recalled a worry about my own state of health. I was making frequent use of cocaine at that time to reduce some troublesome nasal swellings, and I had heard a few days earlier that one of my women patients who had followed my example had developed an extensive necrosis of the nasal mucous membrane. I had been the first to recommend the use of cocaine, in 1885,† and this recommendation had brought serious reproaches down on me. The misuse of that drug had hastened the death of a dear friend of mine. This had been before 1895 [the date of the dream].**

I at once called in Dr. M., and he repeated the examination. This simply corresponded to the position occupied by M. in our circle. But the '*at once*' was sufficiently striking to require a special explanation. It reminded me of a tragic event in my practice. I had on one occasion produced a severe toxic state in a woman patient by repeatedly prescribing what was at that time regarded as a harmless remedy (sulphonal), and had hurriedly turned for assistance and support to my experienced senior colleague. There was a subsidiary detail which confirmed the idea that I had this incident in mind. My patient—who succumbed to the poison—had the same name as my eldest daughter. It had never occurred to me before, but it struck me now almost like an act of retribution on the part of destiny. It was as

---

* I had a feeling that the interpretation of this part of the dream was not carried far enough to make it possible to follow the whole of its concealed meaning. If I had pursued my comparison between the three women, it would have taken me far afield.—There is at least one spot in every dream at which it is unplumbable—a navel, as it were, that is its point of contact with the unknown.

† This is a misprint (which occurs in every German edition) for '1884', the date of Freud's first paper on cocaine.... the 'dear friend' was Ernst von Fleischl–Marxow. STRACHEY

** *Fleischl died in the year 1891. Ed.*

though the replacement of one person by another was to be continued in another sense: this Mathilde for that Mathilde, an eye for an eye and a tooth for a tooth. It seemed as if I had been collecting all the occasions which I could bring up against myself as evidence of lack of medical conscientiousness.

Dr. M. was pale, had a clean–shaven chin and walked with a limp. This was true to the extent that his unhealthy appearance often caused his friends anxiety. The two other features could only apply to someone else. I thought of my elder brother, who lives abroad, who is clean–shaven and whom, if I remembered right, the M. of the dream closely resembled. We had had news a few days earlier that he was walking with a limp owing to an arthritic affection of his hip. There must, I reflected, have been some reason for my fusing into one the two figures in the dream. I then remembered that I had a similar reason for being in an ill-humour with each of them: they had both rejected a certain suggestion I had recently laid before them.

My friend Otto was now standing beside the patient and my friend Leopold was examining her and indicated that there was a dull area low down on the left. My friend Leopold was also a physician and a relative of Otto's. Since they both specialized in the same branch of medicine, it was their fate to be in competition with each other, and comparisons were constantly being drawn between them. Both of them acted as my assistants for years while I was still in charge of the neurological out–patients' department of a children's hospital. Scenes such as the one represented in the dream used often to occur there. While I was discussing the diagnosis of a case with Otto, Leopold would be examining the child once more and would make an unexpected contribution to our decision. The difference between their characters was like that between the bailiff Bräsig and his friend Karl*: one was distinguished for his quickness, while the other was slow but sure. If in the dream I was contrasting Otto with the prudent Leopold, I was evidently doing so to the advantage of the latter. The comparison was similar to the one between my disobedient pa-

---

* The two chief figures in the once popular novel, *Ut mine Stromtid*, written in Mecklenburg dialect, by Fritz Reuter (1862–4). There is an English translation, *An Old Story of my Farming Days* (London, 1878). STRACHEY

tient Irma and the friend whom I regarded as wiser than she was. I now perceived another of the lines along which the chain of thought in the dream branched off: from the sick child to the children's hospital.—*The dull area low down on the left* seemed to me to agree in every detail with one particular case in which Leopold had struck me by his thoroughness. I also had a vague notion of something in the nature of a metastatic affection; but this may also have been a reference to the patient whom I should have liked to have in the place of Irma. So far as I had been able to judge, she had produced an imitation of a tuberculosis.

A portion of the skin on the left shoulder was infiltrated. I saw at once that this was the rheumatism in my own shoulder, which I invariably notice if I sit up late into the night. Moreover the wording in the dream was most ambiguous: *'I noticed this, just as he did. . . .'* I noticed it in my own body, that is. I was struck, too, by the unusual phrasing: 'a portion of the skin was infiltrated'. We are in the habit of speaking of 'a left upper posterior infiltration', and this would refer to the lung and so once more to tuberculosis.

In spite of her dress. This was in any case only an interpolation. We naturally used to examine the children in the hospital undressed: and this would be a contrast to the manner in which adult female patients have to be examined. I remembered that it was said of a celebrated clinician that he never made a physical examination of his patients except through their clothes. Further than this I could not see. Frankly, I had no desire to penetrate more deeply at this point.

Dr. M. said: 'It's an infection, but no matter. Dysentery will supervene and the toxin will be eliminated.' At first this struck me as ridiculous. But nevertheless, like all the rest, it had to be carefully analysed. When I came to look at it more closely it seemed to have some sort of meaning all the same. What I discovered in the patient was a local diphtheritis. I remembered from the time of my daughter's illness a discussion on diphtheritis and diphtheria, the latter being the general infection that arises from the local diphtheritis. Leopold indicated the presence of a general infection of this kind from the existence of a dull area, which might thus be regarded as a metastatic focus. I seemed to think, it is true, that metastases like this do not in fact occur with diphtheria: it made me think rather of pyaemia.

No matter. This was intended as a consolation. It seemed to fit into the context as follows. The content of the preceding part of the dream had been that my patient's pains were due to a severe organic affection. I had a feeling that I was only trying in that way to shift the blame from myself. Psychological treatment could not be held responsible for the persistence of diphtheritic pains. Nevertheless I had a sense of awkwardness at having invented such a severe illness for Irma simply in order to clear myself. It looked so cruel. Thus I was in need of an assurance that all would be well in the end, and it seemed to me that to have put the consolation into the mouth precisely of Dr. M. had not been a bad choice. But here I was taking up a superior attitude towards the dream, and this itself required explanation.

And why was the consolation so nonsensical?

Dysentery. There seemed to be some remote theoretical notion that morbid matter can be eliminated through the bowels. Could it be that I was trying to make fun of Dr. M.'s fertility in producing far-fetched explanations and making unexpected pathological connections? Something else now occurred to me in relation to dysentery. A few months earlier I had taken on the case of a young man with remarkable difficulties associated with defaecating, who had been treated by other physicians as a case of 'anaemia accompanied by malnutrition'. I had recognized it as a hysteria, but had been unwilling to try him with my psychotherapeutic treatment and had sent him on a sea voyage. Some days before, I had had a despairing letter from him from Egypt, saying that he had had a fresh attack there which a doctor had declared was dysentery. I suspected that the diagnosis was an error on the part of an ignorant practitioner who had allowed himself to be taken in by the hysteria. But I could not help reproaching myself for having put my patient in a situation in which he might have contracted some organic trouble on top of his hysterical intestinal disorder. Moreover 'dysentery' sounds not unlike 'diphtheria'—a word of ill omen which did not occur in the dream.*

Yes, I thought to myself, I must have been making fun of Dr. M.

---

* The German words *'Dysenterie'* and *'Diphtherie'* are more alike than the English ones. STRA.

with the consoling prognosis 'Dysentery will supervene, etc.': for it came back to me that, years before, he himself had told an amusing story of a similar kind about another doctor. Dr. M. had been called in by him for consultation over a patient who was seriously ill, and had felt obliged to point out, in view of the very optimistic view taken by his colleague, that he had found albumen in the patient's urine. The other, however, was not in the least put out: *'No matter'*, he had said, 'the albumen will soon be eliminated!'—I could no longer feel any doubt, therefore, that this part of the dream was expressing derision at physicians who are ignorant of hysteria. And, as though to confirm this, a further idea crossed my mind: 'Does Dr. M. realize that the symptoms in his patient (Irma's friend) which give grounds for fearing tuberculosis also have a hysterical basis? Has he spotted this hysteria? or has he been taken in by it?'

But what could be my motive for treating this friend of mine so badly? That was a very simple matter. Dr. M. was just as little in agreement with my 'solution' as Irma herself. So I had already revenged myself in this dream on two people: on Irma with the words 'If you still get pains, it's your own fault', and on Dr. M. by the wording of the nonsensical consolation that I put into his mouth.

We were directly aware of the origin of the infection. This direct knowledge in the dream was remarkable. Only just before we had had no knowledge of it, for the infection was only revealed by Leopold.

When she was feeling unwell, my friend Otto had given her an injection. Otto had in fact told me that during his short stay with Irma's family he had been called in to a neighbouring hotel to give an injection to someone who had suddenly felt unwell. These injections reminded me once more of my unfortunate friend* who had poisoned himself with cocaine. I had advised him to use the drug internally [i.e. orally] only, while morphia was being withdrawn; but he had at once given himself cocaine *injections.*

A preparation of propyl . . . propyls . . . propionic acid. How could I have come to think of this? During the previous evening, before I wrote out the case history and had the dream, my wife had opened a

---

* *Ernst von Fleischl–Marxow. Ed.*

bottle of liqueur, on which the word 'Ananas'* appeared and which was a gift from our friend Otto: for he has a habit of making presents on every possible occasion. It was to be hoped, I thought to myself, that some day he would find a wife to cure him of the habit.† This liqueur gave off such a strong smell of fusel oil that I refused to touch it. My wife suggested our giving the bottle to the servants, but I—with even greater prudence—vetoed the suggestion, adding in a philanthropic spirit that there was no need for *them* to be poisoned either. The smell of fusel oil (amyl . . .) evidently stirred up in my mind a recollection of the whole series—propyl, methyl, and so on—and this accounted for the propyl preparation in the dream. It is true that I carried out a substitution in the process: I dreamt of propyl after having smelt amyl. But substitutions of this kind are perhaps legitimate in organic chemistry.

Trimethylamin. I saw the chemical formula of this substance in my dream, which bears witness to a great effort on the part of my memory. Moreover the formula was printed in heavy type, as though there had been a desire to lay emphasis on some part of the context as being of quite special importance. What was it, then, to which my attention was to be directed in this way by trimethylamin? It was to a conversation with another friend who had for many years been familiar with all my writings during the period of their gestation, just as I had been with his.** He had at that time confided some ideas to me on the subject of the chemistry of the sexual processes, and had mentioned among other things that he believed that one of the products of sexual metabolism was trimethylamin. Thus this substance led me to sexuality, the factor to which I attributed the greatest im-

---

* I must add that the sound of the word 'Ananas' bears a remarkable resemblance to that of my patient Irma's family name.
† [Footnote added 1909, but omitted again from 1925 onwards:] In this respect the dream did not turn out to be prophetic. But in another respect it *was*. For my patient's 'unsolved' gastric pains, for which I was so anxious not to be blamed, turned out to be the forerunners of a serious disorder caused by gallstones.
** This was Wilhelm Fliess, the Berlin biologist and nose and throat specialist, who exercised a great influence on Freud during the years immediately preceding the publication of *The Interpretation of Dreams*, and who figures frequently, though as a rule anonymously, in its pages. STRACHEY

portance in the origin of the nervous disorders which it was my aim to cure. My patient Irma was a young widow; if I wanted to find an excuse for the failure of my treatment in her case, what I could best appeal to would no doubt be this fact of her widowhood, which her friends would be so glad to see changed. And how strangely, I thought to myself, a dream like this is put together! The other woman, whom I had as a patient in the dream instead of Irma, was also a young widow.

I began to guess why the formula for trimethylamin had been so prominent in the dream. So many important subjects converged upon that one word. Trimethylamin was an allusion not only to the immensely powerful factor of sexuality, but also to a person whose agreement I recalled with satisfaction whenever I felt isolated in my opinions. Surely this friend who played so large a part in my life must appear again elsewhere in these trains of thought. Yes. For he had a special knowledge of the consequences of affections of the nose and its accessory cavities; and he had drawn scientific attention to some very remarkable connections between the turbinal bones and the female organs of sex. (Cf. the three curly structures in Irma's throat.) I had had Irma examined by him to see whether her gastric pains might be of nasal origin. But he suffered himself suppurative rhinitis, which caused me anxiety; and no doubt there was an illusion to this in the pyaemia which vaguely came into my mind in connection with the metastases in the dream.

Injections of that sort ought not to be made so thoughtlessly. Here an accusation of thoughtlessness was being made directly against my friend Otto. I seemed to remember thinking something of the same kind that afternoon when his words and looks had appeared to show that he was siding against me. It had been some such notion as: 'How easily his thoughts are influenced! How thoughtlessly he jumps to conclusions!'—Apart from this, this sentence in the dream reminded me once more of my dead friend who had so hastily resorted to cocaine injections. As I have said, I had never contemplated the drug being given by injection. I noticed too that in accusing Otto of thoughtlessness in handling chemical substances I was once more touching upon the story of the unfortunate Mathilde, which gave grounds for the same accusation against myself. Here I was evidently collecting instances of my conscientiousness, but also of the reverse.

And probably the syringe had not been clean. This was yet another accusation against Otto, but derived from a different source. I had happened the day before to meet the son of an old lady of eighty-two, to whom I had to give an injection of morphia twice a day.* At the moment she was in the country and he told me that she was suffering from phlebitis. I had at once thought it must be an infiltration caused by a dirty syringe. I was proud of the fact that in two years I had not caused a single infiltration; I took constant pains to be sure that the syringe was clean. In short, I was conscientious. The phlebitis brought me back once more to my wife, who had suffered from thrombosis during one of her pregnancies; and now three similar situations came to my recollection involving my wife, Irma and the dead Mathilde. The identity of these situations had evidently enabled me to substitute the three figures for one another in the dream.

I have now completed the interpretation of the dream.† While I was carrying it out I had some difficulty in keeping at bay all the ideas which were bound to be provoked by a comparison between the content of the dream and the concealed thoughts lying behind it. And in the meantime the 'meaning' of the dream was borne in upon me. I became aware of an intention which was carried into effect by the dream and which must have been my motive for dreaming it. The dream fulfilled certain wishes which were started in me by the events of the previous evening (the news given me by Otto and my writing out of the case history). The conclusion of the dream, that is to say, was that I was not responsible for the persistence of Irma's pains, but that Otto was. Otto had in fact annoyed me by his remarks about Irma's incomplete cure, and the dream gave me my revenge by throwing the reproach back on to him. The dream acquitted me of the responsibility for Irma's condition by showing that it was due to

---

* This old lady makes frequent appearances in Freud's writings at this period. STRACHEY
† [Footnote added 1909:] Though it will be understood that I have not reported everything that occurred to me during the process of interpretation.

other factors—it produced a whole series of reasons. The dream represented a particular state of affairs as I should have wished it to be. *Thus its content was the fulfilment of a wish and its motive was a wish.*

Thus much leapt to the eyes. But many of the details of the dream also became intelligible to me from the point of view of wish–fulfilment. Not only did I revenge myself on Otto for being too hasty in taking sides against me by representing him as being too hasty in his medical treatment (in giving the injection); but I also revenged myself on him for giving me the bad liqueur which had an aroma of fusel oil. And in the dream I found an expression which united the two reproaches: the injection was of a preparation of propyl. This did not satisfy me and I pursued my revenge further by contrasting him with his more trustworthy competitor. I seemed to be saying: 'I like *him* better than *you*.' But Otto was not the only person to suffer from the vials of my wrath. I took revenge as well on my disobedient patient by exchanging her for one who was wiser and less recalcitrant. Nor did I allow Dr. M. to escape the consequences of his contradiction but showed him by means of a clear allusion that he was an ignoramus on the subject. (*'Dysentery will supervene,* etc.') Indeed I seemed to be appealing from him to someone else with greater knowledge (to my friend who had told me of trimethylamin) just as I had turned from Irma to her friend and from Otto to Leopold. 'Take these people away! Give me three others of my choice instead! Then I shall be free of these undeserved reproaches!' The groundlessness of the reproaches was proved for me in the dream in the most elaborate fashion. I was not to blame for Irma's pains, since she herself was to blame for them by refusing to accept my solution. I was not concerned with Irma's pains, since they were of an organic nature and quite incurable by psychological treatment. Irma's pains could be satisfactorily explained by her widowhood (cf. the trimethylamin) which I had no means of altering. Irma's pains had been caused by Otto giving her an incautious injection of an unsuitable drug—a thing I should never have done. Irma's pains were the result of an injection with a dirty needle, like my old lady's phlebitis—whereas I never did any harm with my injections. I noticed, it is true, that these explanations of Irma's pains (which agreed in exculpating me) were not entirely consistent with one another, and indeed that they were mutually exclusive. The whole plea—for the dream was nothing else—reminded one vividly of the defence put forward by the man who was charged by one of his neighbours with having given him back a borrowed kettle in a damaged condition. The defendant asserted first, that he had given it back undamaged; secondly, that the kettle had a hole in it when he borrowed it; and thirdly, that he had never borrowed a kettle from his neighbour at all. So much the better: if only a single one of these three lines of defence were to be accepted as valid, the man would have to be acquitted.

Certain other themes played a part in the dream, which were not so obviously connected with my exculpation from Irma's illness: my daughter's illness and that of my patient who bore the same name, the injurious effect of cocaine, the disorder of my patient who was travelling in Egypt, my concern about my wife's health and about that of my brother and of Dr. M., my own physical ailments, my anxiety about my absent friend who suffered from suppurative rhinitis. But when I came to consider all of these, they could all be collected into a single group of ideas and labelled, as it were, 'concern about my own and other people's health—professional conscientiousness'. I called to mind the obscure disagreeable impression I had had when Otto brought me the news of Irma's condition. This group of thoughts that played a part in the dream enabled me retrospectively to put this transient impression into words. It was as though he had said to me: 'You don't take your medical duties seriously enough. You're not conscientious; you don't carry out what you've undertaken.' Thereupon, this group of thoughts seemed to have put itself at my disposal, so that I could produce evidence of how highly conscientious I was, of how deeply I was concerned about the health of my relations, my friends and my patients. It was a noteworthy fact that this material also included some disagreeable memories, which supported my friend Otto's accusation rather than my own vindication. The material was, as one might say, impartial; but nevertheless there was an unmistakable connection between this more extensive group of thoughts which underlay the dream and the narrower subject of the dream which gave rise to the wish to be innocent of Irma's illness.

I will not pretend that I have completely uncovered the meaning of this dream or that its interpretation is without a gap. I could spend much more time over it, derive further information from it and discuss fresh problems raised by it. I myself know the points from which further trains of thought could be followed. But considerations which arise in the case of every dream of my own restrain me from pursuing my interpretative work. If anyone should feel tempted to express a hasty condemnation of my reticence, I would advise him to make the experiment of being franker than I am. For the moment I am satisfied with the achievement of this one piece of fresh knowledge. If we adopt the method of interpreting dreams which I have indicated here, we shall find that dreams really have a meaning and are far from being the expression of a fragmentary activity of the brain, as the authorities have claimed. *When the work of interpretation has been completed, we perceive that a dream is the fulfilment of a wish.*

II.

The principal figure in the dream–content was my patient Irma. She appeared with the features which were hers in real life, and thus, in the first instance, represented herself. But the position in which I examined her by the window was derived from someone else, the lady for whom, as the dream–thoughts showed, I wanted to exchange my patient. In so far as Irma appeared to have a diphtheritic membrane, which recalled my anxiety about my eldest daughter, she stood for that child and, behind her, through her possession of the same name as my daughter, was hidden the figure of my patient who succumbed to poisoning. In the further course of the dream the figure of Irma acquired still other meanings, without any alteration occurring in the visual picture of her in the dream. She turned into one of the children whom we had examined in the neurological department of the children's hospital, where my two friends revealed their contrasting characters. The figure of my own child was evidently the stepping–stone towards this transition. The same 'Irma's' recalcitrance over opening her mouth brought an allusion to another lady whom I had once examined, and, through the same connection, to my wife. Moreover, the pathological changes which I discovered in her throat involved allusions to a whole series of other figures.

None of these figures whom I lighted upon by following up 'Irma' appeared in the dream in bodily shape. They were concealed behind the dream figure of 'Irma', which was thus turned into a collective image with, it must be admitted, a number of contradictory characteristics. Irma became the representative of all these other figures which had been sacrificed to the work of condensation, since I passed over to *her,* point by point, everything that reminded me of *them.*

There is another way in which a 'collective figure' can be produced for purposes of dream–condensation, namely by uniting the actual features of two or more people into a single dream–image. It was in this way that the Dr. M. of my dream was constructed. He bore the name of Dr. M., he spoke and acted like him; but his physical characteristics and his malady belonged to someone else, namely to my eldest brother. One single feature, his pale appearance, was doubly determined, since it was common to both of them in real life. . . .

The construction of collective and composite figures is one of the chief methods by which condensation operates in dreams. . . .

The occurrence of the idea of 'dysentery' in the dream of Irma's injection also had a multiple determination: first owing to its phonetic similarity to 'diphtheria' and secondly owing to its connection with the patient whom I had sent to the East and whose hysteria was not recognized.

Another interesting example of condensation in this dream was the mention in it of 'propyls'. What was contained in the dream–thoughts was not 'propyls' but 'amyls'. It might be supposed that a single displacement had taken place at this point in the construction of the dream. This was indeed the case. But the displacement served the purposes of condensation, as is proved by the following addition to the analysis of the dream. When I allowed my attention to dwell for a moment longer on the word 'propyls', it occurred to me that it sounded like 'Propylaea'. But there are Propylaea not only in Athens but in Munich.* A year before the dream I had gone to Munich to visit a friend who was seriously ill at the time—the same friend who

---

* A ceremonial portico on the model of the Athenian one. STRACHEY

was unmistakably alluded to in the dream by the word 'trimethylamin' which occurred immediately after 'propyls'.

I shall pass over the striking way in which here, as elsewhere in dream–analyses, associations of the most various inherent importance are used for laying down thought–connections as though they were of equal weight, and shall yield to the temptation to give, as it were, a plastic picture of the process by which the amyls in the dream–thoughts were replaced by propyls in the dream–content.

On the one hand we see the group of ideas attached to my friend Otto, who did not understand me, who sided against me, and who made me a present of liqueur with an aroma of amyl. On the other hand we see—linked to the former group by its very contrast—the group of ideas attached to my friend in Berlin [Wilhelm Fliess], who *did* understand me, who would take my side, and to whom I owed so much valuable information, dealing, amongst other things, with the chemistry of the sexual processes.

The recent exciting causes—the actual instigators of the dream—determined what was to attract my attention in the 'Otto' group; the amyl was among these selected elements, which were predestined to form part of the dream–content. The copious 'Wilhelm' group was stirred up precisely through being in contrast to 'Otto', and those elements in it were emphasized which echoed those which were already stirred up in 'Otto'. All through the dream, indeed, I kept on turning from someone who annoyed me to someone else who could be agreeably contrasted with him; point by point, I called up a friend against an opponent. Thus the amyl in the 'Otto' group produced memories from the field of chemistry in the other group; in this manner the trimethylamin, which was supported from several directions, found its way into the dream–content. 'Amyls' itself might have entered the dream–content unmodified; but it came under the influence of the 'Wilhelm' group. For the whole range of memories covered by that name was searched through in order to find some element which could provide a two–sided determination for 'amyls'. 'Propyls' was closely associated with 'amyls', and Munich from the 'Wilhelm' group with its 'propylaea' came half-way to meet it. The two groups of ideas converged in 'propyls–propylaea;' and, as though by an act of compromise, this intermediate element was what found its way into the dream–content. Here an intermediate common entity had been constructed which admitted of multiple determination. It is obvious, therefore, that multiple determination must make it easier for an element to force its way into the dream–content. In order to construct an intermediate link of this kind, attention is without hesitation displaced from what is actually intended on to some neighbouring association. *

The Dream of the "Botanical Monograph" by Sigmund Freud March 1898
1.
   I believe . . . that the instigating agent of every dream is to be found among the experiences which one has not yet 'slept on'. Thus the relations of a dream's content to impressions of the most recent past (with the single exception of the day immediately preceding the night of the dream) differ in no respect from its relations to impressions dating from any remoter period. Dreams can select their material from any part of the dreamer's life, provided only that there is a train of thought linking the experience of the dream–day (the 'recent' impressions) with the earlier ones.

DREAM OF THE BOTANICAL MONOGRAPH *I had written a monograph on a certain plant. The book lay before me and I was at the moment turning over a folded coloured plate. Bound up in each copy there was a dried specimen of the plant, as though it had been taken from a herbarium.*

---

* In a letter to Fliess on June 12, 1900 (*see The Origins of Psychoanalysis,* Basic Books, 1954), Freud describes a later visit to Bellevue, the house where he had this dream. 'Do you suppose', he writes, 'that some day a marble tablet will be placed on the house, inscribed with these words? "In This House, on July 24th, 1895 the Secret of Dreams was Revealed to Dr. Sigm. Freud." At the moment there seems little prospect of it.' STRACHEY

ANALYSIS That morning I had seen a new book in the window of a bookshop, bearing the title *The Genus Cyclamen*—evidently a *monograph* on that plant.

Cyclamens, I reflected, were my wife's *favourite flowers* and I reproached myself for so rarely remembering to *bring* her *flowers,* which was what she liked.—The subject of *'bringing flowers'* recalled an anecdote which I had recently repeated to a circle of friends and which I had used as evidence in favour of my theory that forgetting is very often determined by an unconscious purpose and that it always enables one to deduce the secret intentions of the person who forgets. A young woman was accustomed to receiving a bouquet of flowers from her husband on her birthday. One year this token of his affection failed to appear, and she burst into tears. Her husband came in and had no idea why she was crying till she told him that to-day was her birthday. He clasped his hand to his head and exclaimed: 'I'm so sorry, but I'd quite forgotten. I'll go out at once and fetch your *flowers.*' But she was not to be consoled; for she recognized that her husband's forgetfulness was a proof that she no longer had the same place in his thoughts as she had formerly.—This lady, Frau L., had met my wife two days before I had the dream, had told her that she was feeling quite well and enquired after me. Some years ago she had come to me for treatment.

I now made a fresh start. Once, I recalled, I really *had* written something in the nature of a *monograph on a plant,* namely a dissertation on the *coca-plant* [*Ueber Coca,* 1884], which had drawn Carl Koller's attention to the anesthetic properties of cocaine. I had myself indicated this application of the alkaloid in my published paper, but I had not been thorough enough to pursue the matter further. This reminded me that on the morning of the day after the dream—I had not found time to interpret it till the evening—I had thought about cocaine in a kind of day-dream. If ever I got glaucoma, I had thought, I should travel to Berlin and get myself operated on, incognito, in my friend's [Fliess's] house, by a surgeon recommended by him. The operating surgeon, who would have no idea of my identity, would boast once again of how easily such operations could be performed since the introduction of cocaine; and I should not give the slightest hint that I myself had had a share in the discovery. This phantasy had led on to reflections of how awkward it is, when all is said and done, for a physician to ask for medical treatment for himself from his professional colleagues. The Berlin eye–surgeon would not know me, and I should be able to pay his fees like anyone else. It was not until I had recalled this day–dream that I realized that the recollection of a specific event lay behind it. Shortly after Koller's discovery, my father had in fact been attacked by glaucoma; my friend Dr. Königstein, the ophthalmic surgeon, had operated on him; while Dr. Koller had been in charge of the cocaine anaesthesia and had commented on the fact that this case had brought together all of the three men who had had a share in the introduction of cocaine.

My thoughts then went on to the occasion when I had last been reminded of this business of the cocaine. It had been a few days earlier, when I had been looking at a copy of a *Festschrift** in which grateful pupils had celebrated the jubilee of their teacher and laboratory director. Among the laboratory's claims to distinction which were enumerated in this book I had seen a mention of the fact that Koller had made his discovery there of the anesthetic properties of cocaine. I then suddenly perceived that my dream was connected with an event of the previous evening. I had walked home precisely with Dr. Königstein and had got into conversation with him about a matter which never fails to excite my feelings whenever it is raised. While I was talking to him in the entrance–hall, Professor *Gärtner* [Gardener] and his wife had joined us; and I could not help congratulating them both on their *blooming* looks. But Professor Gärtner was one of the authors of the *Festschrift* I have just mentioned, and may well have reminded me of it. Moreover, the Frau L., whose disappointment on her birthday I described earlier, was mentioned—

---

* This *Festschrift* was in honour of Professor Stricker, Director of the Institute of Pathological Anatomy, at which Dr. Gärtner was Assistant, and where Freud had worked in his student days. STRACHEY

though only, it is true, in another connection—in my conversation with Dr. Königstein.

I will make an attempt at interpreting the other determinants of the content of the dream as well. There was *a dried specimen of the plant* included in the monograph, as though it had been a *herbarium*. This led me to a memory from my secondary school. Our headmaster once called together the boys from the higher forms and handed over the school's herbarium to them to be looked through and cleaned. Some small worms—book–worms—had found their way into it. He does not seem to have had much confidence in my helpfulness, for he handed me only a few sheets. These, as I could still recall, included some Crucifers. I never had a specially intimate contact with botany. In my preliminary examination in botany I was also given a Crucifer to identify—and failed to do so. My prospects would not have been too bright, if I had not been helped out by my theoretical knowledge. I went on from the Cruciferae to the Compositae. It occurred to me that artichokes were Compositae, and indeed I might fairly have called them my *favourite flowers*. Being more generous than I am, my wife often brought me back these favourite flowers of mine from the market.

I saw the monograph which I had written *lying before me*. This again led me back to something. I had had a letter from my friend [Fliess] in Berlin the day before in which he had shown his power of visualization: 'I am very much occupied with your dream–book. *I see it lying finished before me and I see myself turning over its pages.*'* How much I envied him his gift as a seer! If only *I* could have seen it lying finished before me!

The folded coloured plate. While I was a medical student I was the constant victim of an impulse only to learn things out of *monographs*. In spite of my limited means, I succeeded in getting hold of a number of volumes of the proceedings of medical societies and was enthralled by their *coloured plates*. I was proud of my hankering for thorough-

---

* Freud's reply to this letter from Fliess is dated March 10, 1898 (see *The Origins of Psychoanalysis*, Basic Books, 1954, Letter 84); so that the dream must have occurred not more than a day or two earlier. STRACHEY

ness. When I myself had begun to publish papers, I had been obliged to make my own drawings to illustrate them and I remembered that one of them had been so wretched that a friendly colleague had jeered at me over it. There followed, I could not quite make out how, a recollection from very early youth. It had once amused my father to hand over a book with *coloured plates* (an account of a journey through Persia) for me and my eldest sister to destroy. Not easy to justify from the educational point of view! I had been five years old at the time and my sister not yet three; and the picture of the two of us blissfully pulling the book to pieces (leaf by leaf, like an *artichoke*, I found myself saying) was almost the only plastic memory that I retained from that period of my life. Then, when I became a student, I had developed a passion for collecting and owning books, which was analogous to my liking for learning out of monographs: a *favourite hobby*. (The idea of *'favourite'* had already appeared in connection with cyclamens and artichokes.) I had become a *book-worm*. I had always, from the time I first began to think about myself, referred this first passion of mine back to the childhood memory I have mentioned. Or rather, I had recognized that the childhood scene was a 'screen memory' for my later bibliophile propensities.* And I had early discovered, of course, that passions often lead to sorrow. When I was seventeen I had run up a largish account at the bookseller's and had nothing to meet it with; and my father had scarcely taken it as an excuse that my inclinations might have chosen a worse outlet. The recollection of this experience from the later years of my youth at once brought back to my mind the conversation with my friend Dr. Königstein. For in the course of it we had discussed the same question of my being blamed for being too much absorbed in my *favourite hobbies*.

For reasons with which we are not concerned, I shall not pursue the interpretation of this dream any further, but will merely indicate the direction in which it lay. In the course of the work of analysis I was reminded of my conversation with Dr. Königstein, and I was brought to it from more than one direction. When I take into account

---

* Cf. my paper on screen memories [Freud's *Collected Papers*, Vol. 5, Ch. 47].

the topics touched upon in that conversation, the meaning of the dream becomes intelligible to me. All the trains of thought starting from the dream—the thoughts about my wife's and my own favourite flowers, about cocaine, about the awkwardness of medical treatment among colleagues, about my preference for studying monographs and about my neglect of certain branches of science such as botany—all of these trains of thought, when they were further pursued, led ultimately to one or other of the many ramifications of my conversation with Dr. Königstein. Once again the dream, like the one we first analysed—the dream of Irma's injection—turns out to have been in the nature of a self–justification, a plea on behalf of my own rights. Indeed, it carried the subject that was raised in the earlier dream a stage further and discussed it with reference to fresh material that had arisen in the interval between the two dreams. Even the apparently indifferent form in which the dream was couched turns out to have had significance. What it meant was: 'After all, I'm the man who wrote the valuable and memorable paper (on cocaine)', just as in the earlier dream I had said on my behalf: 'I'm a conscientious and hard–working student.' In both cases what I was insisting was: 'I may allow myself to do this.' There is, however, no need for me to carry the interpretation of the dream any further, since my only purpose in reporting it was to illustrate by an example the relation between the content of a dream and the experience of the previous day which provoked it. So long as I was aware only of the dream's *manifest* content, it appeared to be related only to a *single* event of the dream–day. But when the analysis was carried out, a *second* source of the dream emerged in another experience of the same day. The first of these two impressions with which the dream was connected was an indifferent one, a subsidiary circumstance: I had seen a book in a shop–window whose title attracted my attention for a moment but whose subject–matter could scarcely be of interest to me. The second experience had a high degree of psychical importance: I had had a good hour's lively conversation with my friend the eye–surgeon; in the course of it I had given him some information which was bound to affect both of us closely, and I had had memories stirred up in me which had drawn my attention to a great variety of internal stresses in my own mind. Moreover, the conversation had been interrupted before its conclusion because we had been joined by acquaintances.

We must now ask what was the relation of the two impressions of the dream–day to each other and to the dream of the subsequent night. In the manifest content of the dream only the *indifferent* impression was alluded to, which seems to confirm the notion that dreams have a preference for taking up unimportant details of waking life. All the strands of the interpretation, on the other hand, led to the *important* impression, to the one which had justifiably stirred my feelings. If the sense of the dream is judged, as it can only rightly be, by its latent content as revealed by the analysis, a new and significant fact is unexpectedly brought to light. The conundrum of why dreams are concerned only with worthless fragments of waking life seems to have lost all its meaning; nor can it any longer be maintained that waking life is not pursued further in dreams and that dreams are thus psychical activity wasted upon foolish material. The contrary is true: our dream–thoughts are dominated by the same material that has occupied us during the day and we only bother to dream of things which have given us cause for reflection in the daytime.

Why is it, then, that, though the occasion of my dreaming was a daytime impression by which I had been justifiably stirred, I nevertheless actually dreamt of something indifferent? The most obvious explanation, no doubt, is that we are once more faced by one of the phenomena of dream–distortion, which ... I [(have)] traced to a psychical force acting as a censorship. My recollection of the monograph on the genus Cyclamen would thus serve the purpose of being an *allusion* to the conversation with my friend. ... The only question is as to the intermediate links which enabled the impression of the monograph to serve as an allusion to the conversation with the eye–surgeon, since at first sight there is no obvious connection between them.... In this ... example there were two detached impressions which at a first glance only had in common the fact of their having occurred on the same day: I had caught sight of the monograph in the morning and had had the conversation the same evening. The analysis enabled us to solve the problem as follows: connections of this kind, when they are not present in the first instance, are woven retrospectively between the ideational content of one impression and that of the other. I have already drawn attention to the intermediate links in the present case by the words I have italicized in my record of the analysis. If there had been no influences from another quarter, the idea of the monograph on the Cyclamen would only, I imagine, have led to the idea of its being my wife's favourite flower, and possibly also to Frau L.'s absent bouquet. I scarcely think that these background thoughts would have sufficed to evoke a dream. As we are told in *Hamlet:*

There needs no ghost, my lord, come from the grave
To tell us this.

But, lo and behold, I was reminded in the analysis that the man who interrupted our conversation was called *Gärtner* [Gardener] and that I had thought his wife looked *blooming*. And even as I write these words I recall that one of my patients, who bore the charming name of *Flora,* was for a time the pivot of our discussion. These must have been the intermediate links, arising from the botanical group of ideas, which formed the bridge between the two experiences of that day, the indifferent and the stirring one. A further set of connections was then established—those surrounding the idea of cocaine, which had every right to serve as a link between the figure of Dr. Königstein and a botanical monograph which I had written; and these connections strengthened the fusion between the two groups of ideas so that it became possible for a portion of the one experience to serve as an allusion to the other one.

I am prepared to find this explanation attacked on the ground of its being arbitrary or artificial. What, it may be asked, would have happened if Professor Gärtner and his wife with her blooming looks had not come up to us or if the patient we were talking about had been called Anna instead of Flora? The answer is simple. If these chains of thought had been absent others would no doubt have been selected. . . .

II.

In view of the very great number of associations produced in analysis to each individual element of the content of a dream, some readers may be led to doubt whether, as a matter of principle, we are justified in regarding as part of the dream–thoughts all the associations that occur to us during the subsequent analysis—whether we are justified, that is, in supposing that all these thoughts were already active during the state of sleep and played a part in the formation of the dream. Is it not more probable that new trains of thought have arisen in the course of the analysis which had no share in forming the dream? I can only give limited assent to this argument. It is no doubt true that some trains of thought arise for the first time during the analysis. But one can convince oneself in all such cases that these new connections are only set up between thoughts which were already linked in some other way in the dream–thoughts. The new connections are, as it were, loop–lines or short–circuits, made possible by the existence of other and deeper–lying connecting paths. It must be allowed that the great bulk of the thoughts which are revealed in analysis were already active during the process of forming the dream; for, after working through a string of thoughts which seem to have no connection with the formation of a dream, one suddenly comes upon one which is represented in its content and is indispensable for its interpretation, but which could not have been reached except by this particular line of approach. I may here recall the dream of the botanical monograph, which strikes one as the product of an astonishing amount of condensation, even though I have not reported its analysis in full.

How, then, are we to picture psychical conditions during the period of sleep which precedes dreams? Are all the dream–thoughts present alongside one another? or do they occur in sequence? or do a number of trains of thought start out simultaneously from different centres and afterwards unite? There is no need for the present, in my opinion, to form any plastic idea of psychical conditions during the formation of dreams. It must not be forgotten, however, that we are dealing with an *unconscious* process of thought, which may easily be different from what we perceive during purposive reflection accompanied by consciousness.

The unquestionable fact remains, however, that the formation of dreams is based on a process of condensation. How is that condensation brought about?

When we reflect that only a small minority of all the dream-thoughts revealed are represented in the dream by one of their ideational elements, we might conclude that condensation is brought about by *omission:* that is, that the dream is not a faithful translation or a point–for–point projection of the dream–thoughts, but a highly incomplete and fragmentary version of them. This view, as we shall soon discover, is a most inadequate one. But we may take it as a provisional starting–point and go on to a further question. If only a few elements from the dream–thoughts find their way into the dream–content, what are the conditions which determine their selection?

In order to get some light on this question we must turn our attention to those elements of the dream–content which must have fulfilled these conditions. And the most favourable material for such an investigation will be a dream to the construction of which a particularly intense process of condensation has contributed. I shall accordingly begin by choosing for the purpose the dream which I have already recorded.

THE DREAM OF THE BOTANICAL MONOGRAPH *Content of the Dream —I had written a monograph on an (unspecified) genus of plants. The book lay before me and I was at the moment turning over a folded coloured plate. Bound up in the copy there was a dried specimen of the plant.*

The element in this dream which stood out most was the *botanical monograph*. This arose from the impressions of the dream–day: I had in fact seen a monograph on the genus Cyclamen in the window of a book–shop. There was no mention of this genus in the content of the dream; all that was left in it was the monograph and its relation to botany. The 'botanical monograph' immediately revealed its connection with the *work upon cocaine* which I had once written. From 'cocaine' the chains of thought led on the one hand to the *Festschrift* and to certain events in a University laboratory, and on the other hand to my friend Dr. Königstein, the eye surgeon, who had had a share in the introduction of cocaine. The figure of Dr. Königstein further reminded me of the interrupted conversation which I had

had with him the evening before and of my various reflections upon the payment for medical services among colleagues. This conversation was the actual currently active instigator of the dream; the monograph on the cyclamen was also a currently active impression, but one of an indifferent nature. As I perceived, the 'botanical monograph' in the dream turned out to be an 'intermediate common entity' between the two experiences of the previous day: it was taken over unaltered from the indifferent impression and was linked with the psychically significant event by copious associative connections.

Not only the compound idea, 'botanical monograph', however, but each of its components, 'botanical' and 'monograph' separately, led by numerous connecting paths deeper and deeper into the tangle of dream–thoughts. 'Botanical' was related to the figure of Professor *Gärtner* [Gardener], the *blooming* looks of his wife, to my patient *Flora* and to the lady [Frau L.] of whom I had told the story of the forgotten *flowers*. Gärtner led in turn to the laboratory and to my conversation with Königstein. My two patients [Flora and Frau L.] had been mentioned in the course of this conversation. A train of thought joined the lady with the flowers to my wife's *favourite flowers* and thence to the title of the monograph which I had seen for a moment during the day. In addition to these, 'botanical' recalled an episode at my secondary school and an examination while I was at the University. A fresh topic touched upon in my conversation with Dr. Königstein—my *favourite* hobbies—was joined, through the intermediate link of what I jokingly called my *favourite flower*, the artichoke, with the train of thought proceeding from the forgotten flowers. Behind 'artichokes' lay, on the one hand, my thoughts about Italy and, on the other hand, a scene from my childhood which was the opening of what have since become my intimate relations with books. Thus 'botanical' was a regular nodal point in the dream. Numerous trains of thought converged upon it, which, as I can guarantee, had appropriately entered into the context of the conversation with Dr. Königstein. Here we find ourselves in a factory of thoughts where, as in the 'weaver's masterpiece',—

> Ein Tritt tausend Fäden regt,
> Die Schifflein herüber hinüber schiessen,

Die Fäden ungesehen fliessen,
Ein Schlag tausend Verbindungen schlägt.*

So, too, 'monograph' in the dream touches upon two subjects: the one–sidedness of my studies and the costliness of my favourite hobbies.

This first investigation leads us to conclude that the elements 'botanical' and 'monograph' found their way into the content of the dream because they possessed copious contacts with the majority of the dream–thoughts, because, that is to say, they constituted 'nodal points' upon which a great number of the dream–thoughts converged, and because they had several meanings in connection with the interpretation of the dream. The explanation of this fundamental fact can also be put in another way: each of the elements of the dream's content turns out to have been 'overdetermined'—to have been represented in the dream–thoughts many times over.

We discover still more when we come to examine the remaining constituents of the dream in relation to their appearance in the dream–thoughts. The *coloured plate* which I was unfolding led to a new topic, my colleagues' criticisms of my activities, and to one which was already represented in the dream, my favourite hobbies; and it led, in addition, to the childhood memory in which I was pulling to pieces a book with coloured plates. The *dried specimen of the plant* touched upon the episode of the herbarium at my secondary school and specially stressed that memory.

The nature of the relation between dream–content and dream–thoughts thus becomes visible. Not only are the elements of a dream determined by the dream–thoughts many times over, but the individual dream–thoughts are represented in the dream by several elements. Associative paths lead from one element of the dream to several dream–thoughts, and from one dream–thought to several elements of the dream. Thus a dream is not constructed by each individual dream–thought, or group of dream–thoughts, finding (in abbreviated

---

* ... a thousand threads one treadle throws,
  Where fly the shuttles hither and thither,
  Unseen the threads are knit together,
  And an infinite combination grows.
Goethe, *Faust,* Part I [Scene 4] (Bayard Taylor's translation).

form) separate representation in the content of the dream—in the kind of way in which an electorate chooses parliamentary representatives; a dream is constructed, rather, by the whole mass of dream–thoughts being submitted to a sort of manipulative process in which those elements which have the most numerous and strongest supports acquire the right of entry into the dream–content—in a manner analogous to election by *scrutin de liste*. In the case of every dream which I have submitted to an analysis of this kind I have invariably found these same fundamental principles confirmed: the elements of the dream are constructed out of the whole mass of dream–thoughts and each one of those elements is shown to have been determined many times over in relation to the dream–thoughts.

CHAPTER 19

Cocainism

1924

Der Kokainismus in Phantastica. Die Betäubenden und Erregenden Genussmittel für Ärzte und Nichtärzte, von Prof. Dr. L. Lewin, 1924, Verlag von Georg Stilke in Berlin.
"Cocainism" from Phantastica; Narcotic and Stimulating Drugs, their use and abuse, by Louis Lewin, 1924.
Translated from the second German Edition by P.H.A. Wirth, Ph.C., B.Sc. (Munich).

Louis Lewin (1850–1929) was one of the writers who criticized Freud's rosy view of cocaine. Lewin, a distinguished German pharmacologist and toxicologist was first to describe the actions of peyote or mescaline in 1888. His book Phantastica *(1924) is a brilliant description of the effects and history of psychotropic drugs. The section on cocaine abuse is printed here. Lewin's proven accuracy in the description of the drug effects might cause one to doubt that cocaine is a pure central stimulant. Ed.*

1. History of Coca and Cocaine

Towards the middle of the sixteenth century the second Council of Lima attempted to restrict the use of coca-leaves by the Peruvians, Chilians, and Bolivians. In canon 120 the drug is described as "a useless object liable to promote the practices and superstitions of the Indians." Political, economic, social, and religious reasons gave rise to this decision. It was arrived at when the use of this substance was extensive and its cultivation was at its height, and partly because coca had contributed, among other causes such as drudgery and malnutrition, to a deterioration of the hygienic condition of the Peruvians. The conquistadors cooperated with the proprietors of mines and plantations; they forced the natives to labour and paid them with coca-leaves. In the years 1560–9 the Government prohibited compulsory labour and the administration of coca because "the plant is only idolatry and the work of the devil, and appears to give strength only by a deception of the Evil One; it possesses no virtue, but shortens the life of many Indians who at most escape from the forests with ruined health. They should therefore not be compelled to labour and their health and lives should be preserved." All these restrictions proved of no avail, and coca became a State monopoly, to pass at the end of the eighteenth century into the hands of private enterprise.

All this relates to that wonderful plant, Erythroxylon coca, which Francesco Pizarro in the year 1533 found in general use as a euphoric when, setting out from San Miguel's Bay, he penetrated with his troops into the interior of Peru. According to an Indian legend narrated by Garcilasso de la Vega the children of the sun had presented

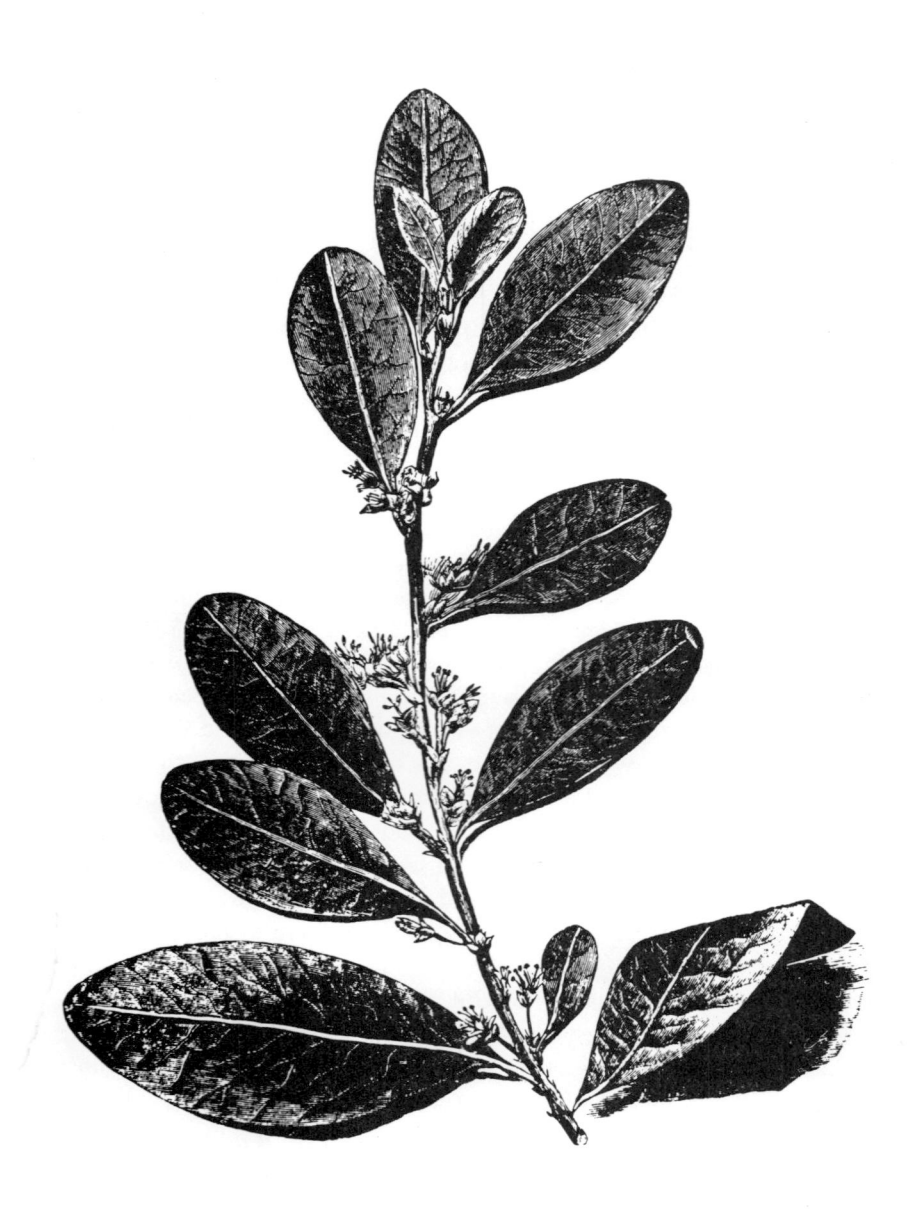

man with the coca leaf after the formation of the empire of the Incas, to "satisfy the hungry, provide the weary and fainting with new vigour, and cause the unhappy to forget their miseries." It is probable, however, that the Indians already cultivated the plant before they formed a federation, and the Incas invented the story of its divine origin in order to reserve it to themselves. They made of it a royal emblem; the queen called herself Mama Cuca, and the priests assisted in upholding the divine honours of the plant by using it in various religious ceremonies. The idols of the time as a sign of divinity were represented with one cheek stuffed with coca leaves. Its use gradually extended to the people, and it was not only applied for supernatural purposes, but for the very worldly object of allowing the plant to act on the organism. Time has changed nothing in this state of affairs, except that the desire for pleasurable sensations now forms the principal motive for the use of the leaves in South America and of cocaine, their derivative, in the rest of the world.

The leaf is chewed mixed with lime or vegetable ashes. The latter, called "lluta" in Aimarà, "llipta" in Keshua, and elsewhere "tonra," are kept in bottle-shaped gourds and extracted with the aid of a needle, the point of which is moistened in the mouth. I possess some preparations which show that these ashes are also found in the form of a circular bluish-grey paste, 4cm in diameter, small pieces of which are added to the leaf. Coca is mainly cultivated in Peru in the Montaña in the departments of Cuzco, Huanuco, Ayacucho, and Puno. In all the deep and hot valleys small plantations can be found. The Keshua and Aymara tribes in Cundinamarca, etc., are consumers of it. In Bolivia, especially in the departments of Cochabamba, Larecaja, and Yungas, in Colombia up to the Gulf of Maracaibo— the Goajiros are addicts—and to a less extent in Ecuador, but only in some valleys of the east slopes of the Cordilleras of Quito, the habit is in vogue. Its use diminishes as we go farther east from the Andes. It has, however, penetrated slightly along the course of the Marañon. The half-castes and the Indian women of the upper reaches of the Amazon all eat *ypadú,* as coca is called in those parts. The women plant the shrub, which reaches a height of ½ to 1½ meters, in a remote spot of the forest. The Marauá Indians on the banks of the Yutahí, and sometimes the Tecunas, Iuri, Passos, and Yauaretés also partake of the drug. The habit, as Koch–Grünberg observed, seems to have spread from the Rio Tiquié over the Papury. In North-Western Brazil the Indians consume coca in incredible quantities. All day long the calabash passes from hand to hand. Such coca eaters can be seen with lumps in their mouths so that their cheeks protrude like knobs. From Bolivia coca has conquered the Argentine. Peru supplies approximately fifteen million, Bolivia eight million kilos of the leaves which when dry furnish up to 1% cocaine, which is prepared in a raw state in the places of production. In the richest mining district of Peru, in Cerro de Pasco alone, fifteen hundred kilos of dry coca leaves are consumed monthly. Coca is also cultivated in Java for the manufacture of cocaine. There the tropical sun develops up to 1.2–1.6% cocaine in the leaves. In India in the district of the Nilgiris the plant also thrives.

In this case, too, consumption regulates production. The enormous development in the use of the drug explains the increase of the annual export shown below:

Coca Leaves

Peru.			Java.		
1877	—	8,000kg	1904	—	26,000kg
1906	—	2,800,000kg	1911	—	740,000kg
1920	—	453,000kg	1912	—	800,000kg
			1920	—	1,700,000kg

The export of raw cocaine increased to the same extent, and for its preparation—according to my personal knowledge—Americans have built large factories in South America.

The cocaine imported into Germany, according to information supplied by the official Bureau of Statistics, amounted to:

1924	—	662kg
1925	—	1,003kg

2. Effects of the Habitual Use of Coca and Cocaine

The disorders which arise from the habitual use of the coca-leaves, which are chewed, and that of cocaine are not the same. The differences are similar to those between opium and morphia. The composition of the two, in fact, is different; in fresh coca leaves there is a fragrant resin and other alkaloids, for instance dextro-cocaine. Experiments which I carried out many years ago with the latter proved that quantities of 0.02–0.04g sufficed to produce in rabbits curious mobile excitation; they continuously ran about in circles and were affected by convulsions and respiratory disturbances.

Nevertheless the use of the leaves and that of cocaine produce very similar results as regards the actual symptoms and final form of the cocaine evil.

Coca is for the coca-eater the source of his greatest delight. Under its influence the troubles of life are forgotten and he experiences in imagination many of the substantial pleasures which reality refuses to give. After breakfast and before going to work he takes some coca from his leather bag and some lime or ashes from his gourd and moulds a fragment, and sometimes lays up a stock of these small lumps. Between 25 and 50g is a moderate daily consumption. While chewing he strives to remain idle. An apathetic feeling of internal peace, from which he cannot be awakened, overcomes him for about an hour. Then he is again capable of work.

The *cocada,* i.e. the duration of the effects of the coca fragment, is his measure of time and distance. It amounts to approximately forty minutes, during which time about three kilometers can be walked or climbed on the plains and two kilometers in hilly districts. Alexander von Humboldt, who explored the Andes in 1802, spoke highly of the degree of endurance which his native guides derived from coca. In recent times European explorers have ascertained by experiment on themselves that the ascent to altitudes of five thousand to six thousand meters is considerably facilitated by coca, and that thanks to the drug the impression of hunger is not felt for a long time by the ill-conditioned body suffering from malnutrition. Experiments carried out years ago in Europe proved that the drinking of an infusion of 12g of coca leaves occasioned, besides a greater frequency of the pulse, palpitation of the heart, faintness, seeing of sparks and *tinnitus aurium,* a feeling of augmented power, and a greater desire for activity. An infusion of 16g of the leaves produced first a strange feeling of isolation from the exterior world and an irresistible urge to use one's strength; then in full consciousness appeared a kind of rigidity with a feeling of the most intense well-being, accompanied by the desire not to make the least movement for the whole day. Finally sleep supervened.

Such was our knowledge of the effects of coca when, in 1885, its active element, cocaine, was introduced into medical science. At that time a morphinistic physician* put forward the unfortunate theory that morphinism could be cured by cocaine. I at once objected, predicting that the only result would be the simultaneous use of both drugs, which I called "twofold craving."[1] This, and even worse, is what in fact happened. Cocaine was soon used by itself as a pleasure-producing agent. At first the doses were small, but they increased up to 1 and 4g, and it is said that they even reached the enormous dose of 8g a day. To believe that this is due to the war is an error; it has only added to the number of addicts persons whose social position had hitherto kept them isolated from its influence. Already in 1901 there were many cocainistic men and women in England, doctors, politicians, and writers. At present the situation is evidently much worse, although morphinism has not been dethroned. In Germany, mainly in the large towns, there are many cocainists in every profession, down to prostitutes and their protectors. In certain bars and restaurants, in the street, etc., cocaine is clandestinely sold, very frequently stolen or adulterated merchandize for which huge prices up to thirty marks are asked and paid. In Berlin there are cocaine dens, both disreputable and dirty and also fashionable and up-to-date establishments. One of these was raided by the police at the beginning of the present year. About one hundred habitués, men and women, from all classes of society, even university and literary men, had gathered there, to lead for a few hours an existence of somnolence and unreality. They spent whole days without taking food, for cocaine anesthetizes the nerves of the stomach, thus preventing

---

* Probably Ernst Von Fleischl-Marxow. *Ed.*

the appearance of any feeling of hunger. They give all that they possess, even indispensable articles of clothing, in order to indulge their mad craving. The most fantastic descriptions of the night side of human life, the sketch of Hogarth representing a party of punch drinkers, and like works which show the vileness of the human individual at a level below that of the beasts, cannot equal in horror the picture of degradation presented by such an assembly in the throes of cocaine.

3. Cocainomania and Its Forms

The possibility of the formation of a habit, even to the extent of very large doses of the plant or the alkaloid if they are progressively increased, the obligation of continuing their use, the agreeable sensations which they produce, and finally the physical and moral misery which results from them; such are the evils which are united in cocainomania, as in morphinism and opium-eating. It is remarkable that as opposed to morphia animals cannot become accustomed to cocaine; they even exhibit an increasing sensibility to the drug. The case is, however, on record, of a monkey which became a cocaine-eater through imitation. Perhaps this can be explained by the anthropoid nucleus. The animal searched the pockets and the cupboards of its mistress for cocaine, which it voraciously consumed. The consequences were the same as in man. Leaving this case out of consideration the tolerance of animals towards cocaine shows that this substance has a quite different character from morphia. Its effects on man confirm this opinion from every point of view. Its action on the brain is very much more violent. A single injection into the gums or under the skin may cause serious troubles of the functions of the brain, for instance mental disorders, illusions and melancholia, which appear after one day and frequently last for weeks or months. The prolonged toxicomaniac abuse brings about by gradual development graver symptoms, the manifestations whereof are apparent among those eager coca-eaters of South America, the *coqueros*. Physically and morally they behave like opium–smokers. A cachectic state appears with extreme emaciation accompanied by a gradual change of demeanor. They are old men before they are adult. They are apathetic, useless for all the more serious purposes of life, subject to hallucinations, and solely governed by the one passionate desire for the drug, besides which everything else in life is of inferior value.

The use of cocaine has consequences which are much more marked and typical, although they present the same character. The method of its introduction into the body is of no importance. There is no other substance which has so many different modes of application. It may be injected subcutaneously, drunk as a beverage in the form of coca wine, cocaine wine or champagne, smoked in cigarettes, thrust into the nose with a brush or employed as snuff, rubbed into the gums or the anus. Every method has its followers. It seems that the greatest number prefer the nasal cavity as the place of application.* Out of twenty-three cocainists, twenty-one chose this method. I know several of these personally, among others an oto-rhinolaryngologist and other scientists, etc. The pursuit of science is not enough to prevent folly. As in the case of morphinism there are instances of husbands perverting their wives to the habit, and mothers their children. In one of the latter cases a morphio-cocainist brought her fourteen-year-old son, within three months, to a daily consumption of 4g of cocaine. But much larger quantities of cocaine are consumed.

I am able to sketch the physical and intellectual life of a cocainist who, like many others, came to me in his misery for help. On account of a facial neuralgia he had frequently taken morphia until a dentist plugged cotton-wool soaked in a 15% solution of cocaine into several carious teeth. From that time onward the need for morphia disappeared. Carious teeth served as receptacles for the cocaine tampons, i.e. places from which the cocaine passed into the blood, and that in abundance. At certain times he pressed these cocaine plugs between the teeth. The greater part of the cocaine passed into the stomach with the saliva. This particular method of application had not existed hitherto but likewise had fatal results. It was introduced in ever-increasing quantities—finally over one gram daily. The unfortunate man's own words were as follows: "With regard to the action of cocaine on my personality, I can honestly declare that the past five

---

* The intense action of cocaine when introduced in this way may be explained by the existence of several arterial and venous systems uniting the nasal cavity with the cavities of the cranium and the corresponding lymphatic channels.

years can be counted among the happiest of my life, and I owe this primarily to cocaine. Nothing can refute this plain fact." His letter of twelve pages terminates with these words: "Time is necessary to bring my conception of the world to a point which is founded on the sentence: God is a substance!" The latter phrase impressively shows in an undisguised fashion the whole effect which cocaine exerts on the brain. The individual is so attached to his periods of delight that everything else, even the future, is despised, although the evils which the approaching catastrophe is absolutely certain to bring with it slowly become apparent even to him.

Will-power diminishes, and indecision, lack of a sense of duty, capricious temper, obstinacy, forgetfulness, diffuseness in writing and speech, physical and intellectual instability set in. Conscientiousness is replaced by negligence, truthful people become liars and the lover of society seeks solitude. One of my patients said he had "lost his amiable smile." The yearning for the narcotic stifles the voice of life and humanity.

The destructive action on the cerebral functions becomes more apparent. The frequent insensibility which often alleviates the misery of the morphinist is completely missing. In contradistinction to the morphinist, the cocainist finds it very difficult to hide his present being behind the mask which society, tradition, and good manners maintain. His internal loss of balance becomes apparent without suppression. Like all narcomaniacs, the cocainist displays a myopia as to his fate, a limitation of his field of vision in the future. He lives only in and for the moment of indulgence of his passion. For him, its slave, it is the best part of the present and the future, even when he is consciously shaken by the force of the toxin. Mental weakness, accompanied by irritability, erroneous conclusions, suspicion, bitterness towards his environment, a false interpretation of things, groundless jealousy, etc., bring about in the individual, now suffering from insomnia, illusions of the senses while fully conscious. Hallucinations of vision, hearing, smell and taste, disturbances in the sexual sphere and the general condition master those who are severely affected. In many cocainomaniacs confusional insanity preceded by general mental disorders, vacancy of mind as in delirium tremens, extreme alarm due to false impressions, set in. A cocainist who had snuffed 3.25g cocaine armed himself for protection against imaginary enemies; another in an attack of acute mania jumped overboard into the water; another broke the furniture and crockery to pieces and attacked a friend.

Abnormal sensations in the peripheral nerves cause the patient to believe there are animals under his skin. The result is frequently self-mutilation, and by a false application of subjective impressions, the mutilation of members of his family, in order to remove the foreign substance from the body. A woman injured herself with needles in order to kill the "cocaine bugs." A man who suffered from twinges and pains in the arms and feet thought he was being forcibly electrocuted. He thought he could see electric wires leading to his body. Attacks of fury and convulsions generally terminate the malady. In the case of a morphinist and cocainist who took of the former 2g and of the latter 8g daily, these attacks were similar to epilepsy, with unconsciousness and no recollection of the fit. In other cases, especially those in which the last dose was excessively increased, spasmodic cramps and convulsive fits may be accompanied by opisthotonus, fever and irregular respiration.

Korsakov's psychosis belongs to one group of mental diseases, cocaine paralysis to another. I have frequently observed, for example in the case of the cocainist described above, a gradual increase in the extent of physical disturbances such as paleness, loss of appetite, extreme emaciation, reduction of urinary excretion, weakness of the sexual functions accompanied by augmented erotic desires, palpitation and irregular activity of the heart, color-blindness, diplopia, disturbances of speech such as stuttering, paraphasia and an irresistible impulse to utter the thoughts, etc. Special symptoms can be ascertained in those cocainists who sniff the drug: eczema and swelling of the nose, especially at its tip, formation of ulcers on the nasal septum and sometimes perforation of the same, morbid changes of the muscles, all kinds of disturbances of the sense of smell, and frequently a modification towards mimicry, unmotivated laughing and a fixed stare.

The end is predetermined. Lucky the cocainist who, shrouded in the darkness of mental derangement, is not conscious of his fatal and tragic destiny. A long time before, many of them have a foreboding of the track along which their passion, owing to the paralysis of their willpower, is relentlessly forcing them. In this respect they behave in the same way as the morphinist, with the difference that the devastation in the cerebral functions occasioned by cocaine is more violent and the inner exclusion of the individual from moral and social life takes place more rapidly and coarsely.

The infringements of law committed by cocainists are numerous and various. Illicit traffic in cocaine, smuggling, the illegal supply of cocaine to cocainists and its unlawful acquisition by addicts have given occasion to many punishments. There are also more serious offences: theft, fraud, forgery, burglary, robbery with violence, committed in order to obtain cocaine or money or goods for its purchase. Criminal offences against the person, such as crimes against morality, murder in a state of cocaine intoxication, etc., have also occupied the courts. Punishment nearly always follows. Nevertheless we cannot allow that these patients are in possession of their free will if we admit at the same time that they obeyed a strong internal constraint, that they were incapable of correctly utilizing new impressions, but that on the contrary these new impressions combined with reminiscences of the past have confused them. It is of no importance in this case whether we consider this state as a permanent disturbance of consciousness or as a transitory morbid state of cerebral activity. If in such an individual a pronounced disposition to talk and perform actions of a megalomaniacal character can be ascertained, then his free will must be denied if the offences of which he is accused contradict his real personality and the actual situation in which he committed the crime. That is, of course, if the deed was quite foreign to his true character and could be explained only by the circumstances. If this is not the case, the criminal is responsible for his actions, but should be recommended to the mercy of the judge.

The cocainist, like the morphinist, is nearly always aroused too late from his delightful state of euphory and somnolence to painful reality. One of them whom I disillusioned wrote to me: "The first impression your letter gave me was that of a sentence of death. It seemed to me as if you considered my case hopeless and myself lost without the possibility of salvation." The determined man pulled himself together, diminished the dose of cocaine, drank a great amount of wine, took veronal—but his fate fulfilled itself as I predicted.

These unfortunate beings lead a miserable life whose hours are measured by the imperative necessity for a new dose of the drug, and with each such dose the tragedy of life and of death takes a step further towards the inevitable end.

Many seek refuge in the only remedy applicable, immediate withdrawal of the cocaine. The statements made above as to demorphinization apply also to cocaine. The acute reaction of deprivation gives rise to symptoms which when viewed from outside seem less serious than those of morphia. Fewer groans and lamentations are uttered, and the craving for the cocaine is less violent. But the real suffering due to the deprivation in the cells of the cerebral cortex is nevertheless serious and varied enough to cause the patient to fear a stay in a sanatorium. It is a question of a stay of a year and more, not merely of a few weeks. But a cure must be effected wherever it is possible. In some exceptional cases only general uneasiness, twitching of the limbs, sickness, perspiration at night and respiratory disturbances occur. Generally palpitations and weakness of the heart, with collapse sometimes accompanied by unconsciousness, vomiting and very occasionally diarrhea set in. States of extreme anguish and hallucinations always occur in this terrible condition. A short time after the withdrawal of the drug, a young woman morphio-cocainist suffered from a maniacal delusion of persecution, and from hallucinations of hearing and smell of a most serious kind. She showed on her arm, for instance, "death spots" (injection scars) which she believed had been made in a mysterious fashion. She imagined she could tell by the odor of her toilet requisites that she was persecuted. She thought she was to be forced to commit suicide, she saw her husband sitting on a tree. In short, she expressed during more than a fortnight all those foolish ideas of which a depraved mind is capable. There were certain days in the meantime when her temper was serene and her occupations those of a normal woman. On the entreaty of the patient and her family she was given another dose of 0.2g cocaine in order to facilitate the withdrawal of the last remainder of morphia, and the old condition returned. The patient made obscene proposals, believed herself persecuted, and this state of sexual excitation, during which she accused her husband of unnatural vices, etc., lasted several days. Gradually her condition improved.

During the period of weaning from the drug, psychotherapy may be combined with the general medical treatment. Unfortunately there are no firm scars of recollection and feeling of the experienced pleasurable sensations which led the cocainist to his addiction and finally into the cocaine pool of infamy. A very small percentage of cocainists recover, the rest relapse.

It is difficult to say whether the international efforts to restrict and regulate the traffic and commerce in cocaine will succeed any better than in the case of morphia. For the reasons I have already discussed, I do not think that fundamental changes will take place in the near future. Even if it were attempted to rationalize or suppress its production by force, other sources of supply and methods of distribution would certainly be found. The prevention of all production is absolutely impossible and out of the question, if only because a substance like cocaine which supersedes all other anesthetics cannot—like morphia—be eliminated.

Nor do I think that its substitute, dextro–psicaine, a synthetic cocaine-isomer which is only half as toxic as the cocaine obtained from coca-leaves, will be of any help, since the supposition that this product, like the other cocaine-isomers, is free from euphoric effects has proved erroneous.

During recent years I have seen among men of science frightful symptoms due to the craving for cocaine. Those who believe they can enter the temple of happiness through this gate of pleasure purchase their momentary delights at the cost of body and soul. They speedily pass through the gate of unhappiness into the night of the abyss.

CHAPTER 20

Freud Looks Back:
Biography and Autobiography

From *An Autobiographical Study* by Sigmund Freud.
Translated by James Strachey.

From *The Letters of Sigmund Freud*, edited by Ernst L. Freud.

Freud gives the following account of the discovery of local anesthesia and his own interest in cocaine in An Autobiographical Study (1935): Ed.

In the autumn of 1886 I settled down in Vienna as a physician, and married the girl who had been waiting for me in a distant city for more than four years. I may here go back a little and explain how it was the fault of my fiancée that I was not already famous at that early age. A side interest, though it was a deep one, had led me in 1884 to obtain from Merck some of what was then the little-known alkaloid cocaine and to study its physiological action. While I was in the middle of this work, an opportunity arose for making a journey to visit my fiancée, from whom I had been parted for two years. I hastily wound up my investigation of cocaine and contented myself in my book on the subject with prophesying that further uses for it would soon be found. I suggested, however, to my friend Königstein, the ophthalmologist, that he should investigate the question of how far the anesthetizing properties of cocaine were applicable in diseases of the eye. When I returned from my friends, Carl Koller (now in New York), whom I had also spoken to about cocaine, had made the decisive experiments upon animals' eyes and had demonstrated them at the Ophthalmological Congress at Heidelberg. Koller is therefore rightly regarded as the discoverer of local anesthesia by cocaine, which has become so important in minor surgery; but I bore my fiancée no grudge for her interruption of my work.

In a letter to Fritz Wittels, Freud recorded the discovery of local anesthesia and the subsequent dispute over attribution as follows: Ed.

To FRITZ WITTELS

Semmering, Villa Schüler
August 15, 1924
Dear Mr. Wittels

Today I received the English translation of your book about me and looked into it here and there. This is the reason for my writing.

You know my attitude to this book; it has not become friendlier. I still maintain that someone who knows as little about a person as you do about me is not entitled to write a biography about that person. One waits till the person is dead, when he cannot do anything about it and fortunately no longer cares.

I cannot compare the English edition with the German, for I didn't bring the latter with me (and the same applies to the Nietzsche). You have apparently made use of my corrections. Certain passages strike me as additions, but this may be the result of a faulty memory. Other passages again gave me the opportunity to admire, if not exactly to envy, your facility.

A biographer should at least attempt to be as conscientious as a translator. *Traduttore = traditore,** says the proverb! I realize that the circumstances have made this especially difficult for you, with the result that omissions occur which distort certain facts, lead to outright mistakes, and so on.

For instance, in the cocaine story by which, for reasons unknown to me, you set such great store. The whole analogy with Brücke's eye discovery collapses if one takes into account what you didn't know (but perhaps should have known?)—i.e., that I guessed its usefulness for the eye, but for private reasons (in order to travel) had to drop the experiment and personally charged my friend Königstein to test the drug on the eye. On my return I realized that he had done a bad job, had dropped the project, and that another man, Koller, had become the discoverer.

The reader would also have gained a different impression of my attitude to Koller's discovery had he been told, which indeed you couldn't have known, that Königstein (it was *he,* not I, who so deeply regretted having missed winning these laurels) then claimed to be considered the codiscoverer, and that both Königstein and Koller chose Julius Wagner *and myself* as arbitrators. I think it did us both honor that each of us took the side of the opposing client. Wagner, as Koller's delegate, voted in favor of recognizing Königstein's claim, whereas I was wholeheartedly in favor of awarding the credit to

---

* "Translator = traitor."

Koller alone. I can no longer remember what compromise we decided on.

. . . You will have realized long ago that I am not pleased with the success of your book about me. But there it is, one is a "great man," therefore helpless.

I greet you with the respect due to your powerful position as a biographer and with something of the old sympathy.

Your
Freud

II

CHAPTER 21

"Coca Koller":
Carl Koller's Discovery
of Local Anesthesia

"Carl Koller and Cocaine" by Hortense Koller Becker from *The Psychoanalytic Quarterly* 1963.

Hortense Koller Becker is the daughter of Carl Koller, Freud's colleague and the discoverer of local anesthesia by cocaine. Mrs. Becker's article, written "to straighten the facts about cocaine, Koller and Freud," also provides an important view of the climate of fin-de-siècle Vienna in which Koller and Freud made their landmark studies and discoveries. They worked alongside such medical pioneers as the physiologists Du Bois-Reymond, Brücke and Billroth, the three pillars of the Helmholtz school; the noted embryologist Kölliker; the Nobel Prize-winner, Willem Einthoven, father of the cardiogram, Professors Snellen and Donders, "giants in the fields of optics and physiology" and many others. It was a remarkable time of scientific discovery, revolutionary thought and art, pervasive anti-Semitism and political corruption within the declining Austro-Hungarian Empire.

Although often at odds with Freud's most authoritative biographers, Jones and Bernfeld, Mrs. Becker's account serves as a uniquely relevant footnote to the widely-recounted histories of Freud, Vienna and the period. The previously unpublished letters of Freud to Carl Koller lend a sense of immediacy to the drama of an era that produced, in addition to Freud, Koller and the other "giants" of medicine such major pioneers in science and culture as Viktor Adler, Arnold Schonberg, Adolf Loos, Oskar Kokoschka, Ernst Mach and Ludwig Wittgenstein. Ed.

It was like a red-hot needle in yer eye whilst he was doing it. But he wasn't long about it. Oh no. If he had been long I couldn't ha' beared it. He wasn't a minute more than three quarters of an hour at the outside.[1]

Thus, an old man described his cataract operation to Thomas Hardy and his wife on their visit to Dorsetshire in 1882.

It takes little imagination to picture the situation before the advent of local anesthesia, particularly in ophthalmology. Operations upon the eye were especially difficult, and for them general anesthesia was unsatisfactory. It was not administered as skilfully as it is today; retching and vomiting often followed which might seriously damage the eye, and the patient's conscious cooperation was frequently necessary. A long, delicate operation upon the sensitive eye demanded the greatest fortitude on his part, but the doctor too was under heavy strain, for he had to work with utmost speed on a tiny surface, with sight itself frequently at stake, torn perhaps by irritation or pity according to the patient's behavior which he had to control at the same time.

Local anesthesia in surgery is now so commonplace that it is hard to realize the suffering we have been spared since September 15, 1884, when a young Viennese doctor [had] a brief paper [he had written], barely two sides of a sheet, [read for him] at a medical meeting in Heidelberg, and thus inaugurated the era of local anesthesia. The young man was Dr. Carl Koller, my father, whose long life ended on this side of the Atlantic in 1944. Later, after my mother's death, I found myself confronted with his papers which she had saved, the accumulation of some seventy-five years.

As I plowed my way through papers and pamphlets, letters, photographs, and medals, I began to regret that I had not questioned him more about the background of his discovery and his colleagues. I wondered what his life had been like in that other world, during that great period of scientific flowering which was to grow so rapidly in every direction and to make inevitable the present immensely complex system of specialization. It was a period when it was possible for one man to possess almost fully the medical knowledge of his time.

The bare facts I knew, to be sure, for they came to my attention late in my father's life when he was repeatedly honored. An exceedingly modest man, he despised general publicity as unworthy and unscientific, as indeed did most of his colleagues. It was assumed that their work belonged only in the annals of medicine, forming a small part of that mighty foundation which safeguards our health, lessens pain and fear, and, above all, is part of the sum of pure knowledge. They had an almost holy respect for this search after knowledge, for which not even the most brilliant intuition sufficed, if it was not followed by most painstaking and accurate research. Many of these men were eccentric, arrogant, and self-willed, and might ride roughshod over our modern concepts of "adjustment," "integration," and "social attitude," but in their work they were disciplined to lay down their pride and to see the destruction of their most cherished, long-held theories in the light of their own careful, objective research.

When I was young, being less high-minded than he and rather fond of glory, I well remember my disappointment when, with his usual contempt for publicity, my father refused to be 'profiled' in The New Yorker or have the history of his discovery broadcast on the air. Then why, when he can no longer forbid it, should I break that wished-for silence? That is a long story and the one I hope to tell here.

As I made my way through drawers and closets, reducing long-loved possessions to a list, I thought the questions which had begun to fill my mind had come too late, but by a strange chance they were still to be answered, and one by one the pieces of the puzzle dropped into place. It came about in this way.

I pulled the lid off a large, dog-eared carton and saw it was heaped to the top with neatly tied, brown paper parcels, variously labeled in my father's small, well-formed handwriting, "Vienna 1880–1884," "January 6th, 1885," "Göttingen 1885," "Utrecht 1885–1887," etc. I ran for the scissors and cut the strings that had been tied over seventy-five years before by his skillful surgeon's fingers. There, fresh as the day they were written, on linen paper still strong and white, in cramped, highly individualistic script, appeared many famous names. There were the physiologists, Du Bois-Reymond and Brücke, also Billroth (a devoted friend of Brahms), all three pillars of the Helmholtz school which had such profound effect on the scientific work of that day. There were Kölliker, the noted embryologist, Sigmund Freud as well as his friend and associate, Josef Breuer, and the diminutive Professor Samuel Ritter von Basch, to whom the ill-fated Emperor Maximilian handed his ring minutes before his execution in a wild, foreign land. As young medical students, Gaertner, Freud, Wagner von Jauregg, and my father often watched that ring on the doctor's hand, while he fired their imagination with stories of his Mexican adventures. There were Oskar Hertwig and that kindest of men, the Nobel prize winner, Willem Einthoven, father of the cardiogram. Here were Professors Snellen and Donders, giants in the fields of optics and physiology, along with many others. Here, too, amid medical papers, slipped into the manuscript of my father's first communication at Heidelberg, was a tissue-thin envelope that had held those very grains of cocaine with which he had first experimented and demonstrated its usefulness in surgery.

As I leafed through those hundreds of papers and letters, the student days in old Vienna came alive again, with their *Kneipen* and *Singvereine,* student manifestoes, and expeditions into the lovely countryside. Pages and pages were filled with plans, hopes, disappointments, poetry, and even girls.

How articulate they all were, how much they had to say which, I suppose, would today have found its way over the telephone and vanished forever. My father was fond of the gloomy, romantic poetry of Lenau—*"Zu viele Raben."* ("Too many ravens"), complained Freud—and of inquiries into the riddle of life. *"Du sprichst immer so schwere Sachen"* ("With you everything has to be so deep"), Freud teased him. Of the fanciful humor that made Alice in Wonderland his favorite book and of his mordant sarcasm the letters, of course, tell nothing. After all, there were none of his among them.

My father was born in 1857 in Schüttenhofen which was then in Austria and is now in Czechoslovakia, and he died in New York in 1944. His lifetime encompassed most of the great discoveries of modern medicine: asepsis, anesthesia, vaccines, antibiotics, and, of course, local anesthesia. He used to say that he was born in the Middle Ages, for in Schüttenhofen water was then still drawn from the village well, and the enormous speed-up of communication and technology had not begun. And he lived well into the Atomic Age. I remember when Sir Ernest Rutherford first smashed the atom in 1919—or to put it more scientifically accomplished the first artificial transmutation—how awed I was as he tried to explain to me the significance of this inevitable step in the growth of human knowledge. Before he died the first atom bomb was being constructed at Los Alamos.

My grandfather, Leopold Koller, a business man in Teplitz, moved to Vienna with his family when his young wife died and his only son Carl was a small child. A man who revered knowledge, he was deeply interested in the education of his children, was very just and high-minded, but austere and distant. Having grown up in a period of revolution and social change, he was one of those Jews who made the difficult break from ritual and dietary laws, although he never ceased to regard himself entirely as a Jew. My father therefore had no formal religious education and was haunted as he grew older by the hopelessness of that loss which was expressed in poetry and prose by men like Matthew Arnold and John Stuart Mill. The conflict of science and religion resolved itself for many into a terrible scepticism, and the verses I now found, by a contemporary poet, Carl Thomas, which my father had clipped from a Teplitz newspaper when he was nineteen, reflected this thinking. "What of fame?" asked the poet, "What of glory? What even of knowledge itself? The end and the answer must be nothingness."

From private tutoring, instruction at some point by the Jesuit fathers, whom he ever after deeply admired, and after the *Akademisches Gymnasium,* he started with some uncertainty upon his career in 1875. For a year he studied jurisprudence and then in 1876 finally turned to the study of medicine at the University of Vienna.

The University and its adjunct, the *Allgemeine Krankenhaus,* or General Hospital, where my father later interned, were manned by such noted teachers as Professor Arlt, Brücke, Ludwig, Meinert, Billroth, Mauthner, and many others. Its teaching was profoundly influenced by the great deterministic Helmholtz school of thought (since Brücke as well as Billroth were two of its pillars), which had far-reaching effects on scientific thinking then as well as for a long time to come.

Continuing my search through the carton, I picked up a card covered with the tiny, disciplined writing of another founder of that school, Du Bois-Reymond, in whose laboratory my father worked for a while. And this recalled a letter he wrote in 1936, some fifty years later, in which he tried to explain determinism to me.

He [Du Bois-Reymond] was quite a celebrity of that age. He made famous studies of the electric eels and rays of South America and had been the Rector of Berlin University, and his oration on that occasion, *Ignorabimus,* drawing the limits of human knowledge quite in the line of Kant, was a classic. I believe it is today. He rode the horse of causality, stating among other things that, if it were possible to know the set-up of things and forces, one would be able to foretell the future with mathematical precision. Of late the atomic physicists and especially the "quantum boys" have been assailing causality, claiming that an atom could change its mind and go a way other than which it is headed. Whereas the strict causality law does away with free will, the "quantum boys" have re-established free will, which is in harmony with our own feelings, but not necessarily correct by any means.[2]

And again in 1941 at the age of eighty-four, in an even lighter vein:

You don't need to think that the difference of opinion which came to a head when discussing the causes which make a dog elevate one hind leg when making use of a hydrant or lamp post is something new, and invented by you and me. It represented two great schools of philosophy, that of the Empirics (which is dead and buried) and of the Nativists, which is very much alive, and which latter has as an extravagant outgrowth the race theories of the Nazis. These two schools of philosophy had it out on the grounds of physiological optics. The great Helmholtz led the Empirics and the much less known Hering, the Nativists. There are no Empirics left any more (except you).

Organisms work the way they are constructed without any benefit of experience. Dr. X, although I hate to quote him in this connection, said, "A hospital works the way it is constructed.' With which he meant it would work smoothly if kitchens, pantry, and laundry are in the right place.[3]

So much for the philosophy underlying the scientific work at the University, reduced, of course, to primerlike terms. That University and the associated General Hospital, despite brilliant teachers, in many ways afforded a frustrating experience for lofty-minded young men with any thought of an academic future. Competition was keen, the requirements difficult, and examiners at times merciless and sarcastic, but these might be considered just and proper obstacles. There were worse things than matching knowledge against knowledge: favoritism, corruption, and the necessity for pulling strings and playing politics utterly at odds with the idealism of most of these proud, aspiring young scientists. Beside these, for men like Freud or my father there was anti-Semitism, an evil-smelling vine that twined about the whole social structure of Vienna, choking so many green hopes to death.

Within the University the strength of anti-Semitism was perhaps heightened by a kind of race consciousness and nationalism which was linked to the German learning of the time. Germany was considered the true source of intellectual life. The non-Germanic peoples of Austria were considered less educated, less cultivated, and inferior, and even some of the great professors preached that this learning, developed by German thought, should be disseminated by those of German blood. True, I had but to look at the letters before me to see that, though the obstacles to promotion for a Jew were aggravated and a professorship was almost out of the question, Jewish students might still, as individuals, have close friendships with and receive inspiration from these unusual teachers, as my father did from Billroth, Ludwig, Stricker, and the others. We must not interpret the situation entirely by its fearful but logical conclusion in the blood bath of World War II.

The letters, therefore, were filled with many problems, as was natural in the crucial years when young men must decide their future. Among them was a series from three students who appeared to see a great deal of one another and whose letters about each other and the same happenings formed a tantalizingly incomplete but continuous story. These were Rosanes, Freud, and the brilliant and charming Lustgarten, who was a particularly close friend of Freud as well as of my father, and served as my father's second in a duel with an anti-Semitic colleague of which I now read for the first time.

Two of the letters written by Freud, when he was twenty-four and my father twenty-three, were about an old bugbear that has not changed much in the last seventy-five years—examinations. One of its most trying forms at the University was the oral *rigorosum* which, while considered a preliminary medical examination, could be taken even after studies were completed. The letters were written to my father on successive days and though the first of them sounds high-spirited and gay, it was not necessary to read the second to find out that its writer was ill and exhausted. This the handwriting showed plainly as it grew more and more erratic and difficult to decipher.

Vienna, 23 July, 1880
Dear Friend:

I no longer believe in earthly justice, for I can now obediently announce to you that I did not fail; on the contrary, I managed to pass with considerable distinction (*per minora*).* I don't know the kind of debacle for which the gods are actually sparing me, but this time they visibly held their sheltering hands over me. Before we turn to more interesting matters, listen to me like a good fellow while I tell you how it all happened. I am very happy about it; what is there to

---

* *per minora*—for less important subjects.

delight in, except for what comes one's way undeservedly? Perhaps one might even say that all men are proud only of distinctions they do not deserve. (Addition to the philosophical aphorisms in Stricker's diaries on General Pathology, in instalments.*)

So I sat in travail with the fateful eve of examination approaching (*eref* examination, as they said in olden times†) and noticed that I still had all the material in front of me. So I decided to forget about pharmacology, of which I had learned narcotics, and to repeat this worthy subject quietly after vacation. But on Wednesday afternoon, twenty-four hours before the decision, I thought it over again; the fiendish laughter of Hell yelled in my ears, the clamor in Israel was great, and my best friends sang the dirge, "Tell it not in Askalon. Publish it not in the streets of Gath," which was sung at the death of Saul and Jonathan. So I decided to delve for twelve more hours into the depths of pharmacology; and as this thought oppressed me, I went for a walk for several hours. It took several hours because I met young Zuckerkandl,** one of the most intelligent and pleasant people whom one might meet. I have to be brief. I could, to be sure, run through the little Binz.†† But in pathological anatomy I have studied only the "general" [part] and of internal medicine only the lung and infectious diseases. This was now a very serious matter. This joke might cost me 17 fl 50 and six months, as well as alienating the regard of Lustgarten*** and Schwarz (you notice I don't put you in the same category). After a short collapse I went forth to the battlefield determined to defend my life in every possible way and to keep un-

---

* Salomon Stricker (1834–1898), professor of general and experimental pathology at the University of Vienna. Joking reference to Stricker's lectures on General and Experimental Pathology which appeared at the time in instalments.
† Reference to Jewish holidays which always start on the preceding evening (*eref—eve*).
** It probably was Otto Zuckerkandl (1861–1921), later professor of urology at the University of Vienna, whom Freud calls the young one, in contrast to his older brother, Emil Zuckerkandl (1849–1910), professor of anatomy.
†† Karl Binz (1832–1913), professor of pharmacology at the University of Bonn, Freud refers here to *Grundzüge der Arzneimittellehre* of Binz. First edition 1866, twelfth edition, 1894. Possibly Freud had the sixth edition (1879) in mind.
*** Dr. Sigmund Lustgarten (1857–1911), instructor (Assistant) at the Chemical Institute, later at the Department of Dermatology at the University of Vienna.

restrainedly quiet in pharmacology. The nearness of battle exerted its usual stimulating effect on me. I was lively, bold, and confident. From Sigmund* I got an "Excellent" in no time for a clinical presentation of measles. Now came the Schlemil historicus.† With his usual lack of skill he questioned me on one subject only, brain hemorrhages. We had a lively debate. I could hardly use the most commonplace abstractum without his saying, "This is not correct, this is a phrase," etc. I replied, "I did not speak without thinking." "Think it over again and you will understand it yourself," he said.

[No signature]

Vienna, 24 July, 1880
Dear Friend:

I had intended to burden you with a detailed account, but fatigue and feeling sick have not let this develop further than the torso which I don't want to withhold from you.

I am very sad to omit everything interesting, but I can't do otherwise for early tomorrow morning I am going to the Semmering with my sister Rosa for the last three days of vacation. But I don't want to leave you too long in doubt of my fate.

Total result: "Excellent" in pathological anatomy, general pathology, gastroenterology.

"Satisfactory" in four others. In pharmacology it may be announced that I did not miss a single question, but I could not avoid giving the impression of having learned nothing, as it always took me a long time before I could compose the right answer. With Stricker I would have had another "excellent" had I not described a *Dämpfung*** as "triangular," when it should have been "square." I am as glad as I am tired. Of our friend Stricker I shall report later.

For the present I wish you the smallest number of encounters, the biggest possible number of rendezvous, sheer *Solo Pagat, Ultimo*

---

* Dr. Karl Sigmund, Ritter von Hanor (1810-1883), since 1869 professor of dermatology and syphilology at the University of Vienna.
† Unlucky fellow, apparently Freud's nickname for one of the examiners.
** An area of dullness in percussion.

Valat,* and assure you that it will give me great pleasure to answer further letters of yours after I have recovered my strength.

With warm greetings
Your friend
Sigm. Freud

The pathological laboratory, with the inscription *Indagandis causis et sedibus morborum,* housed two buildings that were to be of the greatest importance in my father's work. One was the chemical laboratory presided over by Professor Ludwig, who had himself been assistant to the renowned Bunsen at Heidelberg, and who more than any other influenced my father's scientific development. The other was Stricker's pathological laboratory, devoted chiefly to animal experimentation. Here along with my father worked his friends, Gaertner, Freud, Spina, and Wagner von Jauregg, who later received the Nobel prize for his treatment of general paresis, in which he induced a fever by inoculating his patient with malaria plasmodium. Here my father studied circulation, respiration, and glandular secretions, employing many different poisons, and it was this work that prepared him for the discovery which is the subject of this text. Here, as he plunged into the search for pure knowledge, he was to have the most satisfying scientific experience of his life.

It was a time, as I have said, before the age of specialization. But in the field of embryology this had already taken place, though the number of embryologists was very small. My father became absorbed in a then much disputed question, the origin of the mesoderm, or middle germ layer, of the chicken embryo. At a certain stage in the development of the embryo, the mesoderm appeared as though out of nowhere and it was a mystery how this came about. At the age of twenty-two, my father did not stumble upon the solution but reasoned it out, and his papers on the subject, published in 1879[4] and 1881, created a stir in the small world of embryology. If one may judge by the letters, the young researcher found himself in the midst of an international correspondence. Not only the great histologist

---

* Winning hands in the old Austrian card game, tarok.

Kölliker, but other men prominent in the field, B. Benecke, Leo Gerlach, Edouard van Beneden of Belgium, and F. M. Balfour of England, to name a few, sent him their work and reviewed their scientific problems with him. He was honored by having his findings incorporated into the impressive *Festschrift* for Kölliker,[5] and they then found a place in the textbook of the Embryology of Man and Mammals by Oskar Hertwig,[6] one of the most highly regarded and authoritative books in the field at the time. Many of the letters were addressed to the *"Hochwohlgeborener Herr Professor"* in ignorance of the age and status of the young scientist. This discovery, although of no significance to the general public, seemed to my father a greater scientific achievement than his discovery of local anesthesia, which had such important effects on the history of medicine and surgery. Perhaps this was the happiest time of his life. He had received recognition in his chosen scientific field, and above all he had been privileged to experience the pure and divine joy that comes when a man finds himself, as Einstein, I believe, somewhere describes it, after much thought upon a new plateau of human knowledge.

It was my father's teacher in ophthalmology at the University, Professor Arlt, who pointed out to his students the need for a local anesthetic in eye surgery. This idea inspired my father, who now wished to go into the field of ophthalmology and hoped, by some important contribution in that field, to win one of the two assistantships in ophthalmology at the University. So he set to work upon this problem.

"Up to 1884," he wrote Dr. Chauncey Leake in 1927, "the only method of local anesthesia known and not very frequently practiced was the Richardson ether spray, which acts by freezing and was used for subcutaneous abscesses and for similar operations of short duration. The immediate cause of my approaching the question of local anesthesia was the unsuitability of general narcosis in eye operations —eye operations were formerly being done without any anesthetic whatever."[7]

And he added in a paper which resulted from Dr. Leake's suggestion: "I therefore began to experiment in local anesthesia of the eye with a view to surgery—performing a great many experiments upon animals. Thus I tried chloral, bromide, and morphine and other substances, but without success and gave up these experiments for the time being. Although these experiments had been unsuccessful they had the good effect that my mind was prepared to grasp the opportunity whenever I should encounter a real anesthetic."[3]

A quantity of photographs slid about among the piles of letters as I probed, and one inscribed to my father, was of a young man with a noble forehead, great intelligent eyes, and an expressive face. This was von Fleischl-Marxow, one of the two assistants of the famed Brücke. This charming man with a fantastically brilliant mind suffered from a disease so painful that it had driven him to morphine addiction. Ironically his terrible agony was a most important link in the chain of events that was later to relieve so much of the world's pain—the use of cocaine as a local anesthetic.

Cocaine is the alkaloid derivative of the coca leaf—which was not separated from the leaf until 1855. The story of coca is very long and old, and there is space to mention only a few of the men who contributed to the knowledge of it. They must be thought of as individual trees in a forest.

The coca plant had been known from early times to the Indians of Peru and, from the time of Pizarro, had found a place in the literature. It was considered by the Incas a living representation of the god, and the fields where it grew were thought to be holy. "Travelers in South America," wrote my father, "on the high plateaus of the Andes in Peru and Bolivia brought back many tales of its mysterious properties." In 1700 the poet Cowley wrote of how the god Varicocha gave man the nourishing leaves which enabled him to endure long hunger and heavy labor.

In 1847 Prescott wrote:

This is a shrub which grows to the height of a man. The leaves when gathered are dried in the sun and being mixed with a little lime, form a preparation for chewing much like the betel nut of the East. With a small supply of this cuca in his pouch and a handful of roasted maize, the Peruvian Indian of our time performs his wearisome journeys day after day without fatigue, or at least without complaint. Even food the most invigorating is less grateful to him than his loved narcotic. Under the

Incas it is said to have been exclusively reserved for the noble orders. If so, the people gained one luxury by the conquest.[9]

Actually the conquistadors feared the power that lay in the control of the divine plant by one group, so that the second Council of Lima, October 18, 1569, three hundred and fifteen years before its present medical use was discovered, issued a decree against its exclusive use by one class. And after that period it was used so generally and extensively that it constituted a most important item of Spain's colonial trade. Indeed, the December 22, 1884 issue of the Medical Record remarks, "At the present day the laborers of the whole of South America continue the use of coca."

About the year 1863 in Paris, a young French chemist, Angelo Mariani, concocted a medicine from an infusion of imported coca leaves in wine, and *vin* Mariani, Mariani elixirs, Mariani lozenges, and Mariani teas soon became enormously popular, especially in America. Mariani became a standard and respected name, users were warned against imitators, and his products were endorsed by the most distinguished doctors such as W. Oliver Moore, de Wecker, and Charles Fauvel, who recommended them for a wide variety of uses. Mariani himself said of his wine, "It nourishes, fortifies, refreshes, aids digestion, strengthens the system, it is unequaled as a tonic, it is a stimulant for the fatigued and overworked body and brain, it prevents malaria, influenza, and wasting diseases." Dr. J. Leonard Corning wrote the following endorsement:

Of Vin Mariani I need hardly speak as the medical profession is already aware of its virtues. Of all the tonic preparations ever introduced to the notice of the profession, this is undoubtedly the most potent for good in the treatment of exhaustive and irritative conditions of the central nervous system.[10]

Though manufactured in France by a Frenchman, this remedy was used most widely in America. I noticed, however, that the Viennese pharmacist, Dr. August Vogl,[11] under whom my father studied and whose library was used by Freud for reference, highly recommended a cocaine tea which he himself brewed, and which he had been using for several years, adding sugar and cream, in preference to Russian tea! About the coca leaf infusions, one apparently could not say enough; but in regard to the chewing of leaves there were occasional warning notes. At the end of Prescott's passage on coca he says, "Yet with the soothing charms of an opiate, this weed so much vaunted by the natives, when used to excess, is said to be attended with all the mischievous effects of habitual intoxication."[12] A footnote adds:

> A traveler (Poeppig, noticed in the Foreign Quarterly Review)[13] expatiates on the malignant effects of the habitual use of the cuca as very similar to those produced on the chewer of opium. Strange that such baneful properties should not be the subject of more frequent comment with other writers! I do not remember to have seen them even adverted to.[14]

Although Gardeke first extracted the active principle of the coca leaf in 1855 and named the alkaloid erythroxylon,[15] its present name came a little later. My father wrote:

> In 1858, the Austrian government sent the frigate *Novarra* on an expedition encircling the globe. Dr. Scherzer, not a medical man, but a trade expert, who was sent on this expedition to study trade opportunities, took a quantity of the leaves and gave them to the great chemist Wöhler, at the University of Göttingen, Germany. Dr. Wöhler had his assistant, Dr. Albert Niemann, extract the active principle. He found this to be an alkaloid and named it cocaine.[16]

Now it had been known from earliest observation that the chewing of coca leaves made the lips and tongue numb (that is to say it numbed the mucous membrane of those parts), and this fact was also observed in the alkaloid cocaine almost as soon as it was separated from the leaf. In 1862 Professor Schroff, in a paper read before the Viennese Medical Society, pointed out that cocaine numbed the tongue, narrowed the peripheral arteries, and widened the pupils by its action via the bloodstream or when applied locally. Nor was he the only one to have experimented upon the eye. These facts were commented upon by Mantegazza in 1859, De Marles in 1862, the Spaniard Moréno y Maiź in 1868, and by many others. In 1879 von Anrep, at the Pharmacological Institute at Würzburg, wrote a comprehensive experimental paper in which he also described the locally numbing effects of cocaine and even the dilation of the pupil upon local application, and he suggested that this drug might some day become of medical importance. "Strangely enough," commented G. F. Schrady in an editorial in the Medical Record of November 8, 1884, "Anrep did not note that the conjunctiva was insensible, or if so did not appreciate the significance of this fact."

In the textbook on pharmacology which my father studied at the University, he had underlined the following passage which appears in the article dealing with the coca plant:

> Local effects: Injection under the skin as well as painting the mucous membrane, for example, the tongue—brings about the loss of feeling and pain. 15 minutes after painting it Anrep was incapable of distinguishing sugar, salt and sour at the treated spot. Even the needle pricks could no longer be felt there, whereas the other unpainted side reacted normally. The loss of sensibility lasted between 25 and 100 minutes.
>
> [The article concludes with] Therapeutic Uses: Up to now cocaine has not found any medical use. But on account of its powerfully stimulating effects on the psyche, respiration, and the heart, and also on account of its anesthetizing effect upon the mucous membrane, it might deserve experimental trial in quite a number of diseases. [Relative to the therapeutic use of the coca leaves:] There have been some experiments but no trustworthy ones over an extended period. They are, however, sold commercially and highly recommended for all possible needs.[17]

Probably the general effects of cocaine were so striking that its numbing of the mucous membrane was disregarded, although this characteristic had been generally observed and was uniform. As a matter of fact, anyone with medical training who had studied the alkaloid and learned that it numbed the mucous membranes of the tongue and lips now had sufficient information to reason out this discovery. It was certainly very strange, with this fact repeatedly noted, with experimentation already performed upon the eye itself, with a result of such importance only a short step away, that this discovery should not have been made by any of the brilliant scientists who experimented with cocaine over a period of twenty-five years. Even my father, his mind prepared by his search for a local anesthetic in surgery several years earlier, was not immediately aware of the significance of this attribute. And it was not until he had the drug in his own possession and had noted its effect upon himself, that the numbing of the mucous membrane of the lips had sufficient impact to distract him from the purpose for which he was directly experimenting. This, as we shall see, was to test its general physiological effects for his friend, Freud.

Yet such is often the course of scientific discovery. To translate Mephistopheles' warning to Faust, which Freud quotes in his autobiography in another connection: "It is vain that you seek scholarly knowledge all about you; for every man learns only what he can."[18]

It was not chance that the man who had been previously searching for a local anesthetic in surgery was the first to realize that the Peruvian herb was his answer. My father wrote: "Just as the fact that sulphuric ether produced sleep and insensibility to pain had been known for a long time before Morton demonstrated successfully that this state could be utilized for the painless performance of operations, so the fact that cocaine locally applied paralyzed the terminations and probably the fibres of the sensitive nerves had been known for twenty-five years before it came into the hands of someone interested in and desirous of producing local anesthesia for the performance of operations."[19]

Although cocaine had been the subject of interested research from the time the crystal erythroxylon was separated from the leaf (Dr. Herman Knapp[20] stated in 1884, "There is an extensive earlier literature on coca and its alkaloids"), it had many ups and downs and was repeatedly abandoned especially in England and continental Europe as of no practical value. Freud later wrote that its neglect there might have arisen from the lack of uniformity and unreliability of its manufacture, and that these might have been responsible for the contradictory and inconclusive experimental results, as well as its scarcity and high price. Whatever the reasons, it had fallen into disrepute and was little spoken of at this particular time. Freud was undoubtedly acquainted with cocaine in a general way, since he probably studied the same textbook as my father, and it will be recalled that in his letter he mentioned that he had studied narcotics. But now his attention was redirected to it, and this time with the keenest interest, by at least two articles. In one, Aschenbrandt[21] described the remarkable effects of cocaine upon Bavarian soldiers during the fall maneuvers, how with its help they were able to endure hunger, strain, fatigue, and heavy burdens. The other, by W. H. Bentley in the *Detroit Therapeutic Gazette* (one of sixteen articles on the subject published there which Freud had read), described the use of cocaine in the treatment of morphinism by withdrawing morphine and substituting cocaine. There existed in the United States quite a literature on the use of cocaine in this way. Freud now began to harbor the hope that it might be possible to relieve the suffering of his friend, Fleischl, with this interesting drug. "The circumstances under which Freud became interested in cocaine," my father recounted, "were the following: It happened at that time that a young physiologist of great prominence and promise, an unusually brilliant and attractive man, was being treated for morphinism by Dr. Josef Breuer, assisted by one of my colleagues, Dr. Sigmund Freud, the neurologist, later founder of the school of psychoanalysis.[22]

"As assistant to the pathologist, von Rokitansky, he [Fleischl] had infected his thumb and in the amputated stump neuromata had developed, so that in consequence of the unbearable pain he had fallen a victim to the morphine habit. Dr. Breuer and Dr. Freud tried to break the morphine habit by substituting cocaine for morphine and in their plan they failed, so that their patient became a cocainist instead of a morphinist, probably the first of these unfortunates in Europe. And many a night have I spent with him watching him dig imaginary insects out of his skin in his sensory hallucinations."[23]

Dr. Breuer was my grandfather's family physician and was deeply admired by my father, who described him as almost Christlike in character and charity, wise, restrained, lofty in spirit, with that rare balance between the inquiring, intuitive mind and thorough, objective appraisal and research. "Well-known among other things," said my father, "for his work on the semicircular canals with the physiologist, Hering." Of course he is better known to the general public for his early work with Freud, which is the first chapter in the story of psychoanalysis.

Freud and my father had known each other for four or more years. They belonged to at least one circle of friends Paneth, Schnabel, Emil Wahler, Lustgarten, Rosanes, and many others, as the letters before me attest. They planned excursions together into the lovely countryside of Vienna and played tarok, an old-fashioned, four-handed card game, at the sidewalk cafés. I even came upon one card written by Freud to my father arranging such a game, but complaining about the unreliability of Lustgarten, who often defaulted at the last minute. The sentiment *En cas de doute, abstiens-toi* ("In case of doubt—don't!"), attributed to St. Augustine, which dashed so many of my impulsive childhood schemes, came from the plaque which hung over Freud's desk at the *Allgemeine Krankenhaus*. Occasionally they wandered down some scientific bypath together, as I see from a letter written to me by my father in 1933:

> Good for you, that you have discovered Graetz's *History of the Jews*. It was a standard work already when I was a very young man. It was in 1883 when a (perhaps the first) electrical exhibition was held in Vienna. It was in the Rotunda on the Prater, the only building that was left standing from the great exhibition of 1873. To profit as much as possible from this electrical exhibition, we, Lustgarten, Freud, and I, studied a textbook on electricity and its appliances, very well and lucidly written by Professor Graetz, Professor of Physics at the University of Munich. This Professor Graetz was or is the son of the Graetz who wrote the history of our people. Since we are talking about electricity and the 1883 exhibition, one of the exhibits did not look like much but it was fraught with History, Science, and Fate. It was a surveyor's compass that looked to be and was a galvanometer of the size of a very small alarm clock. And under it was the legend: "With this *Bussole* Hans Christian Oersted discovered in 1820 that electric current deflects the magnetic needle." In other words he had discovered electromagnetism 63 years before that exhibition, and there were already dynamos and all sorts of instruments and appliances to foreshadow the "electric age" with all its developments from your electric door-buzzer to the telegraph, cable

trolley, and electric R.R. which came from that discovery and that *Bussole*.... When I studied at Göttingen in 1885 and tried to follow the track which the mathematician Gauss had made, I happened to stroll into the P. O. and there was a small marble slab with the inscription: "Here in 1830 the Professors Gauss and Weber plied the first electric telegraph between the physical laboratory and the astronomical observatory." They evidently used Oersted's method, after they had agreed on the meaning of the deflections. Up until this day the cable uses the deflection of the needle when the current is closed for an alphabet. Morse, as you see, did not invent the telegraph, but by inventing the Morse alphabet made the telegraph possible and practical.[24]

Freud, who hoped to marry in the near future and therefore needed more than ever to get on with his career and make a name for himself (little dreaming in those anxious and uncertain days how brilliantly he was to succeed), began to hope that cocaine might be the means toward this end.... [He] now began to harbor the hope that it might be possible to relieve the suffering of his friend, Fleischl, with this interesting drug.... He became more and more interested in its general physiological effects, and the more he tested it the more he became convinced of its miraculous powers. It now seemed possible to him that with its apparent harmlessness, it might not only be used for therapy in morphine addiction but help to increase work output, relieve depressions, contribute to a sense of well-being, and in short become a drug of the greatest usefulness to mankind....

With his enthusiasm, strong personality, and vivid manner of expressing his ideas, Freud made his interest known to his fellow students, among them my father, who was of course, also interested in the treatment of their friend, Fleischl. Freud and my father lived on the same floor of the *Allgemeine Krankenhaus* as interns and saw each other almost daily, they were in the habit of discussing their hopes, disappointments, and work. On more than one occasion Freud asked his assistance in experimenting upon some project, just as he later asked him to undertake experiments with him on the general physiological effects of cocaine. One of these earlier requests, breezily dashed off, has remained among my father's papers.

Freud now set to work to assemble all the known facts about

cocaine in a thorough and colorfully written paper,[25] which had the effect of redirecting the attention of the Viennese doctors to this drug, creating immense general interest and excitement which went far beyond the circle of his friends and fellow students.

This study, twenty-five pages in length, discusses the coca plant, its history, the story of coca leaves in Europe, the action of cocaine on healthy human beings, and its therapeutic uses. The last heading, divided into seven parts, includes the following uses of cocaine: as a stimulant; for digestive disturbances; for the treatment of consumption; as a means of withdrawing alcohol and morphine in cases of addiction; for asthma; as an aphrodisiac; and lastly, its local uses. This may give some idea of the exciting but confusing range of possibilities that had been tried and discarded again and again since the scientific investigation of coca began.

In describing the history of the coca leaf in Europe, Freud wrote: "Since the discovery of cocaine numerous observers have examined the effect of coca on animals and sick and healthy human beings, and some have employed the preparations designated as cocaine, some coca leaves in infusions, and some in the manner in which the Indians use them." Under the heading, Therapeutic Uses, he noted: "To many doctors cocaine seems fated to fill the gap in medical psychiatric treatment, which provides enough means of lowering the heightened excitement of the nerve centers, but knows no means of raising the lowered functioning of these. According to them coca is recommended for the most varying kinds of psychic weaknesses." The paper ends with the following paragraph describing the local uses of coca: "The attribute of cocaine and its salt, the numbing of the skin and mucous membrane with which it comes in contact in concentrated solutions, may lead to other uses especially in *diseases* of the mucous membrane. Following Collin, Charles Fauvel praises cocaine in the treatment of the pharynx, and describes it as *le tenseur par excellence des chordes vocales*. More uses that stem from the anesthetic effect of cocaine might very well develop."

The local numbing [referred to in the final paragraph of *Über Coca*] seemed to suggest to Freud few uses beyond those already observed by von Anrep or mentioned in the textbook of Nothnagel and

Rossbach. A possible usefulness in surgery did not occur to him any more than it had to Mantegazza, Niemann, Wöhler, Schroff, Morena, or any of the other experimenters with cocaine since its separation from the leaf. What seems so obvious today probably escaped him because his goal was so very different; it was one which he was to achieve a long, long time later with tools which he himself would forge.

Immediately after the completion of his paper, Freud left Vienna on a long-anticipated trip to visit his fiancée in Hamburg. Before this, however, his interest in the general physiological effects of cocaine had led him into some experiments in which he had asked for my father's assistance. "We would take the alkaloid internally by mouth and after the proper lapse of time for its getting into the circulation we would conduct experiments on our muscular strength, fatigue, and the like (measured by the dynamometer)," wrote my father.[26]

This is the chain of events which actually placed cocaine in my father's hand and focused his attention on it: Freud's interest in the drug, awakened primarily by the American literature on substituting it for morphine, by which method he hoped to help his suffering friend, Fleischl; the actual purchase of the scarce, expensive product; and the request he made of my father to engage in experiments during the course of which my father was required to take it by mouth. These were the circumstances that prepared the way for his particular discovery, yet cocaine had been handled, taken by mouth, and its effect, even upon the eye, observed for twenty-five years without its usefulness in surgery occurring to anyone. "Upon one occasion," my father said, "another colleague of mine, Dr. Engel, partook of some [cocaine] with me from the point of his penknife and remarked, 'How that numbs the tongue.' I said, 'Yes, that has been noticed by everyone that has eaten it.' And in the moment it flashed upon me that I was carrying in my pocket the local anesthetic for which I had searched some years earlier. I went straight to the laboratory, asked the assistant for a guinea pig for the experiment, made a solution of cocaine from the powder which I carried in my pocketbook, and instilled this into the eye of the animal."[27] The young assistant in Stricker's laboratory, Dr. Gaertner, was the sole witness to my father's discovery and, troubled by the misstatements that in time came to be so often associated with the story, he retold it in a 1919 newspaper of which he was medical editor.

> For the thirty-fifth time the day is approaching on which the discovery was made which brought blessing to mankind and glory to the Viennese school of medicine. The fortunate discoverer, Dr. Carl Koller, is still as active as ever. If I feel obliged to sketch the history of his contribution today, my reason is that already legends have begun to form about the person of the discoverer and the events that took place at the time of the discovery and after, which their subject, living in America, is not able to correct.
> My right to be able to make these corrections in his place stems from the fact that, favored by a lucky chance, I had the good fortune to be the sole witness to the birth of local anesthesia.
> One summer day in 1884, Dr. Koller, at that time a very young man, was engaged in a piece of embryological research. He stepped into Professor Stricker's laboratory, drew a small flask in which there was a trace of white powder from his pocket, and addressed me, Professor Stricker's assistant, in approximately the following words:
> "I hope, indeed I expect, that this powder will anesthetize the eye." "We'll find out about that right away," I replied. A few grains of the substance were thereupon dissolved in a small quantity of distilled water, a large, lively frog was selected from the aquarium and held immobile in a cloth, and now a drop of the solution was trickled into one of the protruding eyes. At intervals of a few seconds the reflex of the cornea was tested by touching the eye with a needle. . . . After about a minute came the great historic moment, I do not hesitate to designate it as such. The frog permitted his cornea to be touched and even injured without a trace of reflex action or attempt to protect himself—whereas the other eye responded with the usual reflex action to the slightest touch. With the greatest, and surely considering its implications, most justifiable excitement the experiment continued. The same tests were performed on a rabbit and a dog with equally good results.
> Now it was necessary to go one step further and to repeat the experiment upon a human being. We trickled the solution under the upraised lids of each other's eyes. Then we put a mirror before us, took a pin in hand, and tried to touch the cornea with its head. Almost simultaneously we could joyously assure ourselves, "I can't feel a thing." We could make a dent in the cornea without the slightest awareness of the touch, let alone any unpleasant sensation or reaction. With that the discovery of local anesthesia was completed. I rejoice that I was the first to congratulate Dr. Koller as a benefactor of mankind.[26]

Although my grandparents lived in comfortable circumstances in Vienna, my father seems to have been estranged from his stepmother at this critical time and was forced to live very poorly indeed on what he was paid as an intern. A few months later there were many warm letters from her as well as from my grandfather, for whom he had the deepest respect and devotion, but at this all-important moment he was painfully poor, indeed so poor that he could not afford to go to the next important scientific meeting which was to be held in Heidelberg. Thus, at his request, it was his friend, Dr. Josef Brettauer of Trieste, who read his paper for him and demonstrated his experiments at the meeting of the Heidelberg Ophthalmological Society on September 15, 1884.[28]

On the eve of the general meeting, Dr. Brettauer appeared before a small group of the staff and some distinguished visitors and gave them, as it were, a preview. With a sort of romantic justice, one of these men was the great Professor Arlt, whose teaching some years before had inspired my father's work. It happened that Dr. Henry D. Noyes of New York, who had been traveling in Europe, also was present. He immediately sent an account of what he had witnessed to the (New York) Medical Record in a letter which was published October 11, 1884. After describing the experiment, Dr. Noyes, who apppeared to have been somewhat surprised at the youth of the doctor who had made such an important discovery, went on to say:

> The application of the muriate of cocaine is a discovery of a very young physician, or he is perhaps not yet a physician but is pursuing his studies in Vienna where he also lives. His name is Dr. Koller. The future which this discovery opens up in ophthalmological surgery and medication is obvious. The momentous value of the discovery seems likely to be in eye practice of more significance than has been the discovery of anesthesia by chloroform or ether in general surgery and medicine.[29]

On October 17, 1884, at the meeting of the *K. K. Gesellschaft der Ärzte* in Vienna, my father was finally able to read his own paper. By this time, however, the news had already spread like wildfire (so great had been the need for this remedy), and experiments were under way all over continental Europe, England, and across the Atlantic, whereever doctors were gathered.

The first paper read at Heidelberg started with the assumption of the general medical knowledge of the properties of cocaine. "It is a well-known fact that the alkaloid cocaine (Erythroxylon coca) makes the mucous membranes of the throat and mouth anesthetic when brought in contact with it—this led me to investigate the action of this agent upon the eye."[30]

In the second paper he mentioned this again and gave a brief history of the observation of this fact:

> From the foregoing it is evident that cocaine has been instilled in the eye in former years, but those phenomena which will be the subject of my present communication have been overlooked. The internal application of cocaine, tried repeatedly, has always been abandoned again. In 1880 Dr. von Anrep published an elaborate experimental paper on cocaine at the end of which he points out that its local anesthetic action may become of importance. . . . Cocaine was brought into the foreground of discussion for us Viennese physicians by the thorough compilation and interesting therapeutic paper of my colleague at the General Hospital, Dr. Sigmund Freud. Starting from the supposition that a substance paralyzing the sensitive terminations of the mucous membrane of the tongue could not greatly differ in its action on the cornea and conjunctiva, I have made a number of experiments in the laboratory of Professor Stricker.[31]

Since I had never known more than the general outline of this discovery nor inquired beyond this, and since my father was the last man to dwell upon his scientific achievements except when he felt an error must be corrected, I was totally unprepared for what I now found in the literature of that time. The enormous excitement leaped like an electric spark across the arc of more than seventy years. The speed with which the news spread seems incredible when we consider the relatively undeveloped stage of communication.

Articles appeared immediately not only in leading medical journals of Europe, England, and America, such as The Lancet, the Medical Record, *Semaine médicale,* etc., but also, day after day, in lay newspapers. Events moved so rapidly and so much experimentation had occurred in the few weeks before the second paper was published that the sale of cocaine was immediately affected. To cite but one instance, from the Medical Record (November 22, 1884, p. 578):

"Dr. Squibb of Kings County said that he had received over 300 letters asking for cocaine immediately after the publication of Dr. Noyes' letter in the Medical Record—the price of the drug was formerly $2.50 per gram (15 gr) but is now about $.50 a grain."

From all over the world letters poured in. Bundles of them lie about me as I write. They asked my father for fuller information, complained about the rise in price, added their own new-found observations, and congratulated him. Some were from the sick and nearly blind, filled with some last, poor ray of hope, some from lay people, some from doctors, and there was one from a cavalry officer, imploring further information so as to save the sight of his favorite horse.

My father was, of course, aware that local anesthesia had more general implications and was not by any means limited to operations on the eye. "I had started from the fact that the drug made the *lips* and *tongue* numb, but I limited myself to the eye, wishing to make a contribution to ophthalmology and also wishing to establish a claim to the much-coveted position of an assistant at one of the large eye clinics. I did, however, directly suggest to my friend, Jellinek [assistant to Schrötter in the laryngological clinic], that he make experiments on the nose, pharynx, and larynx. He reported the results at the same meeting of the *Gesellschaft der Ärzte* (October 17) at which I read my [second] paper."[32]

Jellinek speedily demonstrated the success of operations in these areas. He said: "The experiments I am dealing with here were made after Dr. Koller had told me of his observations in regard to the cornea, and I must offer him my warmest thanks for his help and for leaving the corresponding medical situation (discovery of the usefulness of cocaine in operations on the nose and throat, etc.) to me."[33]

A letter from my father to Dr. W. Oliver Moore, dated November 11, 1884, was subsequently published in the New York Medical Journal in answer to a request for the history of his discovery. After mentioning the fact that the work of Freud had focused his attention on cocaine, it states:

To convince myself of the wonderful effects of the drug upon the system generally, I took a quantity of the alkaloid, placing it on the tongue, and noticed the benumbing influence (this effect was already known to me through books); the idea occurred to me that the influence of cocaine on the terminal nerves of the conjunctiva and cornea should be the same as on the tongue and, if so, would be of the greatest importance, as we had not such a substance that would produce anesthesia without at the same time cauterizing the tissue.

"To Dr. Koller, therefore," adds the Journal, "is due the honor of the discovery and more credit is due him as he arrived at the facts by *reason* and not by accident. . . . Since his announcement of its wonderful anesthetic properties every journal in this and other countries has been filled with enthusiastic accounts of operations not only on the eye but on regions far removed from that organ."[34]

Le Progrès médicale, of November 29, 1884, states: "All medical journals resound at the moment with news of this triumph of healing. It is scarcely two months since Dr. Koller of Vienna published for the first time the happy attribute [of cocaine] as a local anesthetic for the eye—and already publications on the subject are so numerous and the results so uniform that there exists a whole bibliography. . . . As always in such cases one has already taken as reality that which for so long had been only a hope, and one has the thought that cocaine is to be the means of banishing chloroform for operations on the eye."

Dr. Herman Knapp, one of the foremost ophthalmologists in New York, who in his youth had been assistant to the famous, much-loved surgeon, von Graefe, was to become a lifelong friend of my father. He also followed the events of the discovery with intense interest. Already on October 25, 1884 he had published an article in the Medical Record in which he said: "As soon as I read the remarkable communication by Dr. Henry Noyes[35] I procured specimens [of cocaine] from different sources, Dr. E. R. Squibb, Bradley W. Foucar, N. Y., Messrs. Eimer & Amend, N. Y., and looked up many books."

Matters had proceeded with such explosive rapidity—so fast that the sequence of events and even the facts of the discovery had become obscured—that by December Dr. Knapp thought the time had come to summarize them in an orderly account.[36]

"No modern remedy," he wrote, "has been received by the profession with such general enthusiasm, none has been so rapidly popular, and scarcely any one has shown so extensive a field of useful application as cocaine, the local anesthetic recently introduced by Dr. C. Koller of Vienna. Convinced that it will not only continue to prove as valuable as it has hitherto been found, but that its properties will be the subject of numerous scientific researches and clinical observations all over the globe for many years to come, I propose as far as I am able to collect in the following pages what knowledge has thus far been acquired on this highly interesting and important drug. To help the reader in gathering information is, however, not the only object of this paper. I would like it also to act as a stimulus for new investigations. From this standpoint I consider a faithful, unabridged translation of the original paper which Dr. Koller read before the Medical Society of Vienna and published in the *Wiener Medizinischer Wochenschrift,* October 15, 1884, not only as an acknowledgment of a debt of gratitude we all owe to him, but also as an appropriate introduction to the present article."

The translation of my father's paper then follows, and Dr. Knapp continues: "Two weeks before the original of Dr. Koller's paper was published in Vienna, physicians were informed of its substance. Merck's muriate of cocaine being in the N. Y. market, they without delay tried the new anesthetic in every direction, finding for themselves a number of important facts before Dr. Koller's other European publications reached them.

"This occurred in the following way: Dr. Henry D. Noyes of New York, traveling in Europe, sent to the Medical Record a letter published in that journal on October 11, 1884. One of his notes attracted the greatest attention among the oculists of New York and, I dare say, the whole country. It was 'The extraordinary anesthetic power which a two percent solution of muriate of cocaine has upon the cornea and conjunctiva when dropped into the eye.' The cornea and conjunctiva can be touched and rubbed with a probe, a speculum inserted, the conjunctiva grasped with a pair of fixing forceps, and the eye pulled in different directions, without any unpleasant sensations. 'The solution causes no irritation of any kind and its effect disappears in 15 to 30 minutes.' Its remarkable anesthetic property was discovered by a young physician, Dr. Carl Koller, *Secundärarzt* (intern) at the General Hospital of Vienna, only a few weeks before its presentation at the Heidelberg Ophthalmological Congress through Dr. Brettauer. Dr. Koller made a few trials with it. These he had been led to make from his knowledge of the entirely similar effect which it has for some years or more been shown to have over the sensibility of the mucous membrane of the mouth, pharynx, and larynx. The substance makes a clear solution and is found in Merck's catalogue."

The hopes which Freud harboured for cocaine were of such a different nature and so great that when he returned to Vienna to find its use as an anesthetic in surgery the center of medical conversation and excitement, he did not feel at all that he had missed a discovery, but rather that here was more evidence, although only in regard to a side issue, of the potentialities of the drug with which he had become so deeply enamored. Several papers followed his first one, *Über Coca*. Among my father's papers were two of them, inscribed to him by Freud. Across the top of the first one, giving an account of the experiments with the dynamometer in which my father had taken part, Freud had written facetiously, *"Seinem lieben Freunde Coca Koller* [To his dear friend Coca Koller] from Dr. Sigm. Freud." This paper contains the following paragraph: "Last July in Heitler's *Centralblatt für Therapie,* there appeared a study by me of the coca plant and its alkaloid cocaine, which, basically an examination of the information in the literature and my own experiences with it, brought this long-neglected remedy to the attention of the doctors. I may say that the results of this stimulation were unexpectedly quick and complete. While Dr. Königstein undertook at my suggestion to test the pain-deadening and secretion-shrinking effect of cocaine on the *diseased* conditions of the eye, Dr. Carl Koller, my colleague at the hospital, *independently* of my personal suggestion conceived the happy idea of producing a complete anesthetic and analgesia of the cornea and conjunctiva by means of cocaine, *whose anesthetic effect on the sensibility of the mucous membrane had long been known,* [italics added] and further demonstrated the high practical value of

Separatabdruck aus Dr. Wittelshöfer's „Wiener Med. Wochenschrift."
(Nr. 5, 1885.)

Beitrag zur Kenntniss der Cocawirkung.
Von Dr. SIGM. FREUD,
Sekundararzt im k. k. Allgemeinen Krankenhause in Wien.

Im Julihefte des von Dr. Heitler herausgegebenen Centralblattes für Therapie habe ich eine Studie über die Cocapflanze und deren Alkaloid Cocaïn veröffentlicht [1]), welche auf Grund einer Prüfung der in der Literatur enthaltenen Berichte und eigener Erfahrungen dieses lang vernachlässigte Mittel der Aufmerksamkeit der Aerzte empfahl. Ich darf sagen, dass der Erfolg dieser Anregung ein unerwartet rascher und vollkommener war. Während Herr Dr. L. Königstein auf mein Ersuchen es unternahm, die schmerzstillende und sekretioneinschränkende Wirksamkeit des Cocaïns in krankhaften Zuständen des Auges zu prüfen, hat mein Kollege in diesem Krankenhause, Herr Dr. Karl Koller, unabhängig von meiner persönlichen Anregung, den glücklichen Gedanken gefasst, durch das Cocaïn, dessen abstumpfender Einfluss auf die Sensibilität der Schleimhäute seit Langem bekannt ist, [2]) eine vollständige Anästhesie und Analgesie der Cornea und Conjunctiva zu erzeugen, und hat fernerhin den hohen praktischen Werth dieser lokalen Anästhesie durch Thierversuche und Operationen am Menschen erwiesen. In Folge der darauf bezüglichen Mittheilung Koller's an den diesjährigen Kongress der Augenärzte zu Heidelberg ist das Cocaïn als lokales Anästhetikum zur allgemeinen Aufnahme gelangt.

In Fortsetzung meiner Studien über das Cocaïn habe ich nun versucht, die wunderbare Allgemeinwirkung dieses Alkaloids, welche in einer Hebung der Stimmung, der körperlichen und geistigen Leistungsfähigkeit und Ausdauer besteht,

---
[1]) „Ueber Coca", Centralbl. f. d. ges. Therapie, II. Jahrgang, VII. Juli (nicht, wie vielfach fälschlich zitirt wurde: August) 1884.
[2]) Die siebente der von mir für den Gebrauch des Cocaïns aufgestellten Indikationen behandelt die örtliche Anwendung und schliesst mit den Worten: „Anwendungen, die auf der anästhesirenden Eigenschaft des Cocaïns beruhen, dürften sich wohl noch mehrere ergeben."

this local anesthetic through animal experimentations and operations on human beings. As a result of Koller's communication in regard to this in' this year's Congress of Ophthalmologists at Heidelberg, cocaine has been generally taken up as a local anesthetic.[37]

The other paper was a later reprint of Freud's original paper, *Über Coca,* with a few additional remarks. This paper also bears Freud's inscription across the top, *Seinem lieben Freunde Dr. Carl Koller von Dr. S. Freud,* and it is evident here that his hopes were still high that cocaine could yet achieve for mankind those other great services of which he had dreamed. "For the local application of cocaine: This use of cocaine has received universal recognition through its application by Koller to the cornea, through the work of Königstein and numerous others, and assures cocaine a lasting value in medicine. It is to be expected that the internal uses of cocaine will lead to equally happy results, although the present high price is a hindrance to further experiment."[38]

Freud in his *Autobiography* in 1935, forty-one years later, gave the following account of his interest in cocaine: "A side interest, though it was a deep one, had led me in 1884 to obtain from Merck some of what was then the little-known alkaloid cocaine and to study its physiological action. While I was in the middle of this work, an opportunity arose for making a journey to visit my fiancée, from whom I had been parted for two years. I hastily wound up my investigation of cocaine and contented myself in my book on the subject with prophesying that further uses for it would soon be found. I suggested, however, to my friend Königstein, the ophthalmologist, that he should investigate the question of how far the anesthetizing properties of cocaine were applicable in *diseases* of the eye. When I returned from my holiday I found that not he, but another of my friends, Carl Koller (now in New York), whom I had also spoken to about cocaine, had made the decisive experiments upon animals' eyes and had demonstrated them at the Ophthalmological Congress at Heidelberg. *Koller is therefore rightly regarded as the discoverer of local anesthesia by cocaine, which has become so important in minor surgery;* [italics added] but I bore my fiancée no grudge for her interruption of my work."[39]

Time plays strange tricks. In this statement, as always, Freud gives credit for this scientific piece of work where it is due, although, as we know, he had not only spoken to my father about cocaine but had also asked him to engage with him in experimentation with it. There is, however, something in the tone of this paragraph which can be accounted for, not by his feelings at the time of the discovery, when he still expected to reach other even greater results with cocaine, but only by his feelings a few years later, when these hopes were gone and only its value in surgery shone on undiminished. His biographer, Jones, relates that Freud did not "hastily" leave for Hamburg, but that this journey to see his sweetheart, from whom he had been separated for one year, had been planned ever since they had parted. Jones, like Bernfeld, points out what I believe I have demonstrated by the literature of the time, that Freud's real interest, which later led to such brilliant achievements, had nothing to do with local anesthesia in surgery; he did not think of it and time would not have changed this fact.

It is not known what "diseases of the eye" Freud had in mind when he suggested that his friend, Dr. Leopold Königstein, experiment with cocaine. Königstein did so, but no more than the others who had gone before did he grasp the significance of its use as an anesthetic in surgery.

In an article[40] dated October 19, 1934, written to correct various errors in newspaper articles which had appeared in connection with the fiftieth anniversary of the introduction of cocaine as a local anesthetic, my father wrote:

When Dr. Königstein heard that I declared cocaine a perfect anesthetic for eye operations, he said that I was mistaken, and no wonder. He had tried cocaine in various ways, mostly against inflammations, relying on its vasoconstrictor effects. For instance, he tried to cure trachoma and had used alcoholic solutions, so that it would have been impossible to detect any anesthetic effects because they would have been covered by alcoholic irritation. When Dr. Freud came back in the Fall, as he states in his autobiography, he found that not Dr. Königstein, whom he had asked to make experiments on the diseased eye, had found anything of value, but another friend of his, Dr. Carl Koller, to whom he had also spoken about cocaine.

Dr. Königstein regretted very much that he had allowed such an important fact to slip through his fingers, and when I read my paper about cocaine before the *Gesellschaft der Ärzte* October 17, 1884, Dr. Königstein also read a paper from which it appeared that cocaine was an anesthetic, but in which it was not mentioned that I had made the experiments before him. To prevent an unseemly wrangle about priority, Doctors Freud and Julius Wagner von Jauregg made Dr. Königstein insert a letter (*Wiener Medizinische Presse*, Nos. 42 and 43, 1884) to the effect that he conceded the priority of the idea of utilizing the anesthetic properties of cocaine for practical purposes to me. Freud himself has never laid any claim to it . . . .

Two of the letters remain to tell the story of a type of incident all too common in the history of scientific discovery. Deep as was the contempt for the seeking of publicity in the lay world, rightful priorities were something else and were sometimes bitterly contested in the scientific world in which they were claimed. One of these letters was to my father from Freud, who was apparently shocked and astonished by the conduct of his friend:

Dear Friend:

I am aghast at the fact that in K's* published paper there is no mention of your name; and I don't know how to explain it in view of my knowledge of him in other respects; but I hope you will postpone taking any steps until I have talked to him, and that you will, after that, create a situation in which he can retract.

With kind regards
Dr. Sigm. Freud

The other letter was from Königstein, very amicable in tone and assenting to the wording of the withdrawal of his claim to priority, a draft of which was enclosed in Freud's letter. His position was, to say the least, not very strong, since his paper was read at the time of my father's second paper, nearly a month after the first communication at Heidelberg. The relationship between Königstein and my father seems to have been perfectly friendly afterward, for I found later

---

* Leopold Königstein.

notes from Königstein, the first of which complimented him most warmly for his behavior on the occasion of the duel.

Dr. Rossbach, in whose pharmacological laboratory von Anrep had done thorough and original work which was respected and admired by my father, now raised his voice. He had read a review of my father's paper from which he gathered that von Anrep's work had been ignored. My father's answer is given here as a clear, contemporary statement of exactly what he considered his accomplishment to be.

To LEOPOLD KÖNIGSTEIN
Vienna, December 17, 1884
Honored Editor:

I wish to publish the following explanation, after which the "Priority Protest" which appeared in the No. 50, 1884, of your estimable paper, will be found to be groundless.

1) Herr Professor Rossbach makes the reproach, on the evidence of a review he read about my report before the *Wiener Gesellschaft der Ärzte* on October 17, in which he missed the mention of v. Anrep, that I seem to be less concerned with the priority of v. Anrep than with my own.

I have, however, as can be seen from the accompanying reprint of the aforementioned communication, given due credit to the contribution of v. Anrep concerning the knowledge of the anesthetizing effect of cocaine, in the following words: "In the year 1880 Dr. v. Anrep (*Pflügers Archiv. f.d. ges. Phys. 21 Bd.*) published a comprehensive experimental work about cocaine, at the conclusion of which he already pointed out that the local anesthetic effect of cocaine might become of importance."

I must therefore regret very much that Herr Professor Rossbach did not look at the wording of my article (*Wiener Med. Wochenschrift,* 25 Oct. and 1 Nov.).

2) There can be no question of v. Anrep's priority in regard to the anesthetic effect of cocaine on the mucous membrane, since this was already known to the first researcher about cocaine in Europe, Professor Schroff (Cf. *Ztschr. d. K.K. Fes. der Ärzte in Wien,* 1862), as well as to all those that followed. Concerning this there can be no priority claim in favor of v. Anrep as against a later authority. V.

Anrep, to be sure, has made this effect of cocaine the object of a close study.

3) I have never taken credit in regard to the discovery of this useful physiological characteristic of cocaine, although its effect on the cornea was never before attempted. I have only made that step, as Professor Rossbach rightly remarks, to turn well-known or easily deduced effects of cocaine to use in practical medicine, especially in the field of ophthalmology.[41]

As time went on some warning murmurs began to be heard in connection with cocaine, which had been taken up with such enthusiasm since the publication of Über Coca and since its brilliant success in surgery as a local anesthetic. Already in the October 25, 1884 issue of the Medical Record an editorial had stated: "As yet we know little or nothing of its possible poisonous effect in large doses. It is to be hoped that no rashness in experimentation will demonstrate them."

It so happened that in March 1885 in a lecture before the Psychiatric Society, according to Dr. Siegfried Bernfeld,[42] Freud had said, referring to the treatment of morphinists: "I would advise—without hesitation—giving cocaine in subcutaneous injections of 0.03 to 0.05 grms. per dose and not to shrink from an accumulation of doses."

According to Jones and Bernfeld, his biographers, Freud was to reproach himself bitterly for this statement made in the days of hopeful enthusiasm. For as cocaine came more and more into general use, two or three years after the discovery of local anesthesia, it became apparent that cocaine had not been sufficiently tested in respect of some of its other therapeutic uses, and that addiction and even death had occasionally resulted. The praise and credit that had come to Freud for his fine paper and for having reawakened interest in the drug now turned to attack. He was accused of recommending subcutaneous injections without sufficient research and, in addition to the hue and cry about cocaine, was charged with charlatanism and quackery because of his enthusiasm for Charcot's work. It must have been a bitter experience for a sensitive and brilliant man, trained in the tenets of the Helmholtz school, who judged himself by its stern scientific standards, to find himself condemned as reckless and wanting in these very qualities, all the more since his keen desire to help and heal had led to his difficulties. Interestingly, Bernfeld suggests that this was the reason why Freud never again referred to his lecture on subcutaneous injections. He kept no reprint of its publication in his files, and in all the editions of *The Interpretation of Dreams,* as well as in the *Collected Papers* of 1925 and 1948, he gave 1885 (the date of the lecture) instead of 1884 as the date of his cocaine paper. Whatever his unconscious motivation (as suggested by Jones and Bernfeld), if indeed there was any, this was the only date available to anyone using the above works for reference.[43]

Like his friend Freud, who was to fall from the height of his hopes and dreams of establishing himself into years of disappointing struggle, my father was catapulted from the summit of early renown and success into terrible despair. In his case the change came with the utmost rapidity, whereas it was several years before Freud had to acknowledge the withering of his early hopes.

Although my father's name was now on the tongues of doctors all over Europe and America, and the medical publications were full of his discovery, he had in Vienna many enemies as well as friends. He was not only a Jew (in itself a drawback to promotion at the University) but a difficult, tempestuous young man, one who could never be compelled to speak diplomatically even for his own good. His chances of winning the longed-for assistantship in one of the great eye clinics receded further and further while, for all his glory, he stood looking anxiously into the bleak and uncertain future. Then came an incident which very nearly put an end to his young career.

He had served his year of compulsory military training in the Austrian Army in 1876, and I learned from his papers that his rank as a medical officer was first Lieutenant, or *Oberarzt* in the Army Reserve. His sword, rusted in its sheath, was accepted by me as a natural appurtenance to the attic of our brownstone house in New York, and even now the thought of it calls to mind the shelves laden with knicknacks and objects swathed in white covers and the strong odor of camphor. Now as I began to sort through the brown carton, my eye was caught by a bundle labeled "6 January, 1885." This held letters of congratulation that referred to some event which obviously had nothing to do with the discovery of local anesthesia, but I was not yet familiar enough with German script to have anything but a foggy idea of their content. There were some documents of an imposing official appearance and, to my astonishment, a summons to appear before the Vienna police. Following the trail unsuccessfully through yellowed newspapers—here an account of the disastrous Ringtheater fire with its terrible loss of life and lists of victims, there reports of the Dreyfus case, which fascinated my father as it did the Western world, and many, many articles on the discovery of cocaine and the experiments that followed it—I came at last upon the answer in a newspaper article of January 7, 1885 in the *Neues Wiener Abendblatt*.

(Duel) A few days ago in the General Hospital there occurred an altercation that yesterday led to a duel. The following circumstances led to the happening. The sick brought to the institution come to the Admitting Room on stretchers before they are turned over to the doctors who will take care of them, and it is there decided which will be taken at once and which will be examined later. On this particular day there was in charge of the Admitting Room a young doctor, recently much discussed for his scientific achievement, to whom a man with a very seriously injured finger was brought. The young doctor looked at the injured finger and saw that it was constricted too tightly by a rubber bandage so that the circulation was cut off and that there was immediate danger of gangrene. Among the other interns present in the room was a student of Billroth who asked that the patient be designated for Billroth's clinic (some of the patients are immediately assigned to the various clinics from the Admitting Room). The doctor in charge of the Admitting Room made a note of this request and then wanted to loosen the dangerous bandage but the other began to object. Without paying any attention to these objections, the first doctor quickly cut the ring bandage from the finger of the patient. At the same time the second doctor hurled an insult at him that sounded like "Impudent Jew." A resounding box on the ear was the answer to this insult. As a result of this retaliation the second one, insulted by the box on the ear, naturally found himself obligated to send his seconds to his colleague, and the matter finally ended in a sabre duel which took place yesterday. The young doctor who properly did his duty in saving the sick man entrusted to him from imminent danger remained entirely unwounded while the other after a few passes was led away.

The cold official complaint covered several long pages:

The intern in the General Hospital and Lieutenant in the Army Reserve, Dr. Carl Koller, became involved in an altercation on January 4 of the current year with Friedrich Zinner, a doctor and also a Lieutenant in the Army Reserve, during the performance of their duties as Admitting Physicians at the General Hospital. In the course of this altercation there occurred an act of insult first by word and eventually by action.

For this reason Dr. Zinner sent, as his seconds, two doctors, officers of the active Army, to Dr. Koller to notify him of the challenge. The challenge was accepted.

It was agreed to use "Spadones," i.e., honed foils with very thin and light blades. It was further agreed that the fight would go on until one or the other party should be unable to defend himself. There were going to be no bandages and the seconds were not to interfere, i.e., the seconds should not participate in the duel and not fence off certain thrusts as is sometimes customary.

The duel took place on January 6 at the Cavalry Barracks at Josefstadt.

The two defendants had, for the duration of the fight, taken off their coats and were dressed only in their shirts as far as the upper parts of their bodies were concerned. All in all there were three thrusts (or rounds); during the third, Dr. Zinner was wounded on his head and the right upper arm. He was immediately bandaged and taken to the General Hospital.

Then follows a description of the wounds, the head wound being severe.

According to the expert testimony of the medical examiners, the foils used during the duel are able to produce the wounds described if the foils should be used with a considerable expenditure of strength to strike somebody's head and might well result in a deadly wound.

Considering this expert testimony and also considering that Dr. Zinner actually received a severe wound on his head, the foils used during the duel must be considered deadly weapons.

While the defendant Carl Koller refused to answer the questions of the District Attorney, Dr. Friedrich Zinner has described the beginning and the events of the duel as mentioned above. He declares that he felt constrained to make this challenge because otherwise he would have forfeited his officer's rank as *Oberarzt* [Lieutenant] of the Army Reserve.

Behind this duel, which was not the customary affair in which upper-class German students were wont to indulge, lay a long history of anti-Semitism, of small and large humiliations, and age-old hate. The box on the ear delivered by a hotheaded young man seemed to express for his Jewish colleagues their long-suppressed bitterness and resentment. Like a cry of relief, like the release of a long-held breath, letters poured in congratulating my father and rejoicing that one of their number had at last held up his head and answered his attackers like a man. Freud's letter to his fiancée Martha Bernays, while the duel was in progress, expresses some of these feelings.

To MARTHA BERNAYS
Vienna, Thursday, 6 January, 1885
My precious Darling:

In the confusion of the past few days I haven't found a moment's peace to write you. The hospital is in an uproar. You will hear at once what it is all about.

On Sunday Koller was on duty at the Journal, the man who made cocaine so famous and with whom I have recently become more intimate. He had a difference of opinion about some minor technical matter with the man who acts as surgeon for Billroth's clinic, and the latter suddenly called Koller a "Jewish Swine." Now you must try to imagine the kind of atmosphere we live in here, the general bitterness—in short, we would all have reacted just as Koller did: by hitting the man in the face. The man rushed off, denounced Koller to the director, who, however, called him down thoroughly and categorically took Koller's side. This was a great relief to us all. But since they are both reserve officers, he is obliged to challenge Koller to a duel and at this very moment they are fighting with sabers under rather severe conditions. Lustgarten and Bettelheim (the regimental surgeon) are Koller's seconds.

I am too upset to write any more now, but I won't send this letter off until I can tell you the result of the duel. So much could be said about all this.

Your pleasure over the little presents made me very happy; surely Minna wouldn't think that I would confine her to a calendar! The Eliot* is for her, I have reminded them again. As for the money, my little woman, you keep it; Minna has a claim to part of the previous sum; it will be a long time before either of you get more.

Paneth has given me six bottles of very good wine, some of which will go to my family, but some will be drunk by myself and others here in my room. One bottle has gone off today to Koller to fortify him for the fight. I am considering a reckless purchase. For the forty-

---

* Book by George Eliot.

two florins interest from Paneth I am going to buy myself a decent silver watch with a chronograph in the back; it has the value of a scientific instrument, and my old wreck of a thing never keeps proper time. Without a watch I am really not a civilized person. These watches cost forty florins.—I am too impatient to go on writing.

So far my neuralgia injections are working very well; the trouble is I have very few cases. Yesterday I went to see Prof. Weinlechner* and Standhartner,† who gave me permission to use the treatment on all cases of this kind in their department. I hope to learn more soon about the value of the procedure.

I must go now and see if they are back.

All is well, my little woman. Our friend is quite unharmed and his opponent got two deep gashes. We are all delighted, a proud day for us. We are going to give Koller a present as a lasting reminder of his victory.

Farewell, my sweetheart, and write again soon to

Your Sigmund

In the packet of congratulatory letters was one from Freud to my father, written later on the same day.

Vienna, 6 January, 1885

Dear Friend:

I have missed spending the evening with you. After the vehement excitement of the last days I felt the need to unburden my heart to two of the dearest people, Breuer and his wife. You may guess what we were talking about, and what Breuer's comment was. It would give me great pleasure if you would accept my offer to use the intimate term *du* as an external sign of my sincere friendship, sympathy, and willingness to help. I hope that the shadows which seem to threaten your life at present will soon vanish and that you will always be what you have been in these last weeks and days, a benefactor to mankind and the pride of your friends.

Your Sigm. Freud.

---

* Dr. Joseph Weinlechner, professor of surgery at the University.
† Dr. Josef Standhartner, professor at the University of Vienna.

Only from then on did the letters use this intimate *du*—those were indeed formal times. The only other facts I have since been able to unearth are that my father was pardoned (the pardon was among his papers), that he had never had the slightest experience in dueling, and had managed to take just one hasty lesson, and that his seconds were his friends, Dr. Lustgarten and Dr. Bettelheim, the regimental surgeon. No doubt he never wished to recall the anguish of those days. A box on the ear may very well be a reflex action, but a duel in which the object is to injure or be injured is quite another thing. What thoughts must have filled his mind for those forty-eight hours before the duel? How terrible it must have been not only to dread his own maiming or death but the almost equally horrible alternative, to injure another. What a conflict there must have been in the soul of a physician who, if he is worth his salt, dedicates his whole soul to cherish and fight for life, not to destroy it.

The events of the next few months are unknown to me. Perhaps this duel crystallized the difficulties which, because he was a Jew, hampered his career. One thing is certain; during this time it became apparent that any hopes of promotion in the University, of which the hospital was a part, were quite vain. An article written in 1899 gives one a sense of how unfavorable the situation was. It appeared in a small Viennese periodical in answer to an inquiry as to the whereabouts of Dr. Carl Koller and was entitled University Negligence!

"Dr. Koller is at the moment one of the busiest ophthalmologists of New York. After completing his studies he was for some time intern at the clinic of Professor Weinlechner and settled an affair in which he was involved in the course of his service in a manner as praiseworthy as it was gallant—so that Professor Weinlechner commended Dr. Koller in his reference when he left, most warmly, not only as a doctor but as a man. Dr. Koller, whose first love had always been optics and its science, discovered in his private research, as you correctly brought out, the beneficial effects of cocaine, which was of inestimable value in eye surgery. Cocaine made a triumphal tour through the entire world—Koller, however, was not even able to get so much as an assistant's position in Vienna. Along with the lack of protection that you mention, there was a characteristic of Dr. Koller's that also played a part; namely, Dr. Koller was stiff-necked (stubborn), and a stiff neck paired with real strength of character amidst conditions as you described them hardly served as an impetus to the furthering of a career." The article continued to describe how my father's good friend, Dr. Lustgarten, also was forced to leave Vienna because of some difficulties with the director of the General Hospital. "Both Dr. Koller and Dr. Lustgarten rank in New York as the finest examples of the Viennese school. Creditable as it may be for the latter to be so worthily represented abroad, it must nevertheless be deeply deplored that matters at home should be so ordered that two outstanding doctors in succession must be numbered amongst those who do not count in their own fatherland."[44]

There is a feeling in some of the letters that the period of scientific awakening in Vienna is over and that the orange has been squeezed dry. This disenchantment was reflected not only in Freud's letters, but also in those of Lustgarten, Widder, and others.

So the story went—much fine linen paper covered with helpful suggestions, but the alternatives were hard. It was a bitter experience for my father to find that even with a notable achievement to his credit all doors at home were shut in his face and even in foreign lands, the outlook was none too hopeful. His good friend Le Plat, assistant to another lifelong friend, Professor Ernst Fuchs, wrote warning him away from Paris—for the competition was also keen there and feeling was growing against foreign students coming in to usurp the scarce positions which the French considered rightfully theirs.

Ill and in a pitiable state of hopelessness, my father existed through the days until he was pardoned for his participation in the duel. It was at some time during this period that he literally saw the handwriting on the wall and finally resolved to leave Vienna forever. As he was walking moodily through its streets one day he saw scrawled upon the side of a house these jeering words: *'Die Religion ist uns einerlei / In der Rasse liegt die Schweinerei.'** Up to that moment, he later said, he had felt that anti-Semitism was largely a matter of religious belief, and this was something he considered at least within

---

* 'It is not the religious belief that matters to us/ the swinishness lies in the race itself.'

the scope of comprehension and might still be endured. But these words, written by an unknown hand, illuminated like a flash of lightning the nature of the enemy and a hate with which it was impossible to come to terms.

From Teplitz my father went to study at Göttingen and other seats of learning in Germany and France. Meanwhile, from time to time he corresponded with his friend Freud who, if we judge by his letters, tried in every way to encourage and guide him through his illness and uncertainty.

Vienna, 7 July, 1885

Dear Friend:

I am writing to you in the midst of the vexation and misery of a morning in the Admitting Office, and I am full of the disgust which one acquires in this house.* I spoke with Königstein yesterday who told me about a conversation with Mauthner † that was very funny. He asked M whether he might lecture in his department, because M's appointment can be taken for certain. Upon that M: 'I don't dream of turning my clinic into a *Judenschul*.** No assistant of mine should be a Jew. I won't have any Jewish second assistants either. The Jews don't know anything, they don't understand anything, they should leave this altogether alone. If I take a Jewish assistant and say something to him some day when I am in a bad mood, he will up and leave, whereas a Gentile would have seen to it that everything is smoothed out again', etc., etc.

This was naturally said without any reference to you. You may also deduce from this what can be booked as M's tendency to bluster and to his mischievousness—without malice—but you will retain sufficient reasons to form an unfavorable judgment of your own prospects.

That you should come home now does not seem very sensible to me. You get into bad situations too easily in Vienna and you have not anything to come back for. Stay away as long as you can. Even if you

---
* General Hospital.
† Ludwig Mauthner, first, professor at Innsbruck and then chief of ophthalmology at the *Wiener allgemeine Poliklinik*. He was of Jewish descent.
** Derogatory expression for synagogue.

don't accomplish much there, it is still more than you would do here. And when you are ready, go confidently to America. You will be pleased with this advice.

I did not write you because I did not know what to write. I had run out of ideas and there was nothing better to do than to let the world take its course. Now I still don't know why you never gave me news of yourself for, of course, I am here at your service.

My traveling plans are to go from here to Hamburg on September 1st and to Paris on October 1st. Couldn't we meet? There is a slight chance that I might accompany Fleischl to St. Gilgen.

I send you my warmest greetings and wait to hear from you.

                          Your

                              Dr. Sigm. Freud

Vienna, 14 August, 1885
Dear Friend:

What could you possibly wish to do during these months other than to recuperate like everyone else in beautiful country, good air, and to ride, to climb mountains, and to do anything that will help you to get well?

By the middle of September you could really go to the *Naturforscher Versammlung** in Strassburg. In the first place you are sufficiently human to enjoy the attention you will attract, and secondly there may be a market in which someone would buy you. If you cannot find a post quickly you may have to return to Berlin. I don't know of any better place if you don't want to go to America straight away. You know very well that as long as you have not transformed yourself thoroughly you dare not hope to get on better than before in Vienna. They will forgive you your bluntness but not your irritability.

If you stay in Teplitz I hope to meet you on September 1st (details to follow) at the station of Aussig. But you will have to ride with me for several stops if we hope to get anything out of it. . . .

You will be glad to hear that Rosanes† almost certainly has been

---

* International Meeting of Natural Scientists.
† I. Rosanes, Chief Physician of the Erzherzogin Stefanspital, intimate friend of Freud and Koller.

appointed Surgical Director of a new hospital in Neulerchenfeld. We are so surprised that we can scarcely grasp the good news and only fear that in the eight days before the final decision something may interfere.

Time is heavy on my hands, another 16 days, and what miserable times; my thoughts are somewhere else, I feel physically unwell, even pains, and intellectual bankruptcy, this I hope only temporarily. You will have to put up with someone complaining to you. It is too depressing if only you do the complaining. I send you my heartiest greetings and look forward to hearing from you soon.

Your Dr. Sigm. Freud

My father went to that medical meeting in Strassburg, and I believe it was there that he was "bought in the market," as Freud put it, and became assistant at the *Nederlandsche Gasthuis voor Ooglijder* in Utrecht, presided over by the renowned physiologist, Donders, and his equally famous son-in-law, Snellen, the ophthalmologist. There he worked from 1885 until 1887, busy, fruitful years in the field he loved with associates and superiors whom he could respect and admire. Among his close friends was Professor Willem Einthoven, a man whose genius was combined with the most noble, loving spirit. Years later, when my father introduced his old friend from Utrecht to a meeting in this country, he described how Professor Donders had selected young Einthoven for the chair of Physiology in Leyden when he was only twenty-one or twenty-two and not yet through with his medical examinations, and how Einthoven accepted this immense honor, his heart heavy with conscientious doubts.

A few more letters from Freud help to outline the little I know of the years until my father left the Old World for the New.

Paris, 1 January, 1886
Dear Friend:
I was sitting lonely in my room and translated Charcot, and then pondered over the problems of nerve pathology, but now in spite of the late hour I shall drink to your health and to the success of your work. It is now about a year since I first knew that you were some-

body worthwhile. For the great discoveries are always made by great discoverers. But after our last meeting, I had, as you rightly guessed, given you up, such a pitiful impression did you make upon me. Well, I don't understand it and am not giving out that I understand it, but I rejoice wholeheartedly that matters are going well with you. It cannot all be the result of your improved circumstances, there must also be something spontaneous besides, isn't that so? You will have to give me some credit, little use as I was to you (if I could have been of use, you would have heard from me). Wasn't it my advice that you should look around for a position and, with this in mind, of course, visit the *Naturforscher Versammlung?* Concede this small merit to me, just as with cocaine. I can be all the more happy about it then.

Of your discoveries I understand little, but what I do impresses me immensely. Now that Snellen* and Donders† confirm your opinions, my own point of view can be a matter of indifference to you, but I have always given you credit for the ability to "take lots of pains" and being able to start a subject all over again.

The *"travailler sans raisonner"* belongs to me and not Lustgarten. I found it in Voltaire and had my Martha embroider it for me as a wall plaque. This priority I will not concede. As we are in the midst of complaints and reproaches, let me express my irritation that you wanted to take revenge upon Reuss** without including me. Haven't I always shared everything with you loyally? This frivolous tone is best suited to our present situation. I really should prefer not to predict in earnest, since I do not understand anything about your illness. If you are in a traveling mood, why not undertake a short visit to Paris? If anyone at all, Charcot will be able to give you advice. He is an extraordinary man of unbiased ingenuity and rich experience.

You shall only hear from me when you write. I shall be here for

---

* Herman Snellen, Dutch ophthalmologist. Koller was his assistant in Utrecht, 1885–1887.
† Frans Cornelis Donders, Dutch ophthalmologist and physiologist.
** Professor M. von Reuss, Director of the eye clinic of the General Hospital, who permitted Koller to test cocaine upon the diseased eye in the first weeks of the discovery.

another two months: Rue le Goff, Hôtel Brésil. Keep on writing to me without expecting too much. In my soul there slumbers a project —to look up Dr. Metzger in Amsterdam—if he is worth it and will accept me. Do you know anything about him?

If you should sink into low spirits again—I really think you are cyclic—I do believe that your improved mental efficiency as well as your improved situation will protect you from the low miseries of the last two months. But perhaps you have conquered it for a long period. With warmest greetings I thank you for the pleasure you have thought to give me with your letters.

Happy New Year
Your faithful friend
Sigm. Freud

Vienna, 13 October, 1886
Dear Friend:

With the greatest pleasure I see from your letter what a warm interest you take in me, and I conclude further that a gratifying change has taken place in you since I saw you last at the peak of your illness which, now that I am riper in experience, I can with certainty diagnose as neurasthenia.

I hope to hear more of you immediately, not about sufferings overcome but about present efforts and achievements, and for this reason I yield to the temptation of giving you news exclusively about myself. As a bridegroom one is spoiled for a while into assuming that one is interesting and lovable to others. You are right in thinking that Paris meant the beginning of a new existence for me. I found Charcot there, a teacher such as I had always imagined. I learned to observe clinically as much as I am able to and I brought back with me a lot of information. I only committed the folly of not having enough money to last for more than five months.

On the way back from Paris (to pass over a four-week stay in Berlin which I really spent translating Charcot's new lectures) I settled here rather desperately in rented rooms with service while my small fortune dwindled away rapidly. However, it went better with me than I expected. I shall not analyze whether this was due to Breuer's help, or to Charcot's name, or because I was a novelty. In three and a half months I earned 1100 fl. and said to myself that I could marry if matters continued to improve. A set of circumstances then hastened my marriage; the fact that I could not keep my rooms any longer, my call up to Olmütz for a tour of military duty from August 10th to September 10th, certain family matters, etc.—in short I went from my discharge to Wandsbek* and on September 14th was at last granted my long-cherished wish. Then after a short stay on the Baltic I traveled with interruptions to Vienna; arrived here on September 29th and by October 4th we were already able to announce the start of the practice. My little wife, helped by her dowry and wedding presents, has created a charming home which, however, looks too modest for the noble and splendid rooms of Master Schmidt.†

Only one thing is not going at all in accordance with our wishes; namely, my practice. It is a new beginning and a much more difficult one than the first. But perhaps we shall experience something better soon.

You will see from the reprints mailed at the same time that I have remained loyal to brain anatomy and have entered into close relations with the Russian** whom you brought to my attention. I don't work at home, however, and thank you therefore very much for the microtome you mean to send me. If you want to give me something I need urgently, let it be a perimeter,†† since as a clinician I depend more than anything else on the study of hysteria and one cannot publish anything nowadays without a perimeter.

Now in our next letter we shall leave the person of the undersigned to one side and hear what Dr. Koller is doing.

My wife sends her warmest greetings.

Your Sigm. Freud

Vienna, 1 January, 1887
Dear Friend:

After a long wait to see whether your beautiful but silent present would be followed by a letter, I am using New Year's Day to thank

---

* Wandsbek near Hamburg, where Freud's fiancée lived.
† Stadtbaumeister F. V. Schmidt, the architect of the Sühnhaus, built on the site of the burned–down Ringtheater, in which Freud's first flat was located.
** Liverii Osipovich Darkshevich (1858–1925), Russian neurologist with whom Freud was acquainted and whom he met again in Paris. They published a neurohistological paper together.
†† An instrument for measuring the field of vision.

you very much and to tell you how much pleasure the perimeter (just the thing I wanted)* gave me, as well as the charming picture you gave to my little wife. I shall tell you further in short what there is to say about us; namely, very little. Quiet happiness, as far as social life allows, unsatisfactory wretched practice, continued research in brain anatomy and in the clinical study of hysteria, without a trace of help from the higher-ups. Let's hope that I shall come through in both respects, practice and research, without the aid of these higher-ups. You know how matters stand in Vienna. There is nothing but good news to report of our friends. Lustgarten increases in scientific quality and social status—but that he should put on great airs and become more and more blasé is not what I would wish for him; Rosanes is just as distinguished but shows more sense of humor; Schnabel ridicules them both. Breuer's children are growing up charmingly; he himself is as always much harassed, open to every new idea, kind, and high-minded.

Soon you will get a trifle† from me, a lecture I gave to the *Gesellschaft der Ärzte*.** I thank you for your last paper which I naturally did not understand when I tried to read it. However, I am happy to think what clinical schooling and association with men of good will must have made of you. Otherwise, all I know about you is that you are planning to change Utrecht for Paris for the sake of cuisine (?), and I do not think you would overstep your duty if you would follow up your last amiable but altruistic letter with a more subjective one.

Prosit New Year and best wishes from my wife.

Your Dr. Sigm. Freud

In March 1887 there was a fleeting visit to Vienna, and from his friends Lustgarten, Rosanes, Widder, and Freud came notes arranging for a reunion at the latter's house. The next letter in the series was dated six months later and seems to be an answer, and a decided one, to my father's request for advice on a future plan.

---

* Parenthetic phrase written in English in the original.
† *Beobachtungen einer hochgradigen Hemianästhesia bei einem hysterischen Manne.* (Observations of a Pronounced Hemianesthesia in an Hysterical Male.) *Wiener Mediz. Wochenschrift*, XXXVI, 1886.
** Medical Association.

Vienna, 13 September, 1887
Dear Friend:

You were so kind as to ask for my opinion in regard to a new project for your future. I am flattered but I am giving this to you filled with the sense of the difficulty of offering advice on the question where you should set up practice. Brünn seems an unfortunate idea—a sow's nest, snobbish Jews, the leaders of whom troop to Mauthner and will continue to troop there for a long time to come; and an anti-Semitic gentile population; no intellectual life and all the gossip of a proper provincial town; an ophthalmologist, Plenk, who I believe is in charge of a ward at the hospital, and beside him a colleague in your own specialty, R. A. Schmeichler; conditions as unfavorable as possible to be associated with; just as Widder's predecessor Ignatz Kohn told me. Kohn to be sure is no honeytongue to get along with, but you are not either.

The whole idea does not appeal to me at all and does not seem to be worthy of further investigation. In order to succeed you need the many facets of a big city and its opportunities. If you are in a provincial town and could not get on with a handful of people, you might just as well pack up and leave. Better not go there at all. Your name and your capabilities entitle you to live in a big place. Go to Paris or London and don't get discouraged if at the start there is a slack period in your career. You would also succeed in Holland if you stayed there. Believe me, the choice of place is not important unless you chose one like Brünn where every chance of a future is cut off. I don't know if you have any other reason for being dissatisfied. If you want to stay in Holland, marry a Dutch girl. By the way, tomorrow is my wedding anniversary. I have never regretted it. Matters will never be right with you until you have your own wife and home.

My wife is awaiting her accouchement in 3-5 weeks. I send you my warmest greeting and hope to hear from you soon.

Your faithful
Sigm. Freud

Still undecided about his future, my father nevertheless left Holland and spent several months in London. It was not easy to make the final decision to leave the Old World, and the compass needle wavered before it set the course. For a brief moment he toyed with the idea of sailing as a ship's doctor to Borneo, since distant lands, the wilderness, and its animal life had always attracted him. A letter written to me in 1940, when he was eighty-two, shows that even shortly before he sailed he was still uncertain.

It was 1904. We were at Geneva and M and I went swimming every morning at the Île de Rousseau, where the Rhone issues from Lake Geneva. That place was the most beautiful blue-green water in the whole world. Afterward we went to the Rifflehorn above Zermatt where you have the Matterhorn before you so that you can grasp it. Amongst the guests was also Professor Michel, one of the major lights of ophthalmology, one of those not very numerous, upper-class, affected Germans. He walked with an affected hysterical limp.

This was my second meeting with Michel. My first was in 1888 when I was about to go to America. It was in Würzburg, where there was before Hitler one of the best German universities. I called on Kölliker, who was the first anatomist and embryologist of Germany and all over. He was 70 then and just packing up to go *auf die Gemsen Jagd.* He asked me what I was doing and I answered that I was going to America to practice opthalmology. He was very much astonished and said, *"Ich habe geglaubt, dass Sie Professor der Embryologie in Wien sind* [I thought you were Professor of Embryology in Vienna]." Then hearing of my perplexities, he said, *"Gehen Sie nicht nach Amerika, ich werde Ihnen eine Assistent-Stelle beim Michel verschaffen, dann ist Ihre Laufbahn gesichert* [Don't go to America, I will get you an assistantship to Michel, and then your career is assured]." He sent me to Michel's clinic to get acquainted with him. I went and stayed two days and then returned to Kölliker and told him that I did not like Michel. In retrospect I am touched by the kindness and gentleness of that great man. And so I went to London, stayed three or four months, mostly in the company of Eric Nordenson, and then into the wilderness out of which America was just emerging.

In the end, however, it was a friend in England, Dr. Arthur Ewing, who finally persuaded him to choose America, and in May 1888 he set sail for New York on the S. S. Saale, a ship still equipped with sails.

Separated by an ocean that in those days was very wide, and by time and divergent careers, the correspondence between Freud and my father dwindled. Some time in 1895 a sharp exchange of letters took place over a ridiculous, imagined slight to a female relative of Freud to whom my parents had offered help and hospitality. I think the correspondence stopped at this point. In 1926, however, on one of his trips to Europe my father called upon Freud in Vienna but, alas, he was away at the time and those two old colleagues were never to see each other again.

The next years in the new land were very busy ones: marriage, a family, and establishing the practice which became very large and consumed all his energies.

My father learned to love dearly this new land to which he came— the city of New York, that Baghdad-on-the-Subway with its small O. Henryish, daily adventures; the trout streams of Montana and Colorado (he was an expert dry-fly fisherman); the Western mountain ranges with their aquamarine glacial lakes into which, to my astonishment, he loved to plunge; the virgin forests of Maine where we used to summer. "Mt. Katahdin is without exception the most beautiful mountain that I have ever seen," he wrote, "violet in color, sharply defined in the clear Maine air. Did you ever read the description of it by Thoreau?"

Back of the little inn in the wilderness which we reached by buckboard over bumpy corduroy roads flowed a swift, clear stream over sand and yellow pebbles. I can still see my father instructing my brother in mathematics, a shotgun leaning against the window lest some ducks come winging up that Lazy Tom River.

Of course when he came to this country his work was very well known, but after 1884 he wrote little more on the subject of cocaine. Experimentation had proceeded, as I have already shown, with such speed and in so many directions that the sequence of events was lost sight of. My father was not aware of this until about thirty-five years had elapsed, when more and more frequently misstatements began to appear, almost entirely in the lay press and often coupled with the work of his old friend, Sigmund Freud. Though he had no wish to see his name before the public, my father was surprised on such occasions to see it omitted from the mention of his work, or to have that work so often incorrectly described. It was bewildering to him, I think, to have the facts which had been so widely known and documented in a veritable deluge of print when they occurred, misrepresented so often as the years went by. It is for this reason that I am trying to offer the small slice of truth which it is my privilege to possess. Small as that slice is, it is borne in upon me how difficult it is to know the truth and, when it is known, to impart the knowledge of it, so that one must be amazed that so much in the world is correctly known rather than that there are so many mistakes. I hope my father is right in what he taught us, that what is false is out of harmony with things as they are and must at last be discovered. *"Die Sonne kommt doch an den Tag."**

In 1934 in a letter (to which I have previously referred) to his old friend, Dr. Chauncey Leake, who had requested some further information for a meeting in which my father's work was to be honored, my father wrote: "At the time of my first publication there was no doubt, nor could there be any, that this was the first step in local anesthesia, and a flood of publications in the medical and public press of the world at that time shows it clearly and is accessible of proof. Not only had I asked my friend Jellinek to use the anesthetic in the larynx and nose but, in consequence of the first publication, it was quickly taken up by many others in different fields. In surgery it was first successfully tried by Professor Anton Woelfler, at that time assistant to the famous surgeon Billroth, and only subsequently taken up and developed as Infiltration Anesthesia by Schleich. The historical sequence which was quite clear in the beginning was lost sight of and blurred in the great flood of publications that followed; and so it was said in some of them that I had adapted the use of the new anesthetic to its use in ophthalmology, and in others no mention of my name was made at all, etc."

This state of affairs was further underlined by a letter which my father received in 1939 from his old friend and colleague, Dr. Carl Hamburger, in which he speaks with admiration of Dr. August Bier, one of the foremost surgeons of Berlin, who himself had done im-

---

* "Nothing can keep the sun from rising."

portant work with anesthesia and, undaunted by the Nazi anti-Semitic philosophy, had dared to speak out about the scientific contributions of Jewish doctors.

"Bier," said Dr. Hamburger, "occupied himself with medical history and with philosophy and in the beginning of 1938 published a book[45] wherein, speaking of historical errors in general and anesthesia in particular, he remarked:

" 'Let us see how reliable this particular history is. I select as an instructive example the different opinions which exist about it [anesthesia]. To whom does credit belong for the so valuable practical use of local anesthesia in surgery? Listen as follows to the naked truth that anyone can easily verify. A workable local anesthesia has been known only since 1884 (Koller, Heidelberg, 1884). Only after Koller was this discovery used on all other mucous membranes. It was understandable that general surgery also made use of this glorious remedy.' " Then follows a detailed account of the discovery as already related elsewhere in this paper. " 'These are the historic facts. What, however, does the contemporary history of medicine or even general opinion make of these obvious facts? Let them show me one book of the history of medicine in which the service to medicine of Dr. Koller is worthily pointed out in accordance with its importance. In vain one searches for him under his name in *Der Grosse Brockhaus*.

" 'Who of the general public knows anything of the discoverer of local anesthesia, Koller, and his follower (in general surgery), the modest Braun? The former has even among doctors been completely forgotten.'

"It is very important to be able to point out," Dr. Hamburger commented, "that even in the seventh year of the Nazi regime, the foremost surgeon of Germany wrote: 'None other than the (Jewish) Doctor Koller has contributed the immense service of local anesthesia. What followed were only modifications.' "

Silence had settled down over my father's name in Europe, it is true, and for long years he did not notice or pay any attention to the fact. Every now and then, however, it came to men's minds that there was still living in their midst a man who had made an enormous impact on medicine.

He had been voted an honorary member of the American Physiological and Pharmacological Society, the *Gesellschaft der Ärzte* in Vienna, the *Academia Reale Medica di Roma,* Italy, and the Society of Physicians, Budapest, Hungary. At a Congress in Oxford before he sailed to America, my father had met the ophthalmologist, Dr. Lucien Howe, who, among other important accomplishments, founded a research laboratory for ophthalmological work at Harvard in 1926. He had been present at what Mrs. Howe had called "that historic meeting in Vienna." It was due to the efforts of Dr. Howe that the gold medal of the American Ophthalmological Society was created and the first one presented to my father in 1922.

In 1927 a scroll of recognition was presented to him by the International Anesthesia Society. In 1928 the University of Heidelberg, as a result of agitation by doctors and professors such as Ludwig Cohn, Axenfeld, and others who were disturbed by the lack of recognition, and upon the initiative of his old friend, Professor Fabritius, presented to him the Kussmaul medal in commemoration of the discovery which was first announced in that city.

In January 1930 a gold medal of honor, the first of its kind to be given by the New York Academy of Medicine, was presented to him. In 1934 the American Academy of Ophthalmology and Otolaryngology presented him with another gold medal of honor on the occasion of the fiftieth anniversary of his discovery.

Thus, fifty years after his discovery, unsought recognition came in a sort of awakening from all over the world. Letters and telegrams poured in from all sides, and it seemed as though this would finally reestablish the facts in men's minds. A long article which was a tribute to this discovery[46] revealed to me some hitherto unknown facts. It described how my father was allowed to depart from Vienna, having tangled, I gather, with some to me unknown professor or professors at the University. "Shamefacedly one must admit that Koller has been shown the greatest ingratitude. *Er wurde totgeschwiegen.*"*

In November 1934 there appeared a long article, the reprint of a paper by Professor J. Meller (assistant to my father's life-long friend, Ernst Fuchs), in honor of my father's discovery.[47] It was in the shadow of the approaching storm, with his old enemies no doubt enfeebled or dead, that Vienna at last honored his work.

---

* He was done to death by a conspiracy of silence.

In 1934, also, my father wrote to me:

If you look back of the scenes you see more than from in front. I got a letter from Nordenson (Sweden), who Mother says is the best-looking man she ever met, in which he tells me that he asked Wagenmann, the President of The Heidelberg Ophthalmological Society, to publish a *Festschrift* with my *Vorläufige Mitteilung* [preliminary communication]. But Wagenmann, who is a good friend of mine, had to say it was too late now. Nordenson is naïve or he would have known that the Nazis would not like it. But Wagenmann promised and kept his promise to mention the anniversary in his *Eröffnungsrede* [opening speech]. The next best thing Nordenson could do was to ask Arnold Knapp [the son of Herman Knapp, who first translated my father's paper] to reprint the communication in the issue of the Archives of Ophthalmology, which he did as he had no need to fear the Nazis.[48]

Before me lie the letters of Nordenson and Wagenmann and the proceedings of the meeting at Heidelberg—an amazing document. Dr. Wagenmann, who had begun his career at Göttingen under the ophthalmologist, Thomas Leber (another old friend whose letters, too, were here), had indeed mentioned the discovery in an extraordinary paper at an extraordinary time. From a historical point of view I think it is interesting.

The chairman, Professor Wagenmann, opened the fiftieth meeting of the German Ophthalmological Society with a ringing endorsement of Hitler. But under a bower of flowery prose it became apparent that he had had to bow to government pressure and promise that the constitution of the Society would be changed so that any chairman or delegate must be confirmed by the Ministry of the Interior. And he added that the government's recent emphasis on the study of race hygiene and hereditary diseases must give a new direction to the society's scientific research, which in its particular field must concern itself with hereditary blindness and malformations. Then proceeding to recount the history of the Ophthalmological Society studded with glorious scientific names—Helmholtz, Arlt, Leber, von Graefe, Donders, Axenfeld, and many others—he abandoned his political double talk, described the true ideals of the Society, and dedicated the remainder of his paper to honoring the Jewish doctor.

"Our society was the first scientific society dedicated to the therapy of the eye, and the first one in Germany dedicated to one branch of medicine.... Today we must think gratefully of one other scientific feat that took place fifty years ago at the sixteenth meeting of our society here in Heidelberg. At the first session on September 15, 1884, there was announced for the first time Koller's Preliminary Communication on local anesthesia of the eye. The fact, already known, that the alkaloid rendered the mucous membrane of the mouth and throat numb, suggested to Koller, at that time in Vienna, that he should test its effect on the eye.... Koller, through the introduction of cocaine in the field of ophthalmology, became the discoverer of local anesthesia. We can be proud that the very important fact of local anesthesia grew out of ophthalmology, and that it was here in Heidelberg that the first communication, which was to be of the greatest significance to ophthalmology, took place. The ophthalmologists today no longer can conceive what a blessed effect the introduction of cocaine had for doctors as well as patients. Through this, Koller became the benefactor of mankind, and we all have reason to think of him with gratitude and to give expression of our sincere appreciation. Koller became a member of this society in 1888 and has always been true to it."[49]

My father had indeed been privileged to live in an age of medical awakening almost like a renaissance, to be a discoverer, and to build a life in a new land, highly respected and honored. His long life was spent in the busy and demanding practice of ophthalmology; but he never allowed himself to be closed in by the narrow walls of surgery or of specialization, for he still practiced in the old tradition of the whole man.

But I have always felt that in his heart there was a certain sadness, a feeling that in a way he had missed his calling. His was the mind of a research scientist, and his daring intuitive knowledge and thorough education equipped him for such a career. But pure research is well-nigh impossible for a devoted practicing physician; each way of life is a completely absorbing and jealous mistress. I have always thought that he regretted not having used to best advantage those special gifts with which he was endowed.

My father's mind was unusually clear and incisive until the day he died. I cannot think of any subject within the realm of human knowledge that did not interest him: physics, geography, mountain climbing, astronomy (he once went to Europe primarily to see the first planetarium at Jena), polar expeditions, history, and travel. He dreamed of Tibet, Spitzbergen, Tanganyika, and Alaska until the very end of his life, "but where do I get the time from, and eighty in seven weeks?," and so on and on.

His taste in literature was discriminating and elastic. He read constantly on every imaginable subject, poetry and prose, much of it in French, for that language had always attracted him. His humor could be delightful, whimsical, ironic, or sarcastic with a terrible bite as it fastened on its mark. His choice of words was colorful and had the poet's descriptive precision. The work of which he was proudest and which gave him his most undiluted pleasure was not the discovery of local anesthesia in surgery, but his fundamental research, when he was twenty-two, upon the mesoderm of the chick. I think that his outstanding characteristic, the one which is most often spoken of by those who knew him, was his integrity. Sham and pretense were intolerable to him.

In his obituary in the Archives of Ophthalmology, Dr. S. Bloom wrote: "He was not a calm person, nor had he ever any hesitation about expressing criticism of himself or others if he discovered error. Like all scientifically minded people he despised insincerity in medical practice and often jibed at it. To all with whom he came in contact he was a stimulating personality, always speculating about the unknown and unsolved problems in all lines of endeavor. Friends, colleagues, and patients sensed in him a real person, true, reliable, fearless . . . ."[50]

Over my desk hangs his favorite quotation from Ecclesiastes (IX, 11–12) which my father had typed. I think its broad sweep solaced him—for individual sadness is lost here in the common fate of mankind. It is the old man's submission to that fate which the young man had found so terrible.

"I returned and saw under the sun, that the race is not to the swift nor the battle to the strong, neither yet bread to the wise nor yet riches to men of understanding, nor yet favor to men of skill; but time and chance happeneth to them all."

CHAPTER 22

Freud's Studies on Cocaine

"Freud's Studies on Cocaine" by Siegfried Bernfeld reprinted from the *Journal of the American Psychoanalytic Association*, No. 4, Vol. I, October, 1953.

This article is an authoritative history of Freud's involvement with cocaine. Jones drew heavily on Bernfeld's work for his chapter "The Cocaine Episode" in The Life and Work of Sigmund Freud. *His repetition of Bernfeld's original errors, particularly in translation, has proliferated the confusion about some of Freud's writings on cocaine and subjected Freud to unjust criticism about his enthusiasm for the drug.* Ed.
This paper was submitted by Dr. Bernfeld in a rough draft. He had requested that the paper be returned to him for revision but unfortunately his untimely death prevented this. The manuscript was readied for publication by Mrs. Bernice Engle, of the Langley Porter Clinic, and by Mr. Peter Paret. AMERICAN PSYCHOANALYTIC ASSOCIATION

To the history of Freud's hospital years (1882–1885)[1] belongs a chapter on his advocation of cocaine, a "side interest, though a deep one."[2] In his work with cocaine Freud, for the first time, went his own way. His research under Brücke and Meynert, as well as his work in clinical neurology, for all the talent revealed, for all the originality of detail, was basically conservative. The goals, concepts, methods, the questions asked, the answers given—all were completely within the teaching of admired and loved masters, who inspired him and pressed their stamp of approval on his efforts. The cocaine studies, on the other hand, were not sponsored by anyone. The drug, though isolated from the coca leaves in the year 1859–1860, was hardly known. Those scientists that were acquainted with it generally considered it worthless and at the same time dangerous. Rumors of its benefits were believed to be based on superstitions of wretched Peruvian Indians, accepted by gullible travelers.

In these studies Freud crosses—although only by a few steps—the narrowly drawn boundaries of the sanctioned research field to which he had previously limited himself. It must be considered as his first attempt to break out into full independence. He followed this in the next years with several stronger efforts; but it was not until the latter part of the 1890's that he was capable of pursuing his way completely alone against the "compact majority." The studies also constitute his first scientific encounter with the neuroses, those various forms and degrees of the impairment of happiness and capacity to work, that plagued his friends as well as himself.

The cocaine episode is therefore not only of interest to the biographical consideration of Freud, but also bears directly on the development of psychoanalysis. For both reasons it deserves a thorough and detailed presentation, although it rates only a few lines in the history of pharmacology and medicine.

1. Freud's Monograph "On Coca" (1884)

The reader thumbing through the issue of December 12th, 1883 of the *Deutsche Medizinische Wochenschrift* is arrested by some capitalized words ". . . increase of all mental powers . . . increase of the capacity to endure strain . . . suppression of hunger. . . ." These phrases are not part of a patent medicine advertisement but of a sober and cautious report on observations made by a Dr. Theodor Aschenbrandt* on Bavarian soldiers during fall maneuvers of that year: "The Physiological Effect and the Importance of Cocaine."[3]

It was this paper that stimulated Freud "to study the effect of cocaine on himself and other persons."[4] If he possesses any merit in the matter of cocaine, he says, "it was only that I had believed in Aschenbrandt's report."[5] Aschenbrandt observed six cases, of which the first is typical: "On the second day of the march—it was a very hot day—the soldier T. collapsed from exhaustion. I gave him a tablespoonful of water containing twenty drops of cocaine muriaticum (0,5:10). And about five minutes later T. got up by himself, continued the march for several kilometers to the point of destination; in spite of a heavy pack and the summer heat, he was fresh and in good shape on arrival."[6] Aschenbrandt concluded that cocaine had, in fact, the miraculous effects of which several earlier authors had written.

Freud procured from the source which had served Aschenbrandt—Merck in Darmstadt—samples of the "wonder drug,"[7] and on April

---

* Wittels and Sachs have briefly commented on Freud's cocaine studies; Koller has given several presentations of his point of view; Silverman has written a detailed and vivid, but partly erroneous, fictionalized account. Many writers who have dealt with the discovery of local anesthesia have mentioned Freud, most of them following the passage in the *Autobiography*. Some have exaggerated his achievements. As far as I know, a presentation of Freud's writings on cocaine is to be found only in Maier, Brun, and Jelliffe, who have given brief accounts and evaluations of some of his publications on the subject.

30, 1884 he knew from his own experience that Aschenbrandt and the South American Indians were right. "During a slight depression brought on by fatigue, I took for the first time 0.05 gr. cocaine muriaticum, in 1% water solution.... A few minutes later I experienced a sudden exhilaration and a feeling of ease..."[8] He tried coca a dozen times within the next few months. It never failed him. He always felt this same

... exhilaration and lasting euphoria, which in no way differs from the normal euphoria of the healthy person.... You perceive an increase of self-control, possess more vitality and capacity for work.... In other words, you are simply normal; and it is soon difficult to believe that one is under the influence of any drug.... Long-lasting, intensive mental or physical labor is performed without fatigue.... You are able—on demand—to eat well and without disgust, but you have the clear impression that the meal was not required.... This effect of hardening you against work.... is enjoyed without any of the unpleasant aftermaths which accompany exhilaration through alcoholic means. [And this amazing drug was not habit forming.] Absolutely no craving for further use of cocaine appears after the first, or repeated, taking of the drug; rather you feel a certain unmotivated aversion to it.[9]

Freud tried cocaine on many friends, colleagues, and patients. Always he obtained the same spectacular result, although for the same effect some persons needed much stronger doses than he himself, while others—a very few—showed signs of a short-lived intoxication.

Thus the miracle which the Indians had claimed was simply a fact: "This divine weed, satiating the hungry, strengthening the weak, causing him to forget his misfortune...." did exist.[10] Or in more scientific language: "The effect of coca leaves is not restricted to the Indian race.... Cocaine is the real carrier of the coca effect, which can be produced and employed therapeutically in Europe as well as in South America..."

It seemed quite worthwhile to learn all that there was to know about cocaine. Freud plunged into his usual thorough survey of the literature. The Viennese libraries were of little help, but fortunately the *Index Catalogue* of the Surgeon General's Office in Washington, D.C., had recently progressed to its fourth volume. "The entry 'Erythroxylon Coca' can almost be considered as a complete index of the literature." In the private library of the pharmacologist,

Vogl, he could read enough, so he hoped, ".... to assemble everything worth knowing about coca."

The results of his survey were definitely partial to cocaine. Only a few of the reports based on first-hand experience and on experiments were unfavorable. No concrete damage to the subject nor any unfavorable side effects were observed, but some people

.... after taking cocaine feel uncomfortable, confused, without question toxically influenced. The older Schroff, the first (1863) to test the effect of cocaine, seems among others to have belonged to this group. And this accidental, personal disposition bears part of the guilt of the long-lasting setback that had befallen the alkaloid. [In some other cases cocaine had no effect, due mainly to the quality of the preparation used.] The unfavorable results that were reported soon after the introduction of coca to Europe, the doubtful quality, the rareness and the high cost of the drug, explain this setback of coca in Europe, which in my opinion is an undeserved one.[11]

In the *Detroit Medical Gazette* Freud found reports on the use of cocaine in the treatment of morphine addicts. This made cocaine still more interesting to him since it promised help for an admired friend whose addiction was a long-standing worry to Freud. Von Fleischl (1846–1891),* one of the two assistants to Brücke, a brilliant and

---

* Freud, of course, did not give the name of his patient nor any clues to his identification. In *The Interpretation of Dreams* his cocaine patient is not recognizable, though Fleischl is mentioned by name or otherwise clearly characterized in several of the dreams that deal with cocaine and injections. However, there can be no doubt about the identification. First, Koller, in one of his statements, described one of Freud's patients as a brilliant physiologist who had become a morphine addict because of suffering due to an infection contracted in pathological-anatomy research and to the subsequent formation of neuromata. Second, Exner, in a biographical sketch of Fleischl, alludes vaguely to his drug addiction. Later, in his funeral oration, he specifically mentioned Fleischl's cocainism and morphinism. Third, in the academic circles of Vienna Fleischl's addiction was well known and in my own student years there was still a persistent rumor that Freud had been involved in it. A fourth clue occurs—of all places—in the *St. Louis Medical and Surgical Journal,* 1884. At the end of the English abstract of Freud's monograph one reads: "Prof. Fleischl, of Vienna, confirms the fact that muriate of cocaine is invaluable, subcutaneously injected in *morphinism* (0.05—0.15 grm. dissolved in water); a gradual withdrawal of morphine requires a gradual increase of cocaine, but a sudden abstinence from morphine requires a subcutaneous injection of 0.1 grm. of cocaine. *Inebriate asylums can be entirely dispensed with;* in 10 days a radical cure can be effected by an injection of 0.1 grm. of cocaine 3 times a day. It is evident that there is a direct antagonism between morphine and cocaine."

amiable individual, an inspiring speaker and teacher, as well as a distinguished physiologist, had, at twenty-five while conducting research in pathological anatomy, contracted an infection. An amputation of the right thumb saved him from death. But the continued growth of neuromata required one operation after another. His life became an unending torture of pain and of slowly approaching death, yet his mutilated and aching hand performed experimental work of technical perfection. His sleepless nights he used for studying physics and mathematics. When, with his growing skill, science became an ineffective drug, he took up the study of Sanskrit—and the use of morphine. By the spring of 1884 the second of those withdrawal treatments became necessary, which for the rest of his life had to be periodically repeated. To this suffering friend Freud now recommended an experiment with cocaine. Fleischl's family physician, Breuer,* who was always interested in a new therapeutic approach, seems to have agreed to this suggestion. Thus Fleischl became the first case on the European continent of a morphine addiction cure by coca.

I had occasion [wrote Freud] to observe a sudden withdrawal of morphine together with the use of cocaine on a man who had suffered the most severe abstinence symptoms during an earlier cure. This time his condition was bearable; specifically, depression and nausea were lacking while the cocaine effect persisted.... The patient remained out of bed and quite fit; during the first days he used three decigrams of cocaine muriaticum at a time. After ten days he could do without the medicine.[12]

Thus in the summer of 1884 cocaine seemed to be a very promising, harmless drug, with many possible uses. A forceful invigorant—much stronger than coffee and without the alterations produced by alcohol—it restored in slight depressions optimal health and well-being. It was also a powerful weapon against the needs for food and sleep "which otherwise appear demandingly at certain times of the day, and now are practically obliterated through coca."[13] At the same

---

* Breuer's participation in the treatment is mentioned in one of Koller's statements. It is not possible that Breuer took that part in the treatment attributed to him by Silverman. It seems more likely that Fleischl's withdrawal treatment occurred in Obersteiner's Sanitarium, and under Obersteiner's supervision. However, Breuer, as Fleischl's family physician, had probably been consulted.

time as an "antidote" against morphine, it was worth defending against a few skeptics who had brought it into disrepute. In order to make his and cocaine's case stronger, Freud began to investigate the systemic effects of cocaine with the dynamometer.

Already on the first occasion when he had taken cocaine orally, Freud had observed some numbness of the tongue. Others before him had encountered this anesthetizing property of cocaine, and to Freud this seemed to be a further and very important item on the credit side of coca. He interested his friend Dr. Leopold Königstein —six years his elder and, since 1881, Privatdozent for Ophthalmology—in the study of the uses that could be made of the vascular-constrictive and pain-relieving power of cocaine in the treatment of eye diseases.

At this point the opportunity arose for Freud to visit his fiancée, Martha Bernays, who was living at Wandsbek near Hamburg, and whom he had not seen for over a year. He arranged his notes into a comprehensive monograph, which was concluded on June 18, and sent it to Dr. Heitler for his *Centralblatt*. He discontinued his dynamometer work, left Königstein alone with his experiments, to which he referred in the concluding remark of his paper, and in September 1884 traveled north.

Heitler published the paper *"Über Coca"* in the July 1884 issue of the *Centralblatt*. In it Freud tells the story of the first acquaintance of the conquerors and explorers with the South American coca-leaf chewers and how in 1859 Dr. Scherzer, from the Austrian exploration frigate Novara, brought coca leaves from Peru to America, which were then sent to Nieman, the assistant of Woehler. Nieman succeeded for the first time in isolating an alkaloid, "cocaine," that soon was recognized as the effective agent in the coca leaves, mainly through the animal experiments of Schroff, Sr. Freud then relates how in Germany and Austria, from these early 60's on, sporadic attention was paid to cocaine; how a somewhat greater list of studies was forthcoming in France, while in England only late and very briefly (1874–1876) interest was shown in the new drug. He reports the varied scattered experiences with it and the results of his own observations. A few tentative remarks on his theory of the effects of cocaine are interspersed:

The impression is given as if in such doses the cocaine sensation is produced not so much through direct stimulation, as through the abolition of depressing elements of well-being [*Gemeingefühl*]. It is perhaps permitted to assume that the euphoria of health and well-being is nothing more than the normal state of the healthy brain surface that "knows nothing" of its own organs.[14]

Freud strongly recommends coca for further investigation. According to his own observations it might prove useful:

(a) as a stimulant "in those functional states which we now cover by the name, neurasthenia";
(b) in the treatment of indigestion;
(c) in the withdrawal of morphine.

He mentions as points (d) and (e) its use in a great variety of ailments, for instance, in the treatment of asthma, and (f) as an aphrodisiac. He ends this list and the paper with the paragraph (g):

Local Application of Coca: The property of cocaine and its salines, when applied in concentrated solution, to anesthetize skin and membranous tissues, suggests their possible future use especially in cases of membrane infections. According to Collin, Ch. Fauvel praises cocaine in the treatment of diseases of the pharynx, and describes the drug as "le tenseur des cordes vocales." Some additional uses of cocaine, based on its anesthetic property, will probably be developed in the future.[15]

This monograph is written in Freud's best style. The animated simplicity, the precise and distinctive choice of words—all are present here, in what he would call a "felicitous combination," which is lacking in his brain-anatomical and clinical writings of the same period. To this is added a unique quality which he did not achieve or attempt again in his later writings, a subtle, one might say tender, protective attitude toward his subject, cocaine, evident in the occasional use of slightly unusual words. For instance, instead of a dosage of cocaine, he speaks of a "gift" of cocaine (*Gabe*), or he mentions "the most gorgeous excitement" that animals feel as the effect of an experimental cocaine injection; or he says that "much slander about coca" originates with a certain author. Though an objective report, this paper was charged by such indirect means with a very persuasive undercurrent; and its artistic quality was not the least reason why *"Über Coca"* attracted a great deal of attention during 1884 and 1885. It was generally appraised as the best study of the topic to date. Its few more recent readers, Maier,[16] Brun,[17] and Jelliffe,[18] thought it still very much worth while.

2. Koller's Discovery of Local Anesthesia Through Cocaine (1884)

Freud's monograph was not only generally well received, but immediately on publication had an unexpected and far-reaching side effect—the introduction of local anesthesia into surgery.

At that time, Koller, an acquaintance of Freud, a year and a half younger than he, worked in the General Hospital as an assistant physician in the Ophthalmic Division. In Stricker's Institute for Pathological Anatomy he had taken part in investigations of the mesoderm in the chicken embryo; later he had joined Spina, Gärtner, and Freud in animal experiments concerning the effect of poison on circulatory and glandular functions. His main interests, however, lay in ophthalmology. In his student years when his teacher von Arlt explained to him the "unsuitability of general narcotics, even the great danger of their application in eye operations,"[19] Koller had become deeply interested in the task of finding a local anesthetic for eye surgery. He "began a series of experiments using chloral bromide, morphine, and other substances, but achieved no success and gave up for the time being." However, as he put it almost fifty years later: "I was prepared to grasp the opportunity whenever I should encounter a real local anesthetic." The opportunity presented itself

.... in the summer of 1884 when Freud, who had become interested in the physiologic systemic effects of cocaine, asked me to undertake with him a series of experiments in that direction. So Freud and I used to take the alkaloid internally by mouth and after the lapse of a proper time for its getting into the circulation, we would conduct experiments on our muscular strength, fatigue (measured by the dynamometer) and the like.[20]

In the course of these experiments Koller noticed—as had so many before him—that cocaine when taken by mouth causes the tongue to turn numb. "When I realized that I had in my possession the local anesthetic which I had been previously striving for I went at once to Stricker's laboratory" to test this idea. The exact date when this happened is not known. However, it follows clearly from Koller's own statements that only after the dynamometer experiments were discontinued—when Freud had left for Hamburg, and after his paper on cocaine had been published, and Koller had heard of the ophthalmologist Königstein's experiments—did he, late in August, 1884, realize that cocaine was what he had searched for so long. The discovery came at a very opportune time since he aspired to a position as assistant in the eye department of the University. Nothing could better further his plan than a valuable publication. Gärtner, who calls himself "the only eye witness of the birth of local anesthetics," writes:

One summer day in 1884.... Dr. Carl Koller ran into Professor Stricker's laboratory, pulled a small bottle, containing a trace of white powder, from his pocket and addressed me, as Stricker's assistant, with a speech, the essence of which was: "I hope, indeed expect, that this powder will make the eye insensitive to pain."

"We'll find out about that right away," I replied. A few particles of the substance were dissolved in a small amount of distilled water, a frog was taken out of the frog-container and immobilized by being wrapped in a cloth; then we trickled a drop of the solution on one of his bulging eyes. The reflexes of the cornea were tested in intervals of a few seconds. Nothing unusual happened for about a minute. Then occurred the great, historic moment. The frog allowed his cornea to be touched; he also bore injury of the cornea without a trace of reflex-action or defense. When the drug-treated eye was scratched or pricked he stared at us calmly as if he were quite unconcerned, while the other eye responded with accustomed excitation to the slightest touch. The experiment was continued under the great excitement that the occasion certainly justified. Identical tests were performed on a rabbit and a dog; the results were equally favorable.

One more step had now to be taken; a repetition of the tests on human beings. And that was done. We trickled the solution under each other's lifted eyelids. Then we placed a mirror before us, took pins, and with the head tried to touch the cornea. Almost simultaneously we were able to state jubilantly: "I can't feel anything." We could depress a spot in the cornea without the slightest percept of touch, not to speak of producing unpleasant sensations or reflexes.

With this the discovery of local anesthesia was completed. I am happy to have been the first to acclaim Dr. Koller as a benefactor of mankind. The experiments required no more than one hour.[21]

In great haste Koller wrote a brief preliminary note, dated "in the beginning of September 1884" and since he himself could not afford the trip, had it read by Dr. Brettauer of Trieste—accompanied by impressive demonstrations—at the convention of the German ophthalmologists in Heidelberg on September 15. "The effect was electrical."[22] Within a few weeks numerous cases of successful application of the new discovery were reported all over the world. A month later, on October 17, Koller read a definite and thorough presentation before the Physicians' Society of Vienna. This paper appeared in the Vienna Medical Journal the following week. In the first paragraph Koller remarks: "To us Viennese physicians cocaine has been prominently brought to notice by the thorough compilation and the interesting therapeutic paper of my colleague at the General Hospital, Dr. Sigmund Freud."[23]

Freud returned from Northern Germany in October and found Koller well on the way to world fame; while Königstein was haphazardly trying out cocaine in the treatment of trachoma, iritis and other affections of the eye, and he himself had been relegated to a footnote.

Freud's feelings we cannot know, but we may safely assume that he was disappointed and angry, at least with himself. He hoped to become more than a mediocre physician. He wished to make important contributions to the progress of science. He was striving for recognition from his admired masters, and for higher status in his profession. It was not quite enough to discover and understand what was new to himself; he had to present the experts with real discoveries to justify their attention. But in such matters his own wishes and disappointments did not count. Before each of his publications he searched the literature thoroughly, and whenever he noticed that someone else had been quicker than he, he simply and clearly conceded the fact. Actually he felt himself to be in the possession of such a wealth of new ideas that he had no need to be stingy. When he was forced to give up one or the other ". . . . a fourth and fifth always appear to my prophetic spirit, which thereby becomes frightened like Macbeth before the ghosts of the English kings: 'Will the line stretch out till crack of doom?' "[24] He therefore admitted at once that Koller and not he "had the felicitous thought of producing anesthesia and analgesia of the cornea and the conjunctiva through cocaine,"* and thus not only publicly acknowledged Koller's technical priority, but plainly credited him with the thought and the deed. This discovery he had missed. He knew it; he acknowledged it, and took up his cocaine studies at the point where they had been interrupted by the trip to Hamburg.

Freud, who expected from his friends the same conscientious and generous, or if you like, fatalistic attitude toward priority, found himself forced to insist on it with Königstein. Königstein, so it seems, was really hurt by Koller's discovery. He was a skillful eye surgeon with some research experience in the anatomy and physiology of the eye, but mainly interested in therapy. He was always a doctor first; kind, firm, a little conceited, conscientious and charitable to his patients; he was the man who should have thought of local anesthesia. Less addicted than Freud to the unconditional recognition of facts, his first reaction was to declare Koller in error; his next, to deny Koller's priority. On October 17, when Koller read his paper to the Vienna Physicians' Society, Königstein got up during the discussion and announced that his experiments had shown the usefulness of cocaine in the treatment of certain eye afflictions and in local anesthesia.[25] He did not even mention Koller. Yet from detailed reports[26] of the discussion it is clear that he had been leisurely experimenting with cocaine in the treatment of those diseases in which the vasoconstricting qualities of the drug promised results; and that not before September 15, the date on which Koller's discovery was acclaimed at the Congress in Heidelberg, had he actually begun to try it as a local anesthetic in some animal experiments and on patients in Scholz' Fourth Division in the General Hospital where Freud was then a resident physician. Only a few days before October 15, almost a month later, did Königstein perform a painless enucleation of the eye of a dog—advised by Freud on the technique of the anesthetization. He may, in fact, have thought of such a use for cocaine before, or independently of, Koller; but hazily—just in passing. He did not firmly grasp this idea, and in science as Charcot used to say: "Il faut épouser les idées." Only under strong pressure by Freud, who was

---

* Letter to Dr. Knoepfmacher.

assisted by Wagner-Jauregg, did Königstein, in the publication of his discussion remarks, insert in the last paragraph a reference to Koller, obviously with reluctance, but clear enough to leave Koller as the uncontested discoverer.[27]

Thus the discovery of local anesthesia was not, due to Freud's insistence, followed by an ugly and childish fight—"a rare and model case in the history of pharmacology."[28]

Some subtle and hardly noticed in-fighting did, however, occur between Koller and Freud. In his acknowledgment to Freud, Koller made the bibliographical error of quoting the monograph "Ueber Coca" as published in August 1884. Freud was quick to correct this mistake. He may have felt that the interval between the publication of his paper (July) and Koller's preliminary note announcing the discovery of local anesthesia (beginning of September) was shortened so much that it created the false impression of simultaneity rather than cause and effect. At that time he had not yet developed a scientific theory of parapraxis, but as an alert and sensitive writer he must have felt that some vagueness in Koller's text, together with this error in the footnote, was not the frank, spontaneous, and correct recognition of his own merits in the matter to which he thought himself entitled.* As it turned out Freud's intuition was well founded. Many years later Koller did in fact, in several publications and in (unpublished) memoranda, insist emphatically that in no way had he been influenced by Freud's publication, which, as he said in one place, came out a year after his own discovery.

Wittels, in his biography of Freud, which appeared in 1924, assumes that Freud was greatly troubled by this loss of priority and that he brooded for a long time over the painful question of how it could have happened to him.[29] Commenting on this view Freud wrote to Wittels: "I knew very well how it happened to me. The study of Coca was an allotrion which I was eager to conclude."[30] Twenty-five years before, Freud had expressed himself similarly, though without the Greek word "allotrion," which Gymnasium teachers used with a punitive connotation for everything that detracted from the serious

---

* The neurologist Obersteiner who was very impressed by Freud's work on cocaine seemed to have shared Freud's feelings. He, too, stressed the July date in the introduction to his paper on cocaine.

fulfillment of duty, in favor of a hobby or of mischief. In *The Interpretation of Dreams* (1900) he had explained his failure in these words: "I was not thorough enough."[31]

Scientific achievement as the result of intense and all-excluding concentration on one limited subject used to be one of Freud's favorite topics of discourse,[32] and Koller's case served him as a telling point: Here was a man who had concentrated all his efforts on the one ambition of finding an anesthetic for eye surgery. In contrast, scores of ideas and projects, various emotional and mental interests tempted Freud's attention most of the time, and considerably threatened him in his younger years. Laziness, lack of will power, lack of thoroughness, were his recurrent self-reproaches. By self-discipline he ever so often imposed on himself the duty "to concentrate." He was proud whenever he achieved this restful state—only to feel soon again indomitably distracted by an "allotrion" and disobedient to his self-tyranny.

His pleasure at the achievement of concentration in Meynert's laboratory in 1883 reverberates in his *Autobiography*. When he then, early in 1884, found himself engrossed in the cocaine allotrion, which a few months later he suddenly deserted for his fiancée, one can well understand that he accepted Koller's priority with the feeling that he alone was to blame and had not deserved better.

Yet, there is no indication that Freud would have invented local anesthesia even if he had devoted himself to the study of cocaine with thoroughness and concentration. Freud's thoughts were not on surgery. By vocation a brain anatomist, *faute de mieux* a neurologist, and very reluctantly a physician, he wanted to make the best of his situation. Since he had to be a physician, he wanted to be "a good doctor," one who relieves pain and restores the patient to normal well-being. He did not wish to be the dreaded surgeon, who cuts and hurts cruelly—although for the good of the patient. This attitude of the helpful doctor is well illustrated in a recollection of Freud's:

> One day I was standing in the courtyard of the General Hospital with a group of colleagues .... when another interne passed us, showing the signs of intense pain. I said to him: "I think I can help you," and we all went to my room where I applied a few drops of a medicine which made the pain disappear instantly. I explained to my friends that this drug was

the extract of a South American plant, the coca, which seemed to have powerful qualities for relieving pain and about which I was preparing a publication.[33]

Considering the local anesthetic properties of cocaine, he vaguely saw some probable use for it in the cure of diseases and in the relief of aching mucous membranes. But it did not occur to him to think of it as a possible aid in surgery.

What drew Freud's attention to eye diseases is not known. Shortly after Koller's discovery Freud's father had to undergo a glaucoma operation on one eye. For the son it was a deep satisfaction that his father could enjoy the benefit of cocaine anesthesia. In Freud's presence, Koller administered the cocaine and Königstein performed the operation. Koller made the remark "that on this occasion all the three persons who had been responsible for the introduction of cocaine had been brought together."[34]

Is it not possible that several months before this operation Freud's father had already complained about his eye, and that the worry about his father's health stimulated Freud to think more of eye diseases than of afflictions of other mucous membranes? If that were so it would be quite probable that Freud—whose mind anyhow was not likely to think of surgery—had one more good reason to suppress any thought of operations on the eye. Blindness, loss of an eye, injury to the eyes—all these thoughts touch on anxiety-generating areas of childhood conflicts, especially in connection with the father.

3. Cocaine and Neurasthenia (1885)

The more experiences with cocaine Freud accumulated, the more evident it became to him that the subjective effects of the drug—ranging from euphoria to uneasiness and toxicity—differ vastly in different persons. Freud wished to find a method by which the physiological effects—increased strength and endurance—could be measured and expressed in objective language; from such a "testing method I expected that a real uniformity of the effect of cocaine would be divulged to me."[35] Already before his trip to Hamburg he had tried the dynamometer for this purpose. Some time after his return, at the latest in the beginning of November 1884, he resumed these efforts "of characterizing the coca effect through the behavior of measurable variables."[36] In the investigation, which he carried on through December of that year, he measured the arm-muscle strength by the dynamometer and the reaction time with Exner's neuroamoebimeter. He found that 0.05 to 0.10 gram of cocaine considerably increased the strength of the arm muscles; that this effect at its maximum coincides with the period of euphoria, and that after a slight decrease it persists for several hours. The increase is much greater if cocaine "operates during bad health or reduced motor force."[37] Under cocaine the reaction time is shorter and more uniform though in a less marked degree. This result confirmed his view that the effect of cocaine is "not a direct action on, for instance, the motor-nerve substance or the muscles, but an indirect one, brought about by the creation of an improved over-all state of well-being."

The short paper "Contribution to the Knowledge of the Effect of Cocaine" is the only experimental study that Freud ever published. Although his basic idea is sound and he had a clear concept of what the experimental method could and should do toward the solution of the problem, the experiments were poorly and haphazardly designed, and reported without sufficient precision. Freud had undertaken "repeatedly," as he says, dynamometer readings and reaction-time experiments on himself.*

I realize that such experiments on oneself possess the dubious feature of demanding in the same manner double credibility in the person undertaking them. But for external reasons I had to do it, since none of the individuals at my disposal showed such a regular reaction to cocaine. However, the results of the investigation were also confirmed through my testing of other persons—mainly colleagues.

He added two protocols of the dynamometer experiments and two of the neuroamoebimeter measurements. These protocols, which do not even clearly state the unit (pounds vs. kilograms), could serve as impressive illustrations but not as experimental evidence; they only possess the validity of a preliminary test of the apparatus and of the

---

* Dr. Herzig assisted him in the handling of the neuroamoebimeter.

formulation of the problem. They clearly encouraged a research program. Yet there is no indication that Freud felt the need or even the inclination for an experimental investigation on a proper statistical basis.

Even in this paper, he proved himself to be a remarkable observer. In spite of his poor experimental technique he discovered a fact of basic importance unknown at that time, namely the existence of two independent variables in the curve of muscular strength: "First, that the figures of the motor force of a muscle group indicate regular, moderate variations during the day. Second, that these figures achieve quite different absolute values on different days," depending on the general status of health and well-being. Although the paper carries the title and purpose of a contribution on the effect of coca, Freud was so interested in the side results that he emphasized them rather than the findings on cocaine. But he did not follow them up, apparently because, as he says: "After I had completed these observations, my attention was drawn to a preliminary communication of Dr. M. Buch, which deals with the daily variations of motor force." Thus this short paper that in its first lines concedes priority to Koller ends with a second such admission to Buch—surely a rare case in scientific journals.

The avalanche of publications on cocaine in medical journals, in the newspapers and magazines, which began in October 1884, and continued for several years, was concerned with local anesthesia—this decisive step in man's fight against the horrors of surgery. Koller, not Freud, had guided the investigation in this direction; yet even in the new context Freud's name was mentioned not too infrequently. Though he may have been annoyed by those papers that skipped his work completely, still he was praised in others as the rediscoverer of cocaine. He was asked to give his opinion on the value of Parke's cocaine preparation as compared with that of Merck.[38] An English translation of the main part of *"Über Coca"* appeared in December 1884. His monograph with amendments and supplements was published as a book, *Über Coca,* early in 1885.[39] His experiences and his subsequent recommendations in the treatment of morphine addiction were confirmed by Wallé, Richter, Smidt, Ranke, and others. Freud valued most the confirmation by Heinrich Obersteiner, who enjoyed high repute as a careful student of brain anatomy and neuropathology —he was chief of the newly founded Neurological Institute at the University—and had large facilities for observing morphinists in the private sanitarium which he owned in the hills near Vienna.

Prof. H. Obersteiner [says Freud in reviewing this phase] has, at the Congress in Copenhagen in 1885 reported on the effectiveness of cocaine in morphine withdrawal. However, he made little impression. Only the pamphlets of the chemical company, E. Merck, in Darmstadt, and an extravagant, high-flown paper of Wallé brought the new use of cocaine to the general attention of physicians.[40]

There was one violently objecting voice, that of Erlenmeyer who

... on the basis of a series of experiments ... denied cocaine any usefulness in morphine withdrawal cures, and declared it to be a dangerous drug because of its effect on the vascular innervation. But Erlenmeyer's results rest nevertheless on an obvious error in experimentation, which was immediately uncovered by Obersteiner, Smidt, and Ranke, among others. Instead of following my suggestion and dispensing effective doses (several decigrams) per os, Erlenmeyer had given minimal amounts by subcutaneous injection, and thus attained a fleeting toxic effect from such an—over long duration—ineffective dispensation. For their part, the authors who refuted him announced a full confirmation of my original statement.[41]

Early in 1885 this discussion which Freud's recommendation of the cocaine treatment had initiated was well under way. But its concern was only with one of the benefits that Freud had expected from cocaine. The small though spectacular group of morphinists was not foremost in his mind. He thought more and more of the great masses of functional neurological cases and the neurasthenics. In this spirit he volunteered to present to the Psychiatric Association on March 5, 1885, a paper on the effects of cocaine applied internally. The lecture, published on August 7, 1885[42] summarizes the results of his two preceding publications, and makes new observations. Again he stresses the great individual differences in the subjective effects of cocaine, stating more emphatically than before that only few persons experience, as he does, pure euphoria without alterations. He then concentrates on the psychiatric applications. First, in morphine withdrawal the case of Fleischl is referred to, with the noteworthy addition: "A cocaine addiction did not take place; on the contrary, a growing distaste against the taking of cocaine was unmistakable," which one may assume is due to observations since the spring of 1884. He mentions several other cases under his observation and unrestrictedly recommends cocaine therapy, though "I do know that in some withdrawal cures cocaine did not seem to be helpful, and I expect that differences of individual reactions to the alkaloid will also appear."[43]

But more important to him were the general applications: "Psychiatry is rich in methods that reduce overstimulated nerve action; it is, however, poor in those that can raise the lowered performance." It is therefore desirable to consider the use of cocaine "in such forms of illness, which we interpret as weaknesses and depressions of the nervous system without organic lesion." In fact, some reports had already appeared on its benefits in hysteria, hypochondriacal and depressed states. "On the whole, however, its usefulness in psychiatric practice is still to be proven, and deserves careful testing as soon as the presently unaffordable drug has become cheaper." Although this is the main thought, he must satisfy himself with hope since the literature offered few observations. The use he had made of cocaine on himself and on his few friends did not carry the weight of therapeutic work with patients.

However, his trust in cocaine as a potentially powerful help in the treatment of neurasthenia was based on what that drug had been able to do for him. The reports in the literature impressed him as being quite believable because the drug had brought him—over a period of several months—unfailing relief.

The years between 1882–1885, which he spent in the General Hospital, were not easy ones for Freud. He had given up a scientific career which he had successfully pursued for six years. He was preparing himself for a profession in which the bulk of work bore little attraction for him. He knew that many of his patients would expect relief from their sufferings, but that there was hardly a way known by which to secure such relief. His emotional life was frustrated: separated from his fiancée for years, he felt compelled by his rigorous standards to be satisfied with writing to her and receiving an answer from her every day.

In this situation tiredness, depressed moods, anxieties, worries, indigestion recurred, lowering his happiness and working efficiency. Some of these states might have seemed to him to be somehow connected with his frustrating and disquieting situation; others must have remained mysterious in their origin, their nature, degree, and content. But they all weakened his power of concentration and self-mastery. George Miller Beard's term, neurasthenia, which was then coming rapidly into use in Europe, seemed to explain these symptoms and conditions as the result of tiredness and weakness of a strained and overexcited nervous system. Freud was never afflicted with such weakness for long, but suffered rather recurring spells of several hours' or several days' duration—yet they were too long and too frequent for his impatience. Cocaine, to him, was an almost perfect remedy against his neurasthenic spells. Unlike alcohol it did not produce an artificial, unnatural state of short-lived elation, decreasing at the same time the capacity and inclination to work, and paralyzing the power of self-control. Cocaine simply jacked up mood and capacities from their depressed state to a more normal level. Freud not only enjoyed this effect, but extracted from it an important and highly optimistic insight; the depression of the normal status of well-being must be due to the interference of an unknown central agent, which can be removed chemically. This thought explained to Freud the effect of cocaine on himself, and justified a generalization of his own experience, without the need for cumbersome statistics. In cocaine he thought he possessed not a palliative but a remedy for weakness, depression, and lack of self-control. So equipped he would not stand completely helpless before the complaints of his future patients. It did not occur to him that anyone might use his restored capacities and his increased endurance for purposes other than work.

In retrospect it seems quite significant that in this, his first independent therapeutic effort, Freud was already occupied with the instincts, those periodically appearing imperative needs that originate in our body; that he was searching for means to tame their disturbing power; that already he had conceived—though somewhat vaguely—of a central agent interfering with normal well-being and of its restoration by the removal of the disturber; and that his therapeutic goal was already then what it always remained: the repairing of a depressed ability to be happy, self-controlled, and efficient.

Freud's hopes did not materialize, although the price of cocaine, with a rapidly increasing demand in surgery and dentistry, soon fell to a reasonable level. No one followed his recommendation to investigate the psychiatric potentialities of cocaine. Even Freud himself did not continue experimentation with cocaine as a medicine against neurasthenia. There were strong external reasons why Freud discontinued his active interest: his departure from the General Hospital and his journey to Paris shortly after the publication of his third study on cocaine. When he returned, the beginning of his private practice, his marriage, and the aftermath of Paris—which soon involved him in a conflict with the leaders of the Vienna Medical School—absorbed his time. Yet, there was a more important reason— the entirely unforeseen appearance of a new feature in psychopathology—cocaine addiction.

4. "Craving For and Fear Of Cocaine" (1887)

Fleischl, the "first morphine addict in Europe to be cured by cocaine"[44] in turn became the first cocaine addict in Europe, or one of the first. Koller wrote that he himself had seen Fleischl in terrible physical and mental condition, shaken by paranoid hallucinations that were teeming with white snakes.* Exactly when this event—which was tragic for both Fleischl and Freud—occurred is not known. I think it to be most likely that Fleischl's addiction had begun in the winter of 1884–1885.†

Be that as it may, the alarming appearance of cocaine addiction was reported by Erlenmeyer[45] in May 1886. Already on January 11, Obersteiner had remarked in a paper on intoxication-psychoses "that since the use of cocaine had become frequent, several cases of

---

* Information contained in Dr. M. Silverman's files.
† The related section in Dr. Ernest Jones' Freud biography, which is partially based on unpublished Freud letters, and which through the author's kindness I have had the opportunity of reading in manuscript, bears out this guess.

chronic intoxication had occurred; their status is similar to the alcohol delirium and especially characterized by the hallucination of tiny animals crawling over the patient's skin."[46] During the early months of 1886 a few other such observations were published. But Erlenmeyer was the first who sounded the alarm and described cocaine not only as a dangerous and poisonous drug, but as one that most certainly produced addiction. He condemned its use in the language of a crusader. "Today I count myself fortunate for not having found it possible to recommend the use of cocaine in the morphine withdrawal cure,"[47] he wrote with an eye on Freud. Others followed his lead and within a few months cocaine became a dread word in the German medical literature.

Three years after Freud had first tasted cocaine, the rediscoverer of cocaine found himself the object of more or less veiled accusations of having added to morphine and alcohol "the third scourge of humanity, cocaine."[48] That he who had tried to help, now was accused of having unleashed evil; that the very drug which he had hoped would create his reputation as a healer of neurasthenia now threw doubt on his judgment and loaded him with a reputation of recklessness, contributed to make Freud's first year in practice "the least successful and darkest year"[49] of his life. As he said: "I was occupied with establishing myself in my new profession and with assuring my own material existence as well as that of a rapidly increasing family."[50] In this situation he found himself simultaneously rejected by the leaders of the Vienna Medical School as the propagandist of the foreigner Charcot, and on the national scene accused of the greatest irresponsibility and recklessness. One can well imagine that then, too, as he commented on an earlier crisis of disappointment his "mind, strange to say, was not directed towards the future but instead attempted to improve the past."[51] If only he had not interrupted his work in the summer of 1884, he could now be famous instead of being scoffed at and rejected.

The story of cocaine as Freud tells it in his *Autobiography* reflects this mood forty years later. "In the autumn of 1886 I settled down in Vienna as a physician and married. . . . I may here go back a little and explain how it was the fault of my fiancée that I was not already famous at that early age."[52] And then follows as a flash-back the narration of his cocaine studies, of their interruption by the trip to his fiancée, and of Koller's achievement. He then continues: "I will now return to the year 1886." The regret about the loss of priority that is expressed in this paragraph of Freud's *Autobiography* belongs clearly in the year 1886 and not, as many readers seem to have thought, in 1884.

In July 1887, Freud grasped an opportunity to state his case in a paper "Craving for and Fear of Cocaine," published in the leading Viennese medical weekly.[53]

My experiences with the use of cocaine in certain nervous conditions and the absence of subsequent addiction agree so completely with the reports which a well-known foreign authority, Hammond, has recently made on this subject, that I prefer to translate Hammond's statements rather than to repeat the observations I made in the work "On Coca" and in the paper "Contribution to the Knowledge of the Effects of Cocaine."[54]

Before Freud brings this translation, or rather his abstract of Hammond's paper, he surveys the situation in several paragraphs and explains

how the benefits of cocaine were lost to the morphinists. . . . The patients themselves began to seize on the drug, and to misuse it in the same manner in which they were in the habit of misusing morphine. Cocaine was to be their substitute for morphine; it must have proven itself to be an insufficient substitute, as most morphine addicts quickly reached the enormous dose of 1 Grm. a day in subcutaneous injection. It was now discovered that, used in this way, cocaine is a far more dangerous enemy of a healthy body than morphine. . . . I cannot forego a remark close at hand, which is useful in again ridding the so-called third scourge of humanity, as Erlenmeyer most pathetically labels cocaine, of its horror. That is to say, that all reports on cocaine addiction refer to morphine addicts, individuals who had already succumbed to the demon, whose weakened will power and need for stimulus would abuse any stimulants offered them, and in fact did so. Cocaine has taken no other victims from us, no victims of its own. I have countless experiences with the extended use of cocaine in individuals who were not morphine addicts, and have myself taken the drug for months, without feeling—or hearing of—any special condition similar to morphine addiction, or of a demand for further use of cocaine. On the contrary, more often than I should have liked, an aversion to the drug took place, which caused the discontinuation of its use.[55]

Strange as it may seem today the first cocaine addicts were morphine-cocainists. Most of them were physicians, pharmacists, or doctor's wives, a fact which might be one of the reasons for the almost panic-like reaction of the physicians, as if cocaine by itself would "produce a state very similar to morphine addiction." To Freud this seemed not only an exaggeration but a shift from what he thought to be the main problem in the discussion:

> I believe this one unreliability of cocaine—that one does not know when a toxic reaction will appear—is very closely connected with another with which I must reproach the alkaloid: it is not really known when and in whom an effect is actually to be expected. (I am disregarding, of course, the anesthetic effect.) The clue which can lead to a better understanding of this characteristic might be the following: Cocaine closely has an effect on the innervation of the blood vessels... namely either constricting or dilating.... To me the variable factor, on which the inequality of the cocaine effect depends, seems therefore to lie in the momentary condition and in the lability of the vessel innervation. That excitation of the vessel nerves (or vessel-nerve centers) is very different in different individuals, and that it varies within each, I consider to be absolutely certain. In the lability of the brain-vessel innervation can probably be found one of the main symptoms of the nervous status. Cocaine—if its general effect is created by influencing the circulation of the brain—will have no effect when the vessel *tonus* is stable, but at another time it will create a toxic effect... and in other cases again will produce favorable tonic or hyperemic results. I consequently presume: The reason for the inequality of the cocaine effect lies in the individually different excitation, and in the difference of the conditions of the vessel nerves, on which the cocaine acts. As the degree of this excitation is generally unknown, and since this factor of individual disposition has on the whole been very little considered I feel it is advisable to refrain as far as possible from the use of cocaine in subcutaneous injections in the treatment of internal and nervous maladies.[56]

This paper on "Craving for and Fear of Cocaine" is Freud's last contribution to the topic. It made no impression on his contemporaries. Of course it did not stop the rapid and complete elimination of cocaine from psychiatry, and its slow substitution by new preparations for local anesthesia. This was not merely the result of fear of cocaine, nor did it even stimulate the research into the complex properties of cocaine that Freud had suggested. The paper was probably judged and discarded as the stubborn reiteration of one who could not admit error frankly.

Obviously the paper was written in self-defense against direct or hidden accusations. A remark in the first paragraph indicates the emotional climate in which Freud wrote: "Perhaps it is not superfluous to mention that the morphine-withdrawal cure through cocaine is not something I experienced on my own body, but advice that I gave to another person." As far as I know, this is the only paper of Freud's long writing career in which the personal motive is so much in evidence; though its style and diction are almost as objective as in his other writings. One readily understands that its contemporary readers were inclined to disregard Freud's arguments simply as rationalization. Yet this would not be justifiable today, sixty-four years after its publication. We now can clearly see that Freud was in error on some points, but that his thoughts were amazingly little distorted by the strong impact of his disappointment.

The facts reported in both of his quoted papers were—as he maintained—unimpaired by the appearance of cocaine addiction. The abuse or misuse of a drug in some cases does not exclude its usefulness. In spite of its "evil power," morphine was not eliminated from medical practice. Whatever the strength of his defense motives might be, the observations made on himself and on some of his friends remained as valid in 1887, after the appearance of cocaine addiction, as they had been in 1884. Since he had experienced aversion, rather than a craving for cocaine, habit formation could not—at least not automatically—be the effect of the chemical properties of the drug. For Freud, the rare fact, even the singular fact, always commanded respect, and impelled as much scientific thinking as the conspicuous, statistical sample based on impressive numbers. He would never have originated psychoanalysis without this attitude, but due to it his work was for so long stigmatized as nonscientific. This characteristic regard for the singular fact made him hesitant and skeptical in recognizing that his own reaction to the drug was not the general and not the most significant one.

The panic that the appearance of cocaine addicts had created in Central Europe was no legitimate reason for discontinuing investigation into the pharmacotherapeutic dynamics. By no means was it an appropriate occasion for scientists to express moral outrage. We know today that neither cocaine nor any other chemical, in itself, produces addiction. It is a psychological phenomenon. In the 80's the problem of addiction was approached, if at all, as one of toxicity, specific to certain habit-forming drugs. It was psychoanalysis that several decades later brought the first insight into the nature of addiction and its complex relationship to the effect of the drug. In 1885, when Freud met the problem, he thought of the hunger for stimuli, of the mental weakness, of the lack of self-control as the decisive factors. Freud speaks of addicts with overtones of pity and contempt; but he never stands in awe of those poisons, which were considered by contemporary—and especially German—literature to possess the devilish property of breaking down the power of moral responsibility. In his first acquaintance with the "functional phenomena" he oscillates, so it seems, between moral judgment and objective explanation in neurophysiological terms; between lack of will power or lability of centers. He is, in other words, a contemporary. Yet he refuses to think of habit formation as a direct effect of the poison. This view suits his self-defense in the dispute; it is the more advanced one, nevertheless.

5. A Parapraxis

In his work with cocaine Freud was clearly partial to the internal use of the drug. In the various experiments on himself and on others Freud had always applied it by mouth; to Fleischl he had recommended oral application, and in his paper of 1887 had explicitly warned against subcutaneous injections. Today we fail to see the rationale in his sharp distinction between the harmless oral and the dangerous subcutaneous dispensation. In fact to the spreading of cocainism the injection technique functioned as a brake. Only in the 90's, when oral and nasal applications came into wider use, did the trade in cocaine and thus cocainism assume significant proportions. Whenever Freud defended himself against the reproaches which followed his recommendation of cocaine, he stressed the point that he had not advocated the harmful needle.

Yet in his lecture before the Psychiatric Society in March 1885 referring to the treatment of morphinists he had said: "I would . . . . advise without hesitation . . . . to give cocaine in subcutaneous injections of 0.03 to 0.05 grms. per dose and not to shrink from an accumulation of doses."[57] He does not mention this lecture in his self-defense "Craving for and Fear of Cocaine" in which he quotes as his previous papers on cocaine only his monograph and his dynamometer study.[58] It is not included in the list of his writings that he compiled in 1897.[59] Nor does it appear in any other place in his works. It even seems that he did not keep a reprint of this publication in his files since Brun,[60] who based his bibliography of Freud's prepsychoanalytic writings on Freud's own collection of reprints, does not mention this paper.*

This omission could be a slight matter; an oversight of an excusable expedient of no relevance. But Freud should be measured by his own yardstick and such an omission has its meaning. In 1887, and afterwards, he apparently regretted very strongly that once he had recommended cocaine injections "without hesitation." In 1887, he left out—"dishonestly" as he would call it—this fact; or was it rather an unconscious dishonesty—a parapraxis? If this were so one ought to find an equally "unconscious confession" of it somewhere in Freud's writings. In fact Freud did commit a remarkable error in *The Interpretation of Dreams*. On page 116 he writes of his recommendation of cocaine in 1885—an obvious error. The recommendation actually occurred in 1884 in the paper "Ueber Coca,"† but he did recommend injections in 1885. Wittels noticed this error. Freud commented:

"When I am supposed to have given 1885 as the date of the cocaine experience, I don't know. Suspect an error of the biographer." Yet this

---

* This same fate befell the recommendation of subcutaneous injections for the relief of sciatic pains, which is included in the book edition of *Ueber Coca* as one of several additions written by Freud in 1885.
† Not in the English edition.

date is carried in all the editions of *The Interpretation of Dreams*, as well as in the reprints in the German "Collected Papers" of 1925 and 1948. Only a parapraxis, not a simple printer's error, possesses such power of preservation.

The fragments of his self-analysis that Freud inserted in some of his writings enable us to diagnose pretty closely the kind and strength of those internal fights of which this parapraxis is the scar. Two independent strands of thought are confluent in the regretted and forgotten recommendation of cocaine injections against morphinism; the use of injections in general, and the complex relationship of Freud to his teacher, friend, and patient, Fleischl.

At that time many physicians shared Freud's warning against injections. Hypodermic injections, quite generally, were rarely considered, and then only with some hesitation as if the application, in itself, were somehow uncanny or dangerous. Indeed, it was the fast-spreading use of cocaine as a local anesthetic which has greatly helped to reduce this awe to its rational limitation. Freud often prided himself on his skill and luck with the needle and, for instance, advised Königstein on the finer points of technique. Since Scholz, Freud's chief in the General Hospital, had had an important influence in the early development of the injection technique, it seems quite likely that Freud acquired his skill in Scholz' department. But in Freud's dreams, the source of the more timid attitude that he shared with his contemporaries, and one which is still very much alive in the preconscious of some physicians, appears to be a defense against the symbolic meaning of the procedure which links it with masculine sexual aggression. In Freud's "Dream of Irma's Injection" (1895) this wider topic is associated with memories of the treatment of Fleischl.[61]

Another dream brings to light one important factor in the background of the Fleischl treatment. In July 1882—only two years before his interest in cocaine—Freud had discontinued his work at the Physiological Institute. One of his close friends, Joseph Paneth, highly gifted and devoted to science, had become Freud's successor as teaching assistant (demonstrator) in the Institute. Unhappy about the prospects of slow advancement and uninhibited by any emotional attachment to Fleischl, Paneth in the following years had repeatedly and openly expressed death wishes against Fleischl, the man who blocked his way. This egotism had horrified Freud—as we learn from his dream "In Brücke's Laboratory,"[62] which occurred in 1899 when Fleischl and Paneth were both already dead. Yet until 1882 Freud had been in the same position as Paneth; he, too, had wanted to become an assistant, and in his case also, Fleischl had stood in the way.

.... to be sure, I myself had cherished even more intensely the same wish—to obtain a post which had fallen vacant; whenever there are gradations of rank and promotion the way is opened for the suppression of covetous wishes. Shakespeare's Prince Hal cannot rid himself of the temptation to see how the crown fits, even at the bedside of his sick father.

But Freud had not consciously hoped for Fleischl's possible or near demise. On the contrary, he had judged his chances to be nil and had left the Institute and the scientific career connected with it.

In this context we see that the wish to help Fleischl against his morphine addiction in 1884 had a function in Freud's defense against, and reaction to, his unconscious death wishes. He was trying to help his friend to live longer and to rid him of his weakness. He became Fleischl's successful therapist while Paneth, the villain, was hoping for his end. Yet, as became apparent in 1886, cocaine was an unreliable helper and Fleischl a weakling, who recklessly used the syringe—the teacher who only a few years earlier had impressed Freud "as a man whom he could take as his model."[63]

The coca episode plays its part in several other dreams that Freud interpreted during his self-analysis. For instance in the "Dream of the Botanical Monograph" it appears in connection with Freud's relation to his father, as a part of the dream wish to prove that he is able to do valuable work in spite of the curse of his childhood years: "This boy will never amount to anything."

The disappointment that he soon experienced with cocaine and Fleischl, the accusation that he had not discovered a helpful remedy but rather a tempting poison, that he and his work on cocaine amounted to nothing, the self-reproach that he had once recommended the needle—all this stirred up conflict and guilt. Cocaine, the first topic that he himself—independent of others—chose in order to gain scientific distinction, failed him, and even threatened the independence, which, through marriage and private practice, he was just then attempting to establish.

Each one of these defeats could by itself account for a severe disturbance; their combination could easily confuse the thinking of a gifted young scientist, and might well have distorted or even killed his talent. Yet in Freud's case they manifest themselves only in a bibliographical omission—a parapraxis.

Should one not add that Freud withdrew altogether from the investigation of the psychiatric potentialities of cocaine? We know for certain only that he did not publish any further studies or recommendations of cocaine after July 1887. We do not know when, definitely, he crossed it off the list of his plans.

The irregular effects of cocaine had early intrigued him. They were the motive for the dynamometer studies in 1884, which tried to find a hidden uniformity behind the apparent variety. By March 1885 he had recognized that only in rare cases did cocaine do its job as reliably as it did on himself. In July 1887 his main reproach against cocaine was its unreliability. To understand this puzzle there was then no other way than physiological and pharmacological research, for which Freud had no inclination and, as a neurologist in private practice, without laboratory connections, no proper facilities. He could hardly do anything else than wait until others did the necessary basic research. He turned to different means of helping the neurasthenics.

But we have indications that his interest in cocaine continued to some degree. In the fall of 1887, Freud met Wilhelm Fliess, a physician from Berlin, who at that time was, or a little later became, interested in the medical application of cocaine. During the years of their growing friendship, Freud was intensely interested in the facts that Fliess was discovering by cocainization of the nose. Freud was then experimenting with hypnotism and was trying out new psychological approaches to the neuroses. But he continued to recommend cocainization of the nose to patients, at least until 1895. He happens to cite in *The Interpretation of Dreams* one such incident that had had bad results. On the same occasion he mentions that he himself made good use of this method when his sinuses troubled him.

For many years he apparently continued to have a limited and skeptical interest in the drug. Gradually, however, his psychotherapeutic experiences convinced him that the chemical method of defense against suffering (*Leid*), although the most potent, was for that very reason dangerously noxious; and to the historian of psychoanalysis it is evident that subsequently this conviction served to guide him away from medicinal magic and toward the development of a system of psychological therapy.

III

CHAPTER 23

Sherlock Holmes and Sigmund Freud

"A Study in Cocaine" by David F. Musto, M.D.

I believe this article is a bit of fantasy carefully woven into the solid fabric of historical fact. Whether or not it is fantasy depends on whether the reader has an unshakeable belief in the real existence of Sherlock Holmes. The proposition is so eminently plausible that we must accept that if history is logical Dr. Musto has discovered the origins of psychoanalysis. Ed.

Cocaine stimulated the early careers of two brilliant investigators, Sigmund Freud and Sherlock Holmes. In fact, their common attraction to the euphoric properties of the coca leaf may be more than a coincidence. But whatever the Freud-Holmes relationship, the cocaine episodes in each of their lives reflect the impact of a new psychic drug on literature and science. Some of their admirers may deny or overlook this aspect of their careers, thinking that any association with such a drug can only be an embarrassment. But the international enthusiasm for cocaine which antedated and extended beyond their periods of endorsement makes it unlikely that any fair-minded person will censure them.

The cocaine episode illustrates how easily objective evaluation may be submerged by personal enthusiasm and how remarkably difficult it may be, in spite of vast amounts of evidence, to judge correctly a widely used drug. Perhaps a reason for delay in recognizing limitations lies in the vividness of physicians' experience when they used cocaine on their own bodies. Papers about cocaine abound with rapturous subjectivity; they not only strongly assert that everyone should try it, but also impatiently question the motives of those who disagree.

A description of coca's peculiarities had been carried to Europe in the 16th century by Nicolas Monardes of Spain, but the period of excitement over coca arose chiefly from numerous 19th-century reports.[1] The intense popularization of coca began just after the middle of the last century. Following his stay amongst Peruvian natives, the Italian physician, Paolo Mantegazza, declared that a great new weapon against disease had been providentially located.[2] His description echoed the spirit of similar accounts which more than two centuries previously had introduced to Europe the cinchona bark from the jungles of South America. Cinchona proved a most useful substance, providing the first effective treatment of malaria: perhaps coca would have equally valuable effects.

Warning against coca's excessive use, Mantegazza nevertheless could hardly restrain his fascination and hope. His pamphlet, *Sulle virtu igieniche e medicinali della coca* (1859), attracted wide attention throughout Europe and the British Isles, although the lack of an inexpensive, effective preparation slowed acceptance of the claims. Shortly after Mantegazza's report, the Viennese biochemist Niemann isolated an active principle, cocaine, from the leaves (1859).[3] First scientific reports, however, were unenthusiastic. The noted pharmacologist, Schroff (1862), while not impressed by cocaine's psychotropic properties, did describe its paralytic effects on the frog's nervous system.[4] Schroff's study, a contrast to the vivid description by Mantegazza, slowed the acceptance of cocaine as a miraculous remedy.

In England experimentation led to a similar muted response. On Feb 21, 1874, Dr. E. H. Sieveking announced in a letter to the *British Medical Journal* that he had obtained a chest of coca leaves and invited his colleagues to conduct experiments. Next week the *BMJ* published a letter from Dr. Arthur Leared wishing Dr. Sieveking good luck. Dr. Leared had experimented with a box of leaves a few years previously and found them of no effect: he wondered whether the long sea voyage had affected their potency. Then a few years later the seventy-eight-year-old president of the British Medical Association, Sir Robert Christison, related that after chewing some coca leaves he was able to walk fifteen miles and accomplish other arduous tasks without exhaustion.[5] But balancing this fantastic news, reports that same year from University College, London, recited a sober account of cocaine's inefficacy.[6] Physicians apparently could not agree on the properties of coca.

Closer to the source of the coca leaf, Americans started to report considerable use and promise for the drug. In the decorous pages of the *Boston Medical and Surgical Journal,* Dr. G. Archie Stockwell revealed to the medical profession the possibilities of coca (provided it was not used to excess).[7] The year was 1876 and from Dr. Stockwell's account it appeared that Americans could face their second century of independence with the conveniently vigorous effects of a substance which "never depresses," has "no re-coil," and eliminates fatigue. "The moderate use of coca," he reasonably concluded, "is not only wholesome but frequently beneficial. . . ." He mentioned that there were, of course, those who would detract from the value of the drug or feared an habituating tendency or effect on the personality. He derided the alarmists and chided the simpletons who mistook the effect of mercurialism in the Indians for the toxic symptoms of coca, since many of the Indians suffered from their work in quicksilver mines.

By 1880 Detroit's *Therapeutic Gazette* blossomed with the wonderful effects of coca. From Rockford, Ill., a physician wrote of "a new cure for the opium habit": drug-slaves could substitute coca extract for opium and thereby wean themselves from the poppy's vicious milk; this accomplished they could then stop taking coca.[8] In Kentucky, a Valley Oak physician encouragingly found coca to be a cure for alcoholism. Near the close of 1880, Dr. W. H. Bentley wrote that the coca plant held succor not only for the alcoholic and the dope-fiend but also for those afflicted with a variety of chronic diseases which he believed originated in the nervous system, eg, tuberculosis and dyspepsia. He broadened its reputed usefulness by describing a stubborn case of impotency whose joyous outcome could be attributed only to coca extract.[9] By now the drug was drawing increased enthusiasm. In 1881, Dr. H. F. Stimmel of Chattanooga, Tenn, frankly stated, "to say that I am surprised or astonished at the wonderful, and almost incredible effects of that new remedy [fluid extract of coca] as a nervous stimulant would not adequately express my appreciation of it."[10]

Outside the scientific journals less rigorous reports appeared. The chief source of the nonmedical cocaine literature was a popular magazine, *The Strand* of London, which was the outlet, as the faithful know, for Dr. John Watson's accounts of the exploits of Sherlock Holmes.

Some Sherlockian authorities have argued that Holmes did not use cocaine, that it was either a joke perpetrated on the somber Watson or that at worst it was actually morphine, since Watson describes a pacific Holmes with subsequent "black reactions," perhaps more characteristic of opiates than cocaine. In answer I would agree with

Dr. Eugene F. Carey, former surgeon with the Medical Division of the Chicago Police Department, that it is unlikely that Holmes would jab himself for so many years if there was not something potent in that bottle on the mantel.[11] Also, one cannot argue away the evidence that he claimed to have taken cocaine, and that physician Watson believed him.

On the question why Holmes took cocaine, there is little doubt. "My mind," he explained, "rebels at stagnation. Give me problems, give me work, give me the most abtruse cryptogram, or the most intricate analysis, and I am in my proper atmosphere. I can dispense with artificial stimulants. But I abhor the dull routine of existence." (This statement occurs in *The Sign of the Four* which is dated September 1888 by William S. Baring-Gould. I accept the chronology of Baring-Gould as the most accurate available.)[12]

Holmes had his black moods and prolonged periods of boredom from which he sought relief. This was not, however, evidence of a manic-depressive disorder as is asserted by the Boltax-Astrachan hypothesis (BAH) which will be discussed later.[13] I would suggest that Holmes was treated for his ennui and occasional melancholia by an accepted regimen of cocaine; that when the side-effects began to interfere with his functioning, he gave up the drug; and that after a period away from the paranoiogenic world of the detective, he returned to London, resumed his career, and reached the pinnacle of his success without further resort to drugs other than tobacco.

A brief resumé of canonical references to cocaine reveals that in the first (*A Scandal in Bohemia*), perhaps as late as 1886, Watson refers to Holmes as "alternating from week to week between cocaine and ambition. . . ." By June 1887, Holmes is joking to Watson about his cocaine injections and denying that he has added opium-smoking to his vices (*The Man with the Twisted Lip*). In September of that year (*The Five Orange Pips*) Holmes is described as a "self-poisoner by cocaine and tobacco." In *The Yellow Face*, Holmes, "save for the occasional use of cocaine . . . had no vices" (April 1888). But the use of cocaine seems to have increased during the summer, for in September of the same year (*The Sign of the Four*), Watson observes the injections and writes: "Three times a day for many months I had witnessed this performance." Shortly thereafter, Watson ceases to be a steady observer since he married in May of the following year. Looking back on this period many years later, Holmes refers to a hypodermic syringe as an "instrument of evil" (*The Missing Three-quarter,* 1896), and we can assume that his frequent use of the drug had ended with a three-year hiatus abroad following his disappearance at Reichenbach Falls (May 4, 1891).

Reasons for believing that the cocaine problem reached a critical stage just before the episode at Reichenbach Falls (*The Final Problem*) rest upon an analysis of the case as described by Watson. After Watson married he became seriously concerned about Holmes' condition. This motivated Watson to a most unusual course: he advertised for help. On the 28th of October, 1890, he turned to the *Lancet,* writing an appealing and desperate letter asking for advice on how to cure "a patient" suffering from cocaine-craving.[14] Naturally he signs it with a pseudonym, since all Britain would know who John H. Watson's "patient" would be; the letter is purportedly from "Irene," a name whose significance will not escape any serious student.*

The result of Watson's attempt to wean Holmes from cocaine at

THE LANCET.

LONDON: SATURDAY, NOVEMBER 1, 1890.

COCAINE CRAVING.
To the Editors of THE LANCET.

SIRS,—I have a patient who suffers from cocaine craving. I find it impossible to keep cocaine out of his reach. This habit has brought him into a very low state of health. Perhaps some of your readers might be able to give me some suggestion as to treatment. I have tried the usual remedies in vain. He suffers from great nervousness, sleeplessness, and has become very thin.—I am, Sirs, yours truly,

Oct. 28th, 1890.   IRENE.

---

* "To Sherlock Holmes she is always *the* woman. I seldom heard him mention her under any other name. In his eyes she eclipses and predominates the whole of her sex . . . ," *"A Scandal in Bohemia."*

this junction is not known, but one evening a few months later Holmes unexpectedly enters Watson's consulting room. "It struck me," records Watson, "that he was looking paler and thinner than usual." Holmes startles Watson by immediately requesting that the shutter be closed and bolted. He confides his fear of air guns and warns Watson that soon he will have to leave—by going over Watson's back garden wall. Holmes had two bleeding knuckles following a fight with a ruffian whom he felt had been "sent" to do him in. He asks Watson to come away for a week on the Continent. "Anywhere," pleads Holmes, "it's all the same to me." This talk was out of character for Holmes and his pale, worn face told Watson that his nerves were at their highest tension. There then poured from Holmes a fantastic tale, but one cannot know whether Watson accepted this or only feigned to believe.

To get the full flavor of Holmes' elaborate system, one must read the case in its entirety, but I will give a few examples of his patterns of thought. They have the unusual quality, familiar, however, to clinicians, of explanations whose proof is suggested by the sinister fact that no proof is possible. Holmes was suffering, perhaps, from the side effect of chronic cocaine use which often induces an extremely suspicious cast of mind and leads the sufferer to weave elaborate schemes to explain facts of whose significance only he is aware.

To return to the tête-à-tête in the consultation room—Holmes saw the look of wonder on Watson's face and finally decided to confide to his only friend what was creating such anguish. Note the objective value of his evidence.

"You have probably never heard of Professor Moriarty?" said he.
"Never."
"Ay, there's the genius and the wonder of the thing!" he cried. "The man pervades London and no one has heard of him. That's what puts him on a pinnacle in the records of crime. . . ."

Later Holmes relates his growing suspicions which give an insight into the evolution of his system. "For years past I have continually been conscious of some power behind the malefactor, some deep organizing power which forever stands on the way of the law, and throws its shield over the wrong-doer. Again and again. . . ."

It is too painful to record in all its detail Holmes' "deductions" which explain everything to him (*paranoia moriartii?*).[15] Suffice it to say that all the evidence Watson ever witnesses occurs as he and Holmes leave on a Paris-bound train from Victoria Station. They catch a glimpse of "a tall man pushing his way furiously through the crowd, and waving his hand as if he desired to have the train stopped." Holmes declares that this man is Moriarity, and Watson humoringly agrees, recalling to himself all the "Moriaritys" he has seen trying to catch a train at Victoria Station. As the train gathers speed, Holmes feels comfortable enough to take off his disguise as an aged Italian priest.

Holmes is continually in exuberant spirits, in spite of all his watchfulness. In Switzerland a mysterious fall of rocks, explained by the guide as not uncommon for the season or place, meets with no reply from Holmes although "he smiled with the air of a man who sees the fulfillment of that which he had expected."

As Holmes glances about, fearing the worst, hoping that at least the arch-criminal would die along with him, he tells Watson that his mind is starting to find interest in things other than the criminal world. "Of late," he muses, "I have been tempted to look into the problems furnished by nature." Well he might, for his mind was not functioning well and perhaps the causes for this were to be found not among criminals but in the pharmacology of cocaine and the dynamics of the mind.

Holmes' disappearance at the Reichenbach Falls, as he and Watson pursued a course toward the Austrian border, is well known. It is equally well known that he reappeared on April 5, 1894, almost exactly three years later—having traveled widely, engaged in chemical research, and having no longer a craving for cocaine. His greatest years followed.

Several explanations of Holmes' unusual life style have been presented. For the sake of an exhausting completeness, the Boltax-Astrachan hypothesis (BAH) will now be discussed. As readers of [the *Journal of the American Medical* Association are already] aware, (*JAMA* 196:1094, 1966), Boltax and Astrachan of New Haven advanced the fancy that Sherlock Holmes suffered from a manic-depressive disorder. This pessimistic diagnosis would, in their view, account for his alternating periods of lethargy and activity. This is a startling hypothesis, for it invokes one of the most severe disorders known to psychiatry. It is as if a neurologist thought the probable cause of most headaches was a space-occupying lesion. Other than his alternating moods of moderate degree, Holmes' only possible deviation from mental health might be his views on Professor Moriarity. But, as Dr. George Vash pointed out in contradiction to BAH (*JAMA* 197:664-665, 1966), occasional inertia in a man of creativity is not so unusual and certainly in Holmes' case is far less than would occur in a manic-depressive illness.[16] It is hazardous to make dogmatic clinical judgments on the basis of evidence from the past, and it is especially unwise to advance the severer and rarer ailment as the first explanation of phenomena.

But what else happened between 1891 and 1894? Only conjecture is possible. It was at this time that Sigmund Freud, the Viennese neurologist who originally supported the use of cocaine as a nerve tonic, ceased writing in favor of the treatment. Freud showed great concern for those who had over-used the drug and who, although they might not be termed addicted, suffered from the side effects of its intoxication. Holmes, I suggest, was treated for chronic overuse which had affected the reality-testing aspect of his deductive powers. He was functioning well as a computer, but the data from which his deductions took their origin were not well distinguished from fantasy. His cure probably took the form of rest, abstinence from the drug, and the absorption of his mind in other matters. We can be certain, however, that as he rested, whether in Switzerland or in a pleasant sanatorium in the Viennese suburbs, he talked. And his ideas and especially his methods must have influenced those to whom he spoke. We are accustomed to the attention Holmes paid to the unusual fact, the unraveling of a complicated problem from the noting of a small slip or characteristic. This style of reasoning may have been the gift of Holmes to those who treated him for his temporarily inefficient mental processes.

Sigmund Freud's interest in cocaine was prompted by reading articles in the *Therapeutic Gazette* and especially by the hope held there for its usefulness in curing morphine addiction. In 1883, Freud, while working in Brücke's laboratory, had become a friend of Ernst von Fleischl-Marxow (1846–1891), a brilliant physiologist and physicist. Characteristically, when Freud formed a strong friendship it was extravagantly pursued. "He has always been my ideal," Freud wrote his fiancée, "and I could not rest till we became friends."[17] Again he wrote, "I love him not so much as a human being, but as one of Creation's precious achievements."[18] Fleischl was a morphine addict, occasioned by the severe pain of neuromata at the site of a thumb amputation, and one of Freud's major reasons for securing cocaine from Merck & Co. was the possibility of curing him. In May 1884, about a month after obtaining the drug, Freud was encouraged by the results of some cocaine he had given Fleischl. Its euphoric qualities led Freud to call it a "magical drug," and ever new possibilities occurred to him. In June of 1884 he finished a review article on the subject, "Ueber Coca," which, in summary, confirmed Mantegazza's endorsement of cocaine a quarter-century previous.[19] In it he chided, "At present there seems to be some promise of widespread recognition and use of coca preparations in North America, while in Europe doctors scarcely know them by name."

With the enthusiasm that a few years later he would wholeheartedly devote to hypnotism, Freud found in cocaine an instrument of almost unbelievable curative power. The success of cocaine, though, would not only bring to mankind a precious boon, it would also satisfy several of Freud's own needs. Efficacy of the drug would cure his esteemed friend, fame would bring him a lucrative practice, and the improvement of his financial position would allow him to marry sooner than planned. In such a situation, it was quite difficult for Freud to perceive cocaine's limitations.

To his fiancée Freud described his twenty-five page review article as "a song of praise to this magical substance."[20] He opened with an historical summary of the literature; in the same spirit as the American Stockwell, he struck out at those who "painted a terrible picture" of the effects of coca. A common theme of the physicians who enjoyed the psychotropic effects of cocaine was an impatience with both outright opponents and the undecided whose qualifications spoiled their own pure enthusiasm. Freud's language in his review article is almost mystical; he looks down as from a great height upon the non-users or the ill-users. And in a later article (January 1885) he dismisses the pharmacologist Schroff, who, although he took cocaine (a dozen years before Freud), did not feel enthusiastic; therefore, he "must bear a share of the blame for the setback of the alkaloid at this time [1862]."[21]

Freud's description of the effect coca had on the healthy human body he based upon experiments made on himself and friends:

The psychic effect of cocaine consists of exhilaration and lasting euphoria, which does not differ in any way from the normal euphoria of a healthy person. . . . I have tested this effect of coca, which wards off hunger, sleep, and fatigue and steels one to intellectual effort some dozen times on myself. . . . Opinion is unanimous that the euphoria induced by coca is not followed by any feeling of lassitude or other state of depression. . . . It seems probable . . . that coca, if used protractedly but in moderation, is not detrimental to the body.[22]

The therapeutic uses of coca or cocaine were, in Freud's earliest opinion, multiple and significant. Coca is useful as a stimulant especially in wartime, on journeys, during mountain climbing and on other such expeditions. When used as a stimulant he said,

. . . it is better that it should be given in small effective doses (0.05– 0.10) and repeated so often that the effects of the doses overlap. . . . To be sure, the instantaneous effect of a dose of coca cannot be compared with that of a morphine injection; but on the good side of the ledger, there is no danger of general damage to the body as is the case with the chronic use of morphine.[23]

Freud felt that one of the most important uses of cocaine would be by psychiatrists treating melancholia or neurasthenia. Reports were in some conflict, but he knew of several striking successes. It filled a need for psychiatrists who had many drugs for calming excited persons but heretofore no safe psychic stimulant. He enumerated other uses for cocaine: treatment of digestive disorders of the stomach, cachexia, typhoid fever, phthisis, syphilis and (*pace* Stockwell) mercurialism.

Freud credits Dr. Bentley's report in the Detroit *Therapeutic*

Gazette with demonstrating the use of cocaine as a treatment for morphine and alcohol addiction. Freud elaborated on its antimorphine properties, reaching an extreme claim in this part of his first paper: cocaine was so powerful a specific to morphine-addiction as well as alcoholism that *"inebriate asylums can be entirely dispensed with."* "Über Coca" concluded with brief comments on cocaine's use in asthma, as an aphrodisiac and, lastly, in local applications as an anesthetic. Its anesthetic effects are sketched in only one paragraph, a brevity for which Freud later reproached himself, since Koller's anesthetic application, made public a month after publication of "Über Coca," eventually was the most applauded use of cocaine and remained so for years to come.

As we have already noted, coca and cocaine were received in America with interest and fairly widespread use. By 1885, the Parke-Davis Company had printed a monograph for physicians summarizing medical experience with the various forms of the coca plant. The introduction to this sizable paper captured its message in a few words:

[Coca is] a drug which through its stimulant properties, can supply the place of food, make the coward brave, the silent eloquent, free the victims of alcohol and opium habit from their bondage, and, as an anaesthetic render the sufferer insensitive to pain, and make attainable to the surgeon heights of what may be termed, "aesthetic surgery" never reached before.[24]

Not only could one buy a handy cocaine case with all the instruments for the various applications of cocaine, and over a dozen forms of the substance (e.g., coca cordial), but even cigarettes and cheroots made from the coca leaf. The Parke-Davis Company, needing to establish that their cocaine was as pure as the German variety; had offered Freud the equivalent of twenty-four dollars to test theirs against Merck's. Freud reported that it was just as good, noting only a slightly perceptible difference in taste, all of which "indicate the greatest future for the Parke cocaine" [August 1885].

Freud found himself with a disappointingly small share of fame. The value of cocaine as a cure for morphine addiction became increasingly difficult to maintain. Reports occurred of addiction to cocaine itself. While the battle continued in the scientific columns of medical journals, Fleischl, Freud's beloved friend, rapidly deteriorated into a pathetic victim of cocaine; by April 1885 he was injecting a gram daily. Freud spent many nights sitting by Fleischl, consoling him and trying to treat his varied symptoms.

Although Freud never publicly retracted his broad endorsement of cocaine, he finally withdrew it as a cure for *morphiumsucht*. His final paper on cocaine was published in July 1887, three years after the "song of praise."[25] Erlenmeyer, in an article based upon a series of tests with morphine addicts, had scathingly attacked cocaine as a useful drug.[26] Freud disputed the conclusion, pointing out that Erlenmeyer gave the drug subcutaneously rather than by mouth as Freud at one time had suggested. Then, having exposed Erlenmeyer's "serious experimental error," Freud withdrew cocaine as a cure for the morphine habit on Freud's own grounds: morphine addicts are "so weak in will power, so susceptible" that they take over cocaine as a new stimulant and replace morphine with an even more destructive habit. But, italicizes Freud, *"cocaine has claimed no other, no victim on its own."* In other words, he indicates that if the patient has not been a morphine addict he will not become a cocaine addict. Freud ends his article with extensive supporting statements by W. A. Hammond, abstracted from the *Journal of Nervous and Mental Diseases*[27] (New York, 1886).

Freud had chosen an indomitable enthusiast when he listed William Alexander Hammond (1828–1900) in support of cocaine. Hammond was a leader of the American medical profession, an international authority on neurology, a prolific author, and a powerful personality. Surgeon General of the Army by the age of thirty-five, he had been dismissed from the service by Lincoln in 1864 for irregularities in purchasing policies. But he recovered well from this blow, established himself as one of the most successful neurologists in New York, and in 1879 was returned to the lists of retired army officers following a new investigation. In the latter part of the century he moved to Washington, DC, where he operated a private hospital "for diseases of the nervous system and for those diseases generally in which the Hammond animal extracts are especially useful." He founded the Army Medical Museum, wrote novels and plays, took a serious albeit antagonistic interest in spiritualism, and authored texts on sleep, neurology, and impotency. All this later earned him a description as "the dominant [medical] personality of his time."[28]

By the summer of 1887 Freud's enthusiasm for cocaine may have moderated but not that of General Hammond who, in the fall of that year, delivered a stout defense of cocaine at the annual session of the Medical Society of Virginia.[29] During the question period, some physicians expressed doubts about the safety of cocaine and its value in hay fever. One delegate told of a fellow physician who had become addicted to it. The General counter-attacked. After all he had said about cocaine, he was surprised at the uncertainty of the questioners. Coca was the outstanding specific for "cerebral hyperemia" (one of Hammond's pet ailments), "the most common affliction of the nervous system," brought on by mental exertion or intense emotional disturbance. A claret glass of wine of coca with each meal worked wonders; of course, cocaine was better, for "what is true of the wine is even more true of the active ingredient." Cocaine excelled in melancholia and "hysteria with great depression of spirits." Perhaps the questioner had misunderstood Hammond's denial of the cocaine habit: "He does not wish to be understood as saying there is no such thing as the cocaine habit, but he does say that the habit is very much like that of the coffee habit." To the delegate doubting its efficacy in hay fever, the General victoriously retorted, ". . . so generally valuable is it in that disease that the Hay Fever Association has adopted it as their remedy!"

Proponents of cocaine's uplifting qualities often found it very difficult to back away from their original claims. Freud defended cocaine's value as a stimulant when Fleischl lay incapacitated only a few miles away. While Hammond proclaimed its virtues, another American, Professor William Stewart Halsted, became seriously habituated to cocaine in the course of perfecting it as a local anesthetic.[30] Even while many physicians knew the bad effects of cocaine, the debate dragged on.

Freud published no more on cocaine and its wonderful attributes after 1887. The cocaine experience was a rough one, his friend for whom it had been a hope was worse, and his desire for fame was crushed by the great Erlenmeyer's rebuke that cocaine was the "third scourge of the human race," after opium and alcohol. For Sherlock Holmes, cocaine had ceased to be a problem by the time he returned to London in 1894. The dangers of this "magical drug," however, were not generally accepted for many years.

CHAPTER 24

Illicit Cocaine in America

1972

From *Dealer: Portrait of a Cocaine Merchant* by Richard Woodley.

This excerpt from Dealer *gives the reader a sense of the place of cocaine in contemporary American life. The book is an excellent study of the life of a cocaine merchant and one of the few modern books to cover the subject in an unromanticized and realistic light.* Ed.

Cocaine: white crystalline powder derived from the coca plant native to the Andes Mountains of South America; a powerful central-nervous-system stimulant that is the least-discussed of the so-called "hard drugs," yet is a staple in the diet of entertainers and the favorite of the drug dealers themselves; the most expensive "high" of them all; the King.

In the illegal drug business, cocaine is sold cut in $10 or $20 capsules (a $20 cap is enough for anything from a three-and-three to a six-and-six, depending upon the snort); teaspoons and tablespoons (tablespoons are "quarters"); "pieces," which are four tablespoons, or about an ounce; parts of "keys" (kilograms, 2.2 pounds) from eighths, quarters, halves, all the way to whole keys of pure cocaine, which costs, in New York, anywhere from $14,000 to $20,000.

A dealer is a pusher with status. The pusher is the lowest level of drug peddler, selling the smallest amounts directly to the users on the street. The dealer sells larger "weights" and has some protective layers of personnel between himself and the street.

For reasons of both money and safety, the dealer tries to move up the ladder. Soon, a dealer always hopes, he will be able to generate more business than his own supplier can accommodate, and then the dealer can jump up a step to deal directly with the man his supplier has been buying from. Each step up means there is another shield between the dealer and the street, and the farther from the street—where carelessness, stupidity, violence, and risk are greatest—the more secure the business. As the dealer rises up the ladder, he buys larger amounts, which enables him to handle a purer quality of cocaine, have greater turnover, and deal with fewer and more responsible people.

As with any other business, advancement is largely a function of ambition, wit, and daring. A dealer may deal easy, at a moderate pace to complement income from other—perhaps legitimate—enterprises, or he may deal hard, high-pressure, running at top speed full time to make it quicker. In either category, the cocaine dealer is not a shopkeeper reliant upon random customers drifting in off the street. The dealer must be a discreet and consistent customer for the man above him. Just so with his own clientele, it must be trustworthy. While there is consignment and credit, it is on a short-term basis, and the terms are harshly enforced. It is a business of huge cash flow, and commits the dealer to a delicate balancing act.

Jimmy deals hard, which means that he invests all he has in product, and then must move it quickly to get his money back. Everybody along the line is pressured to move the product quickly, because cash must flow back up the stream in a hurry. Jimmy doesn't always have product on hand, since he himself must have the cash—or most of it—to buy it. When a good customer wants cocaine, Jimmy, now himself a customer, must make a quick connection for purchase, for if he is unable to provide the right quality of coke quickly enough, he risks losing the customer to another dealer. So he doesn't say he can't get it. In the manner of a true salesman, his pitch is always positive. He'll string you along. He can always get what you want. Sure, get right back to you. Sometimes, rather than admit he can't get it—either because he is short on cash or because his supplier is short on product—he will simply become unavailable, go underground much the same as a threatened debtor, and will surface when he has the product. This, along with a loose-schedule life style and care for security, is why communications with him, as with other dealers up and down the line, are undependable. There are some long nights for dealers and customers alike, while at one end of the line a customer waits hungrily for some snorts of coke, and at the other end the dealer searches anxiously for cash or a supplier with cocaine on hand. Neither cash nor product lies around very long. His skillful manipulation of these elements caused Jimmy to suggest from time to time that I call him the "Juggler."

Dealers keep their records various ways. Jimmy keeps a good bit of his business in his head, some in a pocket notebook, some on scraps of paper tucked into his wallet. First names are listed, and beside each is a dollar figure which is that amount owed to Jimmy. Higher up the line, somebody's book has Jimmy's name listed too, with a dollar figure beside it. "Normal" buying and selling keep him hopping. What jams up the whole system and jeopardizes operations for everybody are delinquent accounts. Debtors, therefore, are punished with sometimes dramatic severity.

Recently two doctors, on one of those countless "drug-abuse" seminars on television, concluded that cocaine had "lost its status" among "drug addicts" and that it had been supplanted by "other more effective, less dangerous stimulants" such as the amphetamines.

Perhaps they got their information from a basic medical reference work, *The Pharmacological Basis of Therapeutics,* which states flatly, "Cocaine abuse is now uncommon in Western countries." Or perhaps they were confused by other sources. It *is* true that cocaine has lost its status in the *medical* world. It was perhaps the first, and for many years around the turn of the century the best, local anesthetic, used primarily in dentistry and for ills and surgery connected with the eye, ear, nose, and throat. Today in this country it has almost entirely been replaced by more effective and less toxic anesthetics, the first of which was procaine (under the trade name of Novocain), which was synthesized in 1905.

But illegal cocaine use, on the other hand, is increasing by gigantic leaps. In 1970, for the first time amounts of illegal cocaine seized by the federal government exceeded seizures of heroin. The Bureau of Narcotics and Dangerous Drugs (part of the Justice Department) reports that in 1970, 267.92 kilograms of coke were seized by agents— a 500% increase over amounts seized in 1969, and a 1,200% increase in four years. Over the same four-year period, seizures of heroin have approximately doubled, to 221.79 kilos for 1970.

Some of this increase is due, of course, to increased vigilance on the part of law-enforcement authorities. But federal officials have also been acknowledging since the latter 1960s that illicit traffic in cocaine is increasing. "It seems," a Narcotics Bureau chief told me, "that cocaine is simply being used a lot more every year." The rock-drug culture accounts for much of the increased usage, but there is as well a stunningly broad group of well-known and well-heeled public personalities—particularly in the entertainment field—who are regular users of cocaine.

Illicit use of the drug is severely penalized. Users are subject to the same sentences as those of heroin. Peddlers get up to fifteen years and fines of up to $25,000. And some state laws are even tougher. New York, for example, gives up to life imprisonment. Given the combination of such widespread use and harsh penalties, one might expect sophistication from the experts. But the federal government, while showing increasing concern about the drug, is performing no experimentation on its effects. Unfortunately, cocaine, compared to heroin and marijuana, remains ominously mysterious to the public.

 Several varieties of the brown or green coca bush, reaching heights of between six and eighteen feet, grow both wild and cultivated on the Amazonian side of the Andes at elevations of from four to six thousand feet. It is cultivated as well in the Indies, Ceylon, India, and parts of Africa.
 Some sources trace use of the leaf as a stimulant back fourteen centuries, when the Incas worshiped it, probably because it gave the chewer increased endurance. Chewing coca leaves is still common among the Andean Indians. According to the Justice Department, the total world need for coca leaves to produce legal cocaine for medical use, or flavoring substances for beverages (such as Coca-Cola), ranges between two and five hundred tons. Yet statistics from Bolivia and Peru alone indicate an estimated annual yield of twelve to fifteen thousand tons—most of which is chewed by native Indians. It is estimated that eight million people still chew the coca leaf.
 In a revealing résumé on cocaine and the coca plant, John T. Maher, a Narcotics Bureau official, wrote: "The fidelity of the present day Indians to coca is due to superstitious ideas retained from ancient times and the necessity to survive 'modern' living in South America. The Indian whose meager fare consists of maize, dried meat, and potatoes relies on coca to sustain his strength, in many cases for mere survival. Without the physical fortification of coca, he would not perform the grueling work required in the mines."
 Laws against ingestion of the plant go back centuries also. Christian missionaries saw the devil in the leaf, and four hundred years ago colonialist governments passed laws against chewing coca. Subsequent to imposition of the laws, the use of coca was perceived to increase, rather than the opposite. This result, Maher ingenuously surmises, was "a natural consequence in defiance of prohibitive laws."

Today, importation of leaves and manufacture of cocaine are tightly controlled under federal narcotics laws. Only two companies, the Stepan Chemical Company and Merck & Company, are licensed by the Justice Department to import coca leaves to make cocaine. In 1969, according to Justice Department figures, 268,679 kilos of leaves were imported to produce 1,184 kilos of cocaine—and 884 kilos of that were exported, primarily to European countries where cocaine is more widely used than here as an anesthetic.

For cocaine manufacture, leaves are picked by hand and dried slowly in the sun. Cocaine, produced either as an alkaloid powder or a more water-soluble hydrochloride, results from a complex process of washing and percolating the dried, crushed leaves with solvents and other chemicals. According to the Narcotics Bureau, clandestine laboratories in South America—especially in Peru and Bolivia—are the source of nearly all illegal cocaine. In powdered form, the drug is smuggled into the United States primarily through Miami and New York.

In general, discussion of the "drug problem" tends to be rabid and uninformed. Talk on cocaine is no exception. Cogent answers to the salient questions—How dangerous is cocaine? Is it addictive? How widespread is its use?—are scarce. And there is much authoritative contradiction.

One major problem has been, of course, that talk about "drugs" has lumped together everything from marijuana to heroin, as if central generalizations could be made (the blows struck by Harry Anslinger and his Federal Narcotics Bureau in the 1930s were powerful and have had lasting effect), although lately it has become acceptable to treat marijuana separately and somewhat more lightly. But cocaine and heroin are still almost universally united under the topic of "hard drugs" (a vague term used to imply serious danger) or "narcotics," despite the fact that they are medically and pharmacologically opposites. Indiana University sociology professor Alfred R. Lindesmith wrote in *The Addict and the Law* (1965) that the opiates (opium, morphine, heroin) "are so completely different from such substances as marijuana and cocaine that they cannot intelligently be discussed together with them...."

Unlike the amphetamines—which ironically may turn out to be more dangerous and habit-forming than cocaine—pure cocaine cannot be obtained by a doctor's prescription. In terms of dealing with "hard drugs," this is an important fact. A druggist's normal mark-up for profit on cocaine, were he permitted to sell it to private citizens, would put the price at something like $50 an ounce. A respectable druggist I know, who hasn't been presented a prescription for cocaine solution in ten years (the last was for a patient suffering hemorrhoidal bleeding), was the other day offered $1,000 for an ounce—about the going rate for pure in the underworld.

CHAPTER 25

Proposals for the Evaluation of Cocaine

1974

ADVERTISEMENT The National Institute on Drug Abuse, United States Government. From *Commerce and Business Daily,* January, 1974

On January 17, 1974 The National Institute on Drug Abuse placed the following advertisement in Commerce Business Daily, a listing of government contract requirements. This is a request to institutions who might have the facilities to fulfil the project requirements. The ad may be considered to be a catalog of what we don't know about cocaine. Ed.

Metabolism and Pharmacokinetic Studies on Cocaine in Animals and/or Man

The National Institute on Drug Abuse is soliciting source information from qualified organizations having the capability and facilities to develop and/or implement sensitive and specific analytical methodology for cocaine and its metabolites in biological materials, and to employ appropriate analytic procedures and pharmacological methodology to investigate the metabolic and pharmacokinetic profile of cocaine in animals and/or man. More specifically, this would involve such aspects as the determination of the plasma levels, half-life of cocaine and its major metabolites, the rate of absorption and elimination of cocaine from various routes of administration and in acute and chronically treated animals and/or investigation of these parameters acutely in man. Pharmacokinetic data would be correlated with the onset and duration of measurable pharmacological effects.

To qualify, organizations must give adequate evidence of knowledge and experience in the area of pharmacology, bioanalytic methodology and pharmacokinetic analysis. Additionally, expertise in Phase I human studies may be required. Organizations may reply in the areas of animal and/or human studies. Responses must refer to SS–NIDA–74–13. (RO14)

Acquire Information and Prepare Bibliographic Materials on Drug Abuse Topics

The National Institute on Drug Abuse is soliciting source information from qualified organizations having the capability of developing an advanced alerting mechanism utilizing contacts across

382   Cocaine Papers

the country and other resources to identify information trends for the Clearinghouse. The contractor will then comprehensively search the literature on these trends and will develop 8 annotated bibliographies throughout a twelve-month period.

To qualify, organizations must give adequate evidence of knowledge and experience in developing annotated bibliographies; assessing underground drug information and program contacts, and assessing standard information resources. Responses must refer to SS–NIDA–74–8. (RO14)

Studies on Patterns and Life Styles of Human Cocaine Users/Abusers

The National Institute on Drug Abuse is soliciting source information from qualified organizations having the capability and facilities to investigate non–medical cocaine use/abuse in humans. More specifically, this would involve estimation of extent, duration and frequency to which cocaine is used in conjunction with other drugs, and at what point cocaine use enters the progression and experimentation of human drug abuse. This would entail using representative case design methodologies to characterize typical cocaine users and their life styles.

To qualify, organizations must give adequate evidence of (1) knowledge and experience in the area of social psychological drug use/abuse, (2) clear evidence of research methodologies such as personality clustering procedures, factor analysis, and representative case designs, and (3) access to appropriate and representative samples of cocaine users either by case record or by interview protocols. Submitters should carefully delineate the sources of data to be used in terms of general demographic and epidemiologic characteristics of the users to be studied. Responses must refer to SS–NIDA–74–16. (RO12)

Matched Comparison of Selected Human Cocaine Users

The National Institute on Drug Abuse is soliciting source information from qualified organizations having the capacity and facilities to perform a feasibility study to compare carefully matched human subjects who use cocaine. Specifically, the project would entail locating and then comparing groups of persons who use cocaine via at least two different routes of administration (shooters, chewers and snorters). The subjects to be studied should be matched on basic demographic and epidemiological characteristics, particularly their geographic location either inside the United States or in a foreign country where both forms of cocaine intake are practiced.

To qualify, organizations must give adequate evidence of (1) knowledge and experience in the psychosocial aspect of drug use/abuse, (2) clear documentation of research expertise in similar types of projects, with examples of methodologies used, and (3) availability of data sources with a description of the kinds of data to be collected. Responses must refer to Notice SS–NIDA–74–17. (RO12)

Evaluation of Cocaine on Complex Human Performance

The National Institute on Drug Abuse is soliciting source information from qualified organizations having the capability and facilities to investigate the effects that cocaine has on complex human performance. More specifically, this would involve determining acute dose-response relationships between cocaine and such tasks as vigilance performance, timing behavior, reaction time, pursuit rates, and problem solving. Further, this would involve the tracing of the time course of the drug's effects.

To qualify organizations must give adequate evidence of knowledge and experience in the area of psychopharmacology, behavioral analysis, and psychomotor performance. Additionally, expertise in Phase I human studies would be required. Responses must refer to SS–NIDA–74–11. (RO14)

Evaluation of Cocaine on Aggressive Behavior

The National Institute on Drug Abuse is soliciting source information from qualified organizations having the capability and facilities to investigate the effects that cocaine has on animal aggression. More specifically, this would involve evaluating the dose–response relations between acute and chronic cocaine administration and aggression exhibited by animals in such models as shock–elicited fighting, isolation–induced aggression, predatory aggression, etc. Furthermore, the time course of these effects should be determined.

To qualify, organizations must give adequate evidence of knowledge and experience in the area of psychopharmacology, behavioral analysis, and animal aggression. Responses must refer to SS–NIDA–74–10. (RO14)

Evaluation of Acute Effects of Cocaine in Humans

The National Institute on Drug Abuse is soliciting source information from qualified organizations having the capabilities and facilities to evaluate the acute physiological and pharmacological effects of cocaine by selected routes of administration in a systematic manner. Particular attention should be given to the occurrence of drug related side effects, estimation of the safe dosage range for the compound, and limits and characteristics of toxicity of the compound. Other parameters to be measured include general vital physiology, EKG, EEG, EMG, blood and urine chemistries, gross behavioral effects, etc.

To qualify, organizations must give adequate evidence of knowledge and experience in the area of clinical drug studies with expertise in clinical physiology, biochemistry, pharmacology and psychology. More specifically, they should show knowledge and experience with psychoactive agents and with the methodological approaches used to study their acute effects. Evidence of a review mechanism to insure human subject rights must also be presented. Responses must refer to SS–NIDA–74–16. (RO14)

Synthesis of Labeled Cocaine and its Metabolites

The National Institute on Drug Abuse is soliciting source information from qualified organizations having the capability and facilities to synthesize designated quantities of labeled cocaine which may be labeled with carbon-13, carbon-14, tritium or deuterium, and labeled and unlabeled cocaine metabolites, as requested by the Project Officer. Furthermore, the organization will also be responsible for maintaining the purity and for distributing of the compounds.

To qualify, organizations must give adequate evidence of knowledge and experience in the area of synthesis of labeled compounds of various specific activities. In addition, expertise in designing the synthesis of specifically labeled as well as randomly labeled compounds is essential. Furthermore adequate evidence must be given that the laboratory is suitably registered for the production and handling of Schedule I substances. Responses must refer to SS–NIDA–74–12. (RO14)

Facts and Myths About Human Cocaine Use/Abuse

The National Institute on Drug Abuse is soliciting source information from qualified organizations having the capability and facilities to investigate facts and myths about cocaine use/abuse. More specifically, this would involve an intensive literature search of the professional and lay literature as well as street myths relating to the effects of cocaine use. Moreover this would entail discussion of rituals of use, sharing behaviors, monetary costs, achieved statuses, and the mood states displayed by users both before, during and after use. This project would require sophisticated and broad ranged literature searches.

To qualify, organizations must give adequate evidence of (1) knowledge and experience in the psychosocial aspects of drug use/abuse, (2) clear documentation of research expertise in similar types of projects, with examples of methodologies used, and (3) availability of data sources with a description of the kinds of data to be collected. Responses must refer to SS–NIDA–74–15. (RO14)

Source information previously submitted to this office or any other office will not be considered. Therefore, interested organizations must submit organizational data and background, qualifications of professional personnel, specific experience in the area of the above nine projects, availability of qualified personnel and facilities necessary to undertake the work involved as well as any other pertinent information including samples of work. Samples will not be returned. The above are not requests for proposals. Acknowledgement of receipt of responses will not be made and telephone inquiries will not be honored. Only those sources deemed best qualified for the work under consideration will be invited to submit proposals when and if requests for proposals are initiated. Responses must be submitted within ten days from the date of this publication.

Contracting Officer,
Room 7C–2S,
National Institute on Drug Abuse,
Parklawn Building (7C–2S),
5800 Fishers Lane,
Rockville, MD 20852

Chapter Notes

Introduction

1. Sigmund Freud, *The Cocaine Papers,* A. K. Donoghue and J. Hillman, editors. 1963 Vienna, Zurich; Dunquin Press, 62 pp.
2. J. Murdoch Ritchie, "Cocaine, Procaine and other Synthetic Local Anesthetics," in *The Pharmacological Basis of Therapeutics,* Alfred Gilman and Louis Goodman, editors. 1970 London/Toronto, Macmillan & Company. pp. 371–401.
3. Jurgen Vom Schéidt, "Sigmund Freud und das Kokain," *Psyche,* 1973, Volume 27, pp. 385–429.
4. Louis Lewin, *Phantastica, Narcotic and Stimulating Drugs their Use and Abuse,* 1931 New York, E. P. Dutton & Company. 335 pp.
5. Bo Holmstedt, "Historical Survey," in *Ethnopharmacologic Search for Psychoactive Drugs,* D. H. Efron, B. Holmstedt, and N. S. Kline, editors. 1967 Washington, D.C., Public Health Service, HEW. pp. 3–32.
6. J. J. Moreau de Tours, *Hashish and Mental Illness,* H. Peters and G. G. Nahas, editors. Translated by G. J. Barnett. 1973 New York, Raven Press, 245 pp.
7. Albert Hoffmann, "The Discovery of LSD and Subsequent Investigations on Naturally Occurring Hallucinogens," in *Discoveries in Biological Psychiatry,* F. J. Ayd and B. Blackwell, editors. 1970 Philadelphia, J. B. Lippincott Co. pp. 93–94.
8. Ibid.
9. Gordon Alles, "Some Relations Between Chemical Structure and Physiological Action of Mescaline and Related Compounds," in *Neuropharmacology,* H. A. Abramson, editor. 1959 New York, Josiah Macy, Jr. Foundation. pp. 169–97.
10. Aldous Huxley, *The Doors of Perception.* 1954 New York, Harper & Row Brothers. pp. 65–66.
11. David F. Musto, *The American Disease: Origins of Narcotic Control.* 1973 New Haven, Yale University Press, pg. 7.
12. Sir Arthur Conan Doyle, "The Sign of the Four," in *The Annotated Sherlock Holmes,* W. S. Baring-Gould, editor. 1967 New York, Clarkson N. Potter, Inc. pp. 610–611.
13. Edward M. Brecher and the editors of *Consumer Report, Licit and Illicit Drugs: The Consumers Union Report on Narcotics, Stimulants, Depressants, Inhalants, Hallucinogens, and Marijuana—including Caffeine, Nicotine, and Alcohol.* 1972 Boston, Little, Brown & Company. pp. 33–34.
14. Loc. cit.
15. Frank Berger and J. Potterfield, "The Effect of Anti-anxiety Tran-

388 Cocaine Papers

quilizers on the Behavior of Normal Persons," in *The Psychopharmacology of the Normal Human*. W. O. Evans and N. S. Kline, editors. 1969 Springfield, Ill., Charles C. Thomas. pg. 99.
16. Larry Stein, *Psychotomimetic Drugs*, D. H. Efron, editor. 1970 New York, Raven Press. pg. 343.
17. Jerome Jaffe, "Drug Addiction and Drug Abuse" in L. Goodman and A. Gilman (op. cit). pp. 276–313.
18. W. Golden Mortimer, M.D., *Peru-History of Coca*, "The Divine Plant of the Incas." With an introductory account of the Incas and of the Andean Indians of today. 1901 New York, J. H. Vail Company, XXXI, p. 576.

Chapter One (The Cocaine Episode Part One)

1. Freud, Sigmund, *An Autobiographical Study*. Translated by James Strachey. London: 1935 Hogarth. 137 pp.

Chapter Two (Freud's Sources)

1. *Detroit Therapeutic Gazette*, Vol. I, No. 9. September 15, 1880.
2. *Detroit Therapeutic Gazette*, Vol. I, No. 6, June 15, 1880.
3. *Deutsche Medizinische Wochenschrift*, No. 50, December 12, 1883, pp. 730–32. Translated by Therese Byck.
4. See the *Journal for Pharmacodynamics*, Vol. IV. 1857.
5. See "*Sulle virtu igieniche e medicinali della coca, e sugli alimenti nervosi in generale.*" Milano 1859.
6. W. Z. N. F., III. 28. 1860.
7. *Prager Vierteljahrsschrift*. LXXIX p. 109.
8. Ball de Ther. LXX pg. 175, 28 Fevr. 1866.

Chapter Three (The Cocaine Episode, Part Two)

1. Hanns Sachs, *Freud, Master and Friend*. 1944 Cambridge, Mass: Harvard University. p. 71.

Freud's reference style is frequently inconsistent and often it would be impossible to find the original book or article, without having more information. The references are given here as originally written, and Freud's explanatory footnotes are placed below the text of the articles. A standard reference method was not in use, but Freud's using Detroit Therapeutic Gazette, Detroit, Th.G., Th.G., D.T.G., *and* T.G. *for the same journal, illustrates the haste in which he wrote* Über Coca. *He was using* The Surgeon General's Catalogue *for his reference list which shows the* Detroit Therapeutic Gazette *as* Therap. Gaz., Detroit. Ed.

Chapter Five (Über Coca)

1. O. R. Markham. *Peruvian Barks*, London: 1880.
2. According to Bibra's estimate. *Narcotic Stimulants*, 1885.
3. Weddell. *Voyage dans le Nord de la Bolivie*, 1853.
4. Scrivener, "On the coca leaf and its use in diet and medicine," *Medical Times and Gazette*, 1871.
5. Garcilasso de la Vega. *Commentarios reales de los Incas*. 1609–1617.
6. Christison, "Observations on the effect of cuca, or coca, the leaves of Erythroxylon Coca." *British Medical Journal*, 1876. Bibra. Loc. cit.
7. Mantegazza, *"Sulle virtu igieniche e medicanali della coca."* Milan: 1859.
8. Scrivener. Loc. cit.
9. According to Ullo, whom Bibra copies.
10. *Systema mat. med. brasil.*, 1843.
11. *Essai sur la coca du Pérou*, Thesis. Paris: 1862
12. cf. Fronmüller. "Coca and Cat." *Prager Vierteljahresschrift für praktische Heilkunde*, v. 79, 1863.
13. *Víagem de cidade de Cuzco a de Belem*, 1840.
14. *Expédition dans les parties centrales de l'Amerique du Sud*, 1851.
15. Spix's and Martius' *Journal in Brazil*, 1831.
16. Loc. cit.
17. *Travel sketches from Peru in 1838 and 1842*.
18. Loc. cit.
19. *Journey Round the World*, 1835.
20. *Travels in Peru and India*, 1862.
21. *Journey in Chile, Peru and on the Amazon River*, 1827–32.
22. *Disertacion sobre el aspecto, cultivo, comercio y virtudes de la famosa planta del Peru nombrado Coca*. Lima: 1794.
23. *Historical and descriptive narrative of twenty years residence in South America*. 1825.
24. Fronmüller. Loc. cit.
25. "The Coca Leaf." *Lancet*. 1876.
26. *Disertacion sobre Hayo o Coca*. Lima: 1793.
27. *Memoria sobre la coca*. Lima: 1793.
28. Mantegazza, "Sulle virtú igieniche e medicinali della coca. Memoria onorata del Premio dell'Acqua nel concorso di 1858, estratto dagli Annali Universali di Medicina 1859." A short paper contained in the *Oesterreichische Zeitschrift für praktische Heilkunde*, of the same year.
29. *Annal. d. Chemie u. Pharmac.* 114, and *Vierteljahresschrift für praktische Pharmacie*, 9.
30. *Annalen. d. Chemie und Pharmacie*, 133.
31. Husemann and Higler. *"Plant Substances, etc."* 1884; Girtler. "On Coca, extract of coca and cocaine." *Wiener Med. Wochenschrift:* 1862.

32. "On the physiological effects of cocaine," *Pflügers Archiv,* XXI, 1880.
33. "Preliminary report on cocaine," *Wochenblatt der Gesellschaft der Aerzte in Wien,* 1862.
34. *Recherches Chimiques et physiologiques sur l'Erythroxylon Coca du Pérou,* 1868.
35. "Cocaine and Diabetes," 1872 (Russian).
36. "Contribution to the study of the effects of cocaine on the animal organism." (Russian).
37. "On the physiological effects and the therapeutic use of cocaine," 1872 (Russian).
38. "An experimental inquiry into the physiological action of Theine, etc., etc" *Edinburgh Medical and Surgical Journal,* 1874.
39. "Coca and its alkaloid cocaine," *New York Medical Record,* 1876.
40. Finska läkaresällsk. handl. XX, 1878.
41. "De la coca et de ses véritables propriétés thérapeutiques," *L'Union Médicale,* 1877.
42. "Sur l'action physiologique des feuilles de coca," *Echo Medical Suisse,* 1861.
43. *Essai sur la coca du Pérou,* Thesis, Paris: 1862.
44. "Note sur l'emploi de la coca." *Bulletin de Thérapeutique,* 1866.
45. "Observations on the effect of cuca, or coca, etc." *British Medical Journal,* 1876.
46. "Experiences in connection with the therapeutic use of coca leaves," *Deutsche Klinik,* 1867.
47. J. Collan, *Finska läkaresällsk. handl.* XX, 1878-from *Schmidt's Yearbooks,* 87, 1880.
48. "Erythroxylon coca; its physiological effects, etc." *Boston Medical and Surgical Journal,* 1882.
49. "The physiological effects of *cocainum muriaticum* on the human body and their significance. Observations carried out during the autumn maneuvers of the Third Bavarian Army Corps in 1883," *Deutsche med. Wochenschrift,* December 12, 1883.
50. Loc. cit.
51. Ploss. *Zeitschrift für Chirurgie,* 1863.
52. *Philadelphia Medical and Surgical Reporter,* 1883.
53. *Detroit Therapeutic Gazette,* February 1883.
54. "Review of some of our later remedies." *Detroit, Th.G.,* December, 1880.
55. "Ricerche sperimentali sull'azione fisiologica e terapeutica della cocaina," *Rendiconti del R. 1st Lombardo,* XIV, 1882.
56. *Pharmakologisch-Therapeutisches Handbuch,* Erlangen, 1862.
57. "Communication on coca," by Dr. Josef Frankl, spa doctor in Marienbad. *Zeitschrift der K. Gesellschaft der Aerzte,* 1860.
58. "Erythroxylon coca in the treatment of typhus and typhoid fevers, and also of other febrile diseases." *British Medical Journal,* v. 1 for 1887.
59. *Detroit Therapeutic Gazette,* July, 1880.

60. "Coca Erythroxylon in exhaustion." *Detroit, Th.G.* October, 1880.
61. *Detroit, Th.G.* September, 1880, based on the *Louisville Medical News*.
62. Marvaud. *Les aliments d'epargne.* Paris: 1874.
63. "Physiology of general metabolism." 1881, *Hermann's Handbuch,* VI, 1.
64. "Erythroxylon coca, its physiological effect especially its effect on the excretion of urea by the kidneys." *Boston Med. and Surgical Journal,* 1882.
65. *Comptes rendus de l'Académies des Sciences,* II, 1870.
66. In Marvaud.
67. "Pathology and Treatment in venereal diseases." In *Detroit, Th.G.* February 1884.
68. Loc. cit.
69. "Erythroxylon coca in the Opium and alcohol habits." *D.T.G.* September, 1880.
70. *D.T.G.* November, 1880.
71. J. Brenton, *T.G.* March, 1881; G. H. Gray, from "The medical brief," *T.G.* June, 1881; H. Leforger, Dec. 1872.
72. E. C. Huse, *T.G.* September, 1880; Henderson, *T.G.* February, 1881.
73. R. Taggart, *T.G.* May, 1881; A. F. Stimmel, *TG.* July, 1881.
74. W. H. Bentley, *T.G.* September (18)80; Volum. January 1881; H. Warner, March (18)81; Stimmel, April and July, (18)81.
75. *Travels in Peru and India,* 1862.
76. "The Erythroxylon coca in asthma." *Philadelphia Medical and Surgical Reporter,* 1881.
77. *T.G.,* Dec. 1880.
78. "De la coca et de ses véritables propriétés thérapeutiques." *L'Union médicale,* 1877.

Chapter Eight (Papers on Coca and other Prospects)

1. Vom Schéidt, J. "Sigmund Freud und das Kokain," *Psyche* 27:385–429 (1973).

Chapter Nine (Contributions to the Knowledge of Cocaine)

1. *"Über Coca," Centralbl. f.d. ges. Therapie,* II Vol., VII, July (not August as often incorrectly cited), 1884. [This is a slap at Koller for an error in quoting the date of Freud's *Über Coca*. See Bernfeld, p. 328 this edition. Ed.]
2. *Pflüger's Archive,* VII. Appendix to the article mentioned.
3. "Variations in human muscle strength during the course of the day," *Berlin Clinical Weekly,* No. 28, 1884.

4. *The Influence of Sleep on Human Muscle Strength,* Petersburg 1883.

Chapter Eleven (On the General Effect of Cocaine)

1. Richter, *Zeitschrift für Ther.* No. 7, 1885.

Chapter Twelve (Parke's Universal Panacea)

1. F. E. Stewart, M.D.P.H.G., in *Philadelphia Medical Times,* September 19, 1885.
2. James L. Minor, M.D., in *Medical Record,* February 7, 1885.

Chapter Seventeen (The Cocaine Episode, Part Four)

1. Letter from Freud to Martha Bernays. July 9, 1885.
2. Wallé, *Deutsche medizinische Zeitung,* 1885, No. 3.
3. Erlenmeyer, "Ueber Cocain-sucht," *Deutsche medizinische Zeitung,* May, 1886; reprinted in *Wiener medizinische Presse,* July, 1886, pp. 918–921.
4. Pp. 155–159.
5. *Internationale Klinische Rundschau,* III (1888), 23.
6. Freud, *Gesammelte Werke.* Vol. II/III p. 116, London: Imago 1940–1952.
7. Freud, "Bemerkungen über Cocainsucht und Cocainfurcht," *Wiener medizinische Wochenschrift,* July 9, 1887, p. 929.
8. Unpublished letter from Freud to Martha Bernays. January 7, 1885.
9. Freud, *Gesammelte Werke.* Vol. II/III p. 123.
10. Unpublished letter from Freud to Martha Bernays. May 10, 1886; *Gesammelte Werke.* Vol. II/III p. 245.
11. F. Wittels, *Sigmund Freud: Der Mann,* d. *Lehre,* d. *Schule.* (Vienna: Tal, 1923), p. 21.
12. Letter to Fritz Wittels, December 18, 1923.
13. Private communication.
14. Freud, *Gesammelte Werke,* Vol. II/III p. 116.

Chapter Twenty-One ("Coca Koller")

1. Hardy, Florence Emily, *Early Life of Thomas Hardy,* 1840–1891. New York: The Macmillan Company, 1928.
2. Unpublished letters, documents, contemporary newspaper articles, etc., 1872.
3. Ibid

4. Koller, Carl: *"Beiträge zur Kenntniss des Hühnerkeims in Beginne der Bebrutung." (Von. Stud. Med. Carl Koller aus den Institut für Allgemeine und Experimentelle Pathologie, Wien.) Vorgelegt in der Sitzung am 20 November,* 1879 von. Prof. Stricker, *aus dem Sitzb. der K. Akad. der Wissensch.* III abth.
5. Kölliker, Rudolph Albert, Von: *Die Entwicklung der Keimblatter des Kaninchens. Festischrift zur Feier des 300 jahrigen Bestehens der Julius Maximilians Universitat zu Wurzburg.* Leipzig, 1882.
6. Hertwig, Oskar: *"Lehrbuch der Entwicklungsgeschichte des Menschen und der Wirbelthiere" Jena: Verlag von Gustav Fischer,* 1888.
7. Koller, Carl: Unpubl. let., doc., Op. cit.
8. Koller, Carl: "Personal Reminiscences of the First Use of Cocaine as a Local Anesthetic in Eye Surgery." Read at the Sixth Annual Congress of the Anesthetists of the United States and Canada in Joint Meeting with the *International Anesthesia Research Society,* VII, No. 1, January–February, 1928.
9. Prescott, William, H: "Education-Quipus-Astronomy-Agriculture-Guano-Important Esculents." *History of the Conquest of Peru,* Vol. I Edited by John Foster Kirk. Philadelphia: J. B. Lippincott & Co., 1847 p. 143.
10. Mariani, Angelo: *Coca and Its Therapeutic Application.* New York: J. N. Jaros, 1896.
11. Vogl, August: *"Histologisch-Pharmakognostische Notizen. Separatabdruck aus der Zeitschrift des Allg. Oster." Apothekerverein. Vorantwortl. Redakteur Fr. Klinger, druck von Carl Uberreuter* in *Wien.* n.d.
12. Op. cit.
13. Noyes, H. D.; "A few cursory notes on the Proceedings of the German Ophthalmological Society in the middle of September, this year." *Medical Record,* XXVI, October 11, 1884. p. 417.
14. Prescott, Wm. Op. cit.
15. Knapp, Herman: "On Cocaine and its Use in Ophthalmic and General Surgery." *Arch. Ophthalmology,* XIII, Nos. 3 and 4, 1884.
16. Koller, Carl. "On the Beginnings of Local Anesthesia." Speech before the *Brooklyn Ophthalmological Society,* April 18, 1940.
17. Loc. cit.
18. Freud: *Autobiography.* Translated by James Strachey. New York: W. W. Norton & Company, Inc., 1935.
19. Koller, Carl: *Personal Reminiscenses.* Op. cit.
20. Knapp, Herman. Op. cit.
21. Aschenbrandt, Theodor: "Die Physiologische Wirkung und Bedeutung des Cocain auf den menschlichen Organismus." *Deutsche medizinische Wochenschrift,* No. 50, December 12, 1883. pp. 730–732.
22. Koller, Carl: "Historical Notes on the Beginnings of Local Anesthesia." *J. Amer. Med. Assn.,* XC, No. 211928, pp. 1742–1743.
23. Koller, Carl. Op. cit.
24. Loc. cit.

25. Freud: "Über Coca." *Centralblatt für die gesammte Therapie,* II, No. 7, July, 1884, pp. 289–314.
26. Koller. Loc. cit.
27. Koller, Carl: Untitled paper dated August 1915.
28. Gaertner, J: "Die Entdeckung der Lokalanasthesie." Vienna: *Der neue Tag,* 1919.
29. Noyes, H. D. Op. cit.
30. Koller, Carl: "Über die Verwendung des Cocaine zur Anästhesierung am Auge." *Wiener medizinische Wochenschrift,* XXXIV, Nos. 43 and 44, 1884.
31. Ibid.
32. Ibid.
33. Jellinek, Edmund: "Das Cocain als Anästheticum und Analgeticum fur den Pharynx und Larynx." *Wiener medizinische Wochenschrift,* XXXIV, No. 45–46, November 8, 1884.
34. Koller. Loc. cit.
35. Noyes. Loc. cit.
36. Knapp, Herman. Loc. cit.
37. Freud: "Beitrag zur Kenntniss der Cocawirkung." *Wiener medizinische Wochenschrift,* XXXV, No. 5, 1885.
38. Freud: "Über Coca." Neu durchgesehener und vermehrter Separatabdruck aus dem *Centralblatt für die gesammte Therapie.* Vienna: Verlag von Moritz Perles, 1885.
39. Freud: Auto. Loc. cit.
40. Loc. cit.
41. Koller, Carl: "Cocain als örtliches Anästheticum." *Berlin Klin. Wochenschrift,* XXII, No. 1, 1885, p. 2.
42. Bernfeld, Siegfried: "Freud's Studies on Cocaine," 1884–1887. *J. Amer. Psa. Assn.,* I, 1953, pp. 581–613.
  Jones, Ernest: *The Life and Work of Sigmund Freud.* Vol. I, New York, Basic Books, Inc., 1953.
43. Ibid.
44. Fackel, Die: *Universitats Bummel.* (signed: J. R.) Karl Kraus, Editor. XI, mid-July, 1899.
45. Bier, August: *Die Seele.* Munich: Verlag F. L. Lehmann, 1938.
46. J., Dr: "A Glorious Day in Austrian Medicine." *Der Wiener Tag.* April 29, 1934.
47. Meller, J: "Gedenkworte zum 50 Jahrestage des Vortrages von Dr. Carl Koller über das Kokain," vor der Gesellschaft der Artze in Wien. *Wiener klinische Wochenschrift,* XLVII, No. 44, November, 1934.
48. Loc. cit.
49. Wagenmann, A: "Erste Wissenschaftliche Sitzung," Montag, August 6, 1934. *Bericht uber die 50 Ausammenkunft der Deutschen Ophthalmologischen Gesellschaft in Heidelberg.* Munchen: Verlag J. F. von Bermann, 1934.
50. Bloom, S: Dr. Carl Koller. *Obituary.* Arch Ophthalmology, XXXI, 1944, pp. 344–345.

Chapter Twenty-Two (Freud's Studies on Cocaine)

1. Bernfeld, S. "Sigmund Freud, M.D. 1882–1885," *Int. J. Psa;* XXXII Part 3, 1951.
2. Freud S: (1925) An *Autobiographical Study,* Translated by James Strachey, London: 1935, Hogarth Press.
3. Aschenbrandt, T: "Die physiologische Wirkung und Bedeutung des Cocain insbesondere auf den menschlichen Organismus, Klinische Beobachtungen während der Herbstwaffenübung," 1883 beim 11. Bayer, A. C. 4 Div. 9. Reg. 2. Bat. *Deutsche med. Wochenschr.,* No. 50, 12. Dez., 1883, pp. 730–732.
4. Freud, S: "Ueber die Allgemeinwirkung des Cocains, Vortrag gehalten im psychiatrischen Verein," 5. Marz, 1885, *Med.-chirur. Centralbl.,* XX, No. 32, Wien, 7. August, 1885, pp. 374–376.
5. Ibid.
6. Aschenbrandt, T. Op. cit.
7. Freud, S. (1925) *Auto. study* op. cit.
8. Freud, S: *"Über Coca,"* Centrabl. f. d. ges. *Therapie* (Wien) II, Juli, 1884 pp. 289–314.
9. Ibid.
10. Ibid.
11. Freud, S: "Beitrag zur kenntnis der Cocawirkung," *Wien, Med. Wochenschr.,* XXXV, No. 5, January, 1885 pp. 129–133.
12. Freud, S: *"Über Coca"* Op. cit.
13. Ibid
14. Ibid.
15. Ibid.
16. Maier, H. W: *La Cocäine. Historique-Pathologie-Clinique-Thérapeutique-Defense Sociale,* translated by S. Jankelivitsch, Payot, Paris, 1928, p. 493.
17. Brun, R: "Sigmund Freud's Leistungen auf dem Gebiet der organischen Neurologie," *Schweiz. Arch. Neurol. & Psychiat.,* XXXVII, 1936, pp. 200–207.
18. Jelliffe, S. E: "Sigmund Freud as a Neurologist," *J. Nerv. & Ment. Dis.,* LXXXV, 1937, pp. 696–711.
19. Koller, K: "Personal Reminiscences of the First Use of Cocaine as a Local Anesthetic in Eye Surgery," *Anesthesia and Analgesia,* January–February, 1928 pp. 10–11.
20. Ibid.
21. Gärtner, G: "Die Entdeckung der Lokalanaesthesie," in *Der Neue Tag,* Wien, 1919.
22. Koller, K: "Vorläufige Mitteilung über locale Anaesthesierung am Auge." *Versam. d. Opthal. Gesellschaft,* Stuttgart, XVI, 1884, pp. 60–63.
23. Koller, K: "Ueber die Verwendung des Cocains zur Anaesthesierung am Auge," *Wien Med. Wochenschr.,* No. 43, pp. 1276–1278; No. 44, pp. 1309–1311, 1884. English translation by Knapp: "On

the use of Cocaine to anesthetize the Eye," *Arch. Ophthal.*, December, 1884.
24. Freud, S: "Beitrag zur Kenn. der Coca wirk. Op. cit.
25. *Weiner Medizinische Wochenschrift*, 1884, p. 1287.
26. *Centralblatt f. d. ges. Therapie*, Vol. 2, 1884, pp. 524–526; *Wiener Med. Presse*, Vol. 25, 1884, pp. 1340–1342; 1365–1368; 1377.
27. Königstein, L: "Ueber das Cocain und seine Anwendung," *Monatsblätter des wissenschaftlichen Club in Wien*, Supplement 3, No. 3, 1885.
28. Seeling, M. G: "History of Cocaine as a Local Anesthetic," Letter to the Editor, *J.A.M.A.*, October 11, 1941.
29. Wittels, F: *Sigmund Freud: Der Mann, die Lehre, die Schule*, Wien, 1924.
30. Freud S: "Beitrag zur Kenn. der Coca wirk. Op. Cit.
31. Freud S: *Gessammelte Werk*, Vols. II & XIV, Imago Publishing Company, London, 1942 & 1948.
32. Wittels, F. Op. cit.
33. Sachs, H: *Freud: Master and Friend*, Harvard University Press, Cambridge, 1944.
34. Freud, S: *The Basic Writings of Sigmund Freud*, translated by A. A. Brill, Modern Library, New York, 1938.
35. Ibid.
36. Freud, S: "Beitrag zur Kenn. der Coca Wirk.," Op. cit.
37. Ibid.
38. Freud, S: "Gutachten über das Parke Cocain, in Gutt, Ueber die verschiedenen Cocain-Präparate und deren Wirkung, *"Wien Med, Presse*, XXVI, No. 32, August, 1885, p. 1036.
39. Freud, S: *Über coca, Neu durchgesehener und vermehrter Separat-Abdruck aus dem Centralbl. f. d. ges. Therapie*, Verlag Moritz Perles, Wien, 1885, pp. 1–26.
40. Freud, S: "Bemerkungen über Cocainsucht und Cocainfurcht, mit Beziehung auf einen Vortrag W. A. Hammond's," *Wien. Med. Wochenschr.*, No. 28, 9. Juli, 1887, pp. 929–932.
41. Ibid.
42. Freud, S: "Ueber die allgem. des Cocains, etc. " Op. cit.
43. Ibid.
44. Freud, S: "Bemer. K. über Cocainsuch und Cocainfur., etc." Op. cit.
45. Erlenmeyer, A: "Ueber die Wirkung des Cocain bei der Morphiumentziehung," *Centralbl. d. Nervenheilkunde*, VIII, Juli, 1885, pp. 289–299.
46. Obersteiner, H: "Ueber intoxicationspsychosen," *Wien. Med. Presse*, XXIV, No. 4, January, 1886.
47. Erlenmeyer, A. Op. cit.
48. Ibid.
49. Freud, S: *Gesammelte Werke* Op. cit.
50. Freud, S: *An Auto. Study* Op. cit.

51. Freud, S: Screen Memories, *Coll. Papers,* V, Hogarth Press, London, 1950, pp. 47–78.
52. Freud, S: *An Auto. Study* Op. cit.
53. Freud, S: "Bemer. K. über Cocainsuch. . . ." Op. cit.
54. Ibid.
55. Ibid.
56. Ibid.
57. Freud, S: "Ueber die Allegem. des Cocains . . ." Op. cit.
58. Freud, S: "Bemer. K. über Cocainsucht. . . ." Op. cit.
59. Freud, S: "Inhaltsangaben der wissenschaftlichen Arbeiten des Privatdozenten Sigm. Freud (1887–1897)," *Gesammelte Werke,* I, pp. 461–488.
60. Brun, R: Op. cit.
61. Freud, S: *Gesammelte Werke,* Op. cit.
62. Ibid.
63. Freud, S: *An Auto. Study* Op. cit.

Chapter Twenty-Three (Sherlock Holmes and Sigmund Freud)

1. Monardes, N: *Joyfull Newes out of the Newe Founde Worlde,* translated by John Frampton, London, 1577, reprinted with an introduction by Stephen Gaselee, New York, 1925, A. A. Knopf, 2 vols. vol 2, pp. 31–32.
2. Montegazza, Paolo: *Sulle virtu igieniche e medicinali della coca,* Milan, 1859.
3. Niemann, A.: *Ueber eine neue organische Base in den Coca blattern,* Göttingen, 1860.
4. Schroff, C.: Vorlaufige Mittbeilungen über Cocain, *Wehnbld k. k. Gesell. d. Arzte in Wien,* 18:233, 1862.
5. Christison, R.: Observations on the effects of the leaves of Erythroxylon coca, *Brit. Med. J.,* Lond. pp. 527–531, 1876.
6. Dowdeswell, G. F.: The Coca Leaf. Observations on the Properties and Action of the Leaf of the Coca Plant (Erythroxylon coca), made in the Physiological Laboratory of University College, *Lancet 1:*631–3; 665–7, 1876.
7. Stockwell, G. Archie: Erythroxylon Coca, *Boston Med. & Surg. J. 96:*399–404, 1877.
8. Huse, Edward C.: Coca Erythroxylon: A New Cure for the Opium Habit, *Therapeutic Gazette, N.S. 1:*256–7, 1880.
9. *Op. cit.,* Bentley, W. H.: Erythroxylon Coca, p. 350.
10. *Op. cit.,* Stimmel, A. F.: Coca in the Opium and Alcohol Habits, N.S. 2:132–33.
11. Carey, Eugene F.: Holmes, Watson and Cocaine, *Baker Street Journal 13:*176–181, 195, 1963, p. 180.
12. Baring-Gould, William S.: *Sherlock Holmes of Baker Street, A Life of the World's First Consulting Detective,* New York, 1962, Clarkson N. Potter, Inc., p. 304.

13. Astrachan, B. A. and Boltax, Sandra P.: Letter to the Editor, *J. Am. Med. Assoc. 196:*1094, 1966.
14. Letter to the Editor, *Lancet,* 1 Nov. 1890, p. 957.
15. Baring-Gould, William S., ed., New York, 1967, Clarkson N. Potter, Inc., p. 346.
16. See, Musto, D. F.: Sherlock Holmes and Heredity, *J. Am. Med. Assoc. 196:*165-69, 1966.
17. Vash, George: Letter to the Editor, *J. Am. Med. Assoc. 197:*664-65, 1966.
18. Sigmund Freud to Martha Bernays, 27 June 1882, unpublished letter quoted in Jones, Ernest: *The Life and Work of Sigmund Freud,* Vol. I, New York, 1953, Basic Books, p. 89.
19. Quoted by Jones without date, *op. cit.,* p. 90.
20. Freud, S.: Ueber Coca, *Centralblatt für die gesammte Therapie 21:* 289-314, 1884.
21. Freud to Bernays, 2 June 1884 in Jones, Ernest: *The Life and Work of Sigmund Freud,* Vol. I, New York, 1953, Basic Books, p. 84.
22. Freud, S.: Beitrag zur Kenntniss der Cocawirkung, *Wiener Medizinische Wochenschrift,* Nr. 5. Fünfunddreissigster Jahrgang, pp. 130-133, 1885.
23. Freud, S.: "Über Coca," *Centralblatt für die gesammte Therapie 21:* 289-314, 1884.
24. *Ibid.*
25. Scientific Department of Parke, Davis & Co.: *Coca Erythroxylon and Its Derivatives,* Detroit and New York, 1885, Parke, Davis & Co., 103 pp., p. 4.
26. Freud, S.: Bemerkungen über Cocaïnsucht und Cocaïnfurcht, *Weiner Medizinische Wochenschrift* Nr. 28:929-932, 1887.
27. Erlenmeyer, A.: Ueber die Wirkung des Cocaïn bei der Morphiumentziehung, *Centralbl. d. Nervenheilkunde,* VIII, Juli, 1885, pp. 289-299.
28. Hammond, William A.: Remarks on Cocaine and the So-Called Cocaine Habit, *J. Nerv. & Ment. Dis. 13:*754-759, 1886.
29. Dana, C. L.: Early Neurologists in the United States, *J. Am. Med. Assoc. 90:*1421-1424, 1928. See also, *Dictionary of American Biography* 8:210-211.
30. Hammond, William A.: Coca: Its Preparations and Their Therapeutical Qualities, with some Remarks on the So-called "Cocaine Habit," *Trans. Med. Soc. Va.* pp. 212-226, 1887.
31. Penfield, W.: Halsted of Johns Hopkins, *J. Am. Med. Assoc. 210:* 2214-2218, 1969.

The bibliography is in two parts; the first is a list of Freud's publications on cocaine and the available translations. This lists only the "Cocaine Papers" and not the many other references to cocaine to be found in Freud's works. The second bibliography lists the books and articles with major commentaries on Freud and cocaine. Fictional accounts are excluded. Ed.

Freud on Cocaine

1. *Ueber Coca.* Von Dr. Sigm. Freud, Secundararzt im k.k. Allgemeinen Krankenhause in Wien. Centralblatt für die gesammte Therapie 2:289–314, 1884 Juli.
   Translation in:
   a. *The Cocaine Papers,* Vienna Zurich, 1963, Dunquin Press, pp. 1–26. (Translated by Steven A. Edminster).
   b. *The Saint Louis Medical & Surgical Journal XLVII,* No. 6:502–505, December 1884. (Translated by S. Pollak, M.D.).
2. *Beitrag zur Kenntniss der Cocawirkung.* Von Dr. Sigm. Freud, Sekundararzt im k. k. Allgemeinen Krankenhause in Wien. Wiener Medizinische Wochenschrift. Sonnabend, den 31. Jänner 1885. Nr. 5. Fünfunddreissigster Jahrgang. pp. 130–133.
   Translation in:
   a. *The Cocaine Papers,* Vienna Zurich, 1963, Dunquin Press, pp. 35–41. (Translated by Robert S. Potash, M.D.).
3. *Über Coca.* Von Dr. Sigm. Freud, Secundararzt im k. k. Allgemeinen Krankenhause in Wien. Neu durchgesehener und vermehrter Separat-Abdruck aus dem Centralblatt für die gesammte Therapie. Wien, 1855. Verlag Von Moritz Perles, Stadt, Bauernmarkt Nr. 11. pp. 1–26. *Translation in:*
   a. *The Cocaine Papers,* Vienna Zurich, 1963, Dunquin Press, pp. 1–26 (Addenda, pp. 27–29). (Translated by Steven A. Edminster).
4. *Ueber die Allgemeinwirkung des Cocaïns.* Vortrag, gehalted im psychiatrischen Verein am 5. Marz 1885 von Dr. Sigm. Freud, Medicinisch-chirurgisches Central-Blatt, Nr. 32, pp. 374–375, August 1885.
   Translation in:
   a. *The Cocaine Papers,* Vienna Zurich, 1963, Dunquin Press, pp. 45–49. (Translated by Steven A. Edminster).
   b. *Drug Dependence* 1(5):15–17, October 1970. (Translator unknown).
5. Gutt[macher, H.], Neue Arzneimittel und Heilmethoden. Ueber die verschiedenen Cocaïn-Präparate und deren Wirkung, Wiener Medizinische Presse, pp. 1035–1038. Aug. 9, 1885.

Translation in:
a. Freud, S.: "Opinion on Parke's Cocaine" in *The Cocaine Papers,* Vienna Zurich, 1963, Dunquin Press, p. 53. (Translated by Leona A. Freisinger).
6. *Beiträge über die Anwendung des Cocaïn.* Zweite Serie. I. Bemerkungen über Cocaïnsucht und Cocaïnfurcht mit Beziehung auf einem Vortrag W.A. Hammond's, 1887. Weiner Medizinische Wochenschrift Nr. 28, pp. 929–932.
Translation in:
a. *The Cocaine Papers,* Vienna Zurich, 1963, Dunquin Press, pp. 57–62. (Translated by Leona A. Freisinger).

On Freud on Cocaine

1. Becker, Hortense Koller: "Carl Koller and Cocaine," *Psychoanalytic Quarterly* 32:309–343, 1963.
2. Bernfeld, Siegfried: "Freud's Studies on Cocaine," 1884–1887, *Journal of the American Psychoanalytic Association* 1(4):581–613, 1953.
3. Brown, Charles T.: "Freud and Cocaine," *The Military Surgeon* 114:285–286, 1954.
4. Caldwell, Anne E.: "Origins of Psychopharmacology" from *CPZ to LSD,* Springfield, 1970, Charles C. Thomas, Publisher, pp. 17–20, 141–2.
5. Donoghue, A.K. and Hillman J. (eds.), "Introduction" to *The Cocaine Papers,* Vienna Zurich, 1963, Dunquin Press.
6. Feigenbaum, Aryeh: "Freud and the discovery of the anesthetic properties of cocaine," *Acta Medica Orientalia, Journal of the Israeli Medical Association* 15:201–205, 1956.
7. Jelliffe, Smith E.: "Sigmund Freud as a neurologist," *Journal of Nervous and Mental Disease* 85:696–711, 1937.
8. Jones, Ernest: "The Cocaine Episode" in *The Life and Work of Sigmund Freud,* Vol. I, New York, 1953, Basic Books, Inc., pp. 78–97.
9. Musto, David F.: "Sherlock Holmes and Sigmund Freud, A Study in Cocaine," *Journal of the American Medical Association* 204:125–130, 1968.
10. Musto, David F.: "The American Disease." *Origins of Narcotic Control,* New Haven and London, 1973, Yale University Press.
11. Schusdek, A.: "Freud on Cocaine," *Psychoanalytic Quarterly* 34:406–412, 1965.
12. Vom Scheidt, Jürgen, "Sigmund Freud und das Kokain," *Psyche* 27(1):385–430, 1973.

Biographical Notes

Aschenbrandt, Theodor. A Bavarian military physician who evaluated the effect of cocaine on soldiers in the field.

Bentley, W. H. An American physician from Kentucky who was one of the earliest proponents of the use of cocaine in the treatment of morphine addiction.

Bernays, Martha (1861-1951). Freud's fiancee and later his wife.

von Bibra, Ernst (1806-1878). A physician and geographer who wrote an account of his trip to South America in 1849 describing the use of the coca leaf in Peru and Bolivia.

Billroth, Christian Albert Theodor (1829-1894). Professor of surgery at the University of Vienna, and a pioneer in the fields of antiseptic technique and intestinal surgery. He operated on Fleischl-Marxow's hand.

von Brücke, Ernst Wilhelm (1819-1892). Professor of Physiology at the University of Vienna. One of the leading experimental physiologists of his day and the director of the physiological laboratories in Vienna. Brücke was a scientist Freud admired.

Charcot, Jean Martin (1825-1893). A neurologist in Paris whose work on hypnosis and hysteria stimulated Freud's investigations into the unconscious.

Erlenmeyer, Freidrich Albrecht Adolf (1849-1926). A neuropsychiatrist and the first to use bromide in the treatment of epilepsy. Erlenmeyer was a serious critic of Freud's advocacy of cocaine.

Exner, Siegmund (1846-1926). A neurophysiologist, interested in the physiology of the senses, and a Professor of Physiology in Vienna who developed the device which Freud used to measure reaction time.

von Fleischl-Marxow, Ernst (1846-1891). An assistant in Brücke's laboratory and a brilliant physiologist, he was an important figure in Freud's early medical career. An infection contracted while conducting research in pathological anatomy, resulted in the amputation of his right thumb. In constant pain thereafter he became a morphine addict and was treated with cocaine by Freud.

Fliess, Wilhelm (1858-1928). A nose and throat specialist who was Freud's extremely close friend and correspondent.

Gärtner, Joseph. An assistant in Stricker's laboratory who assisted Koller in the first demonstration of local anesthesia. Gärtner figures in several of Freud's dreams.

Halsted, William Stewart (1852-1922). One of the founders of American surgery, a Professor at Johns Hopkins, and the first to block nerve conduction by a local injection of cocaine.

Hammond, William Alexander (1828-1900). Surgeon General of the Army at age 34, a pioneer in American neurology, and the Professor of Neurology at Bellevue in 1876.

von Jauregg, Julius Wagner (1857-1940). An Austrian physician and psychiatrist who won the Nobel Prize for his work using fever therapy as a treatment for syphilis. A professor of Freud's in Vienna.

Koenigstein, Leopold (1850-1924). An ophthalmologist and colleague of Freud's who became involved in a battle with Carl Koller over the discovery of local anesthesia.

Koller, Carl (1857-1944). The discoverer of local anesthesia.

Lewin, Louis (1850-1929). A Prussian physician, pharmacologist and toxicologist who described the effects of many psychoactive drugs in his book *Phantastica, Narcotic and Stimulating Drugs* (1924).

Lustgarten, Sigmund (1857-1911). Bacteriologist in Vienna, the discoverer of the syphilis bacteria, and one of Freud's teachers.

Mantegazza, Paolo (1831-1910). An Italian physician and anthropologist, also a professor of Anthropology in Florence.

Meynert, Theodor (1833-1892). Professor of Psychiatry in Vienna and a neurologist and anatomist who advocated humane treatment of mental patients.

Monardes, Nicolas (1507-1578). Early Spanish physician and botanist who described the coca plant and its effects.

Morselli, Enrico (1852-1929). Italian psychiatrist working in Turin who published on the effect of cocaine in depression.

Niemann, Albert (1880-1921). German physician who crystallized cocaine and after whom Niemann Pick Disease is named.

Nothnagel, Hermann (1841-1905). A physician and professor of Medicine in Vienna who did research on Addison's Disease.

Noyes, Henry Drury (1832-1900). American physician who introduced the use of cocaine into ophthalmic surgery in the U.S.A. and a professor of Ophthalmology at Bellevue.

Rosanes, I. Chief physician at the Erherzogin Stefanspital and an intimate friend of both Freud and Koller.

Schroff, Karl Damian Ritter (1802-1887). Professor of Pharmacology and Pathology in Vienna and the author of a pharmacology textbook describing cocaine, which Freud used as a reference.

Wöhler, Friedrich (1800-1882). A pioneer German organic chemist who synthesized urea in 1828. Albert Niemann worked in his laboratory.

Index

Index

Academia Reale Medica di Roma, 316
The Addict and the Law, 378
Addiction, *see* alcohol, cocaine, morphine, opium etc.
Adler, Viktor, 263
Aggression, and cocaine, 383
Alcohol, xxxvii, xxxviii, 16, 64, 86, 128-9, 143, 144, 172, 187, 189-91, 324, 341, 343, 370
Alcoholism, 52, 69, 80, 87, 118, 282, 367
Alice in Wonderland, 268
Les aliments d'epargne, 55
alkaloid cocaine, vxiii, 8, 77, 121, 128
action, 255
Alles, Gordon, xxii
Allgemeine Krankenhaus, see General Hospital, Vienna
America, 305
American Academy of Ophthalmology and Otolaryngology, 316
American Neurological Association, 145
American Ophthalmological Society, 34
American Physiological and Pharmacological Society, 315
American Psychoanalytic Association, 324
Amphetamine, xxii, xxxvi, xxxviii, 377
and cocaine, xxxiv ff.
psychotogenic, xxx
v. cocaine, 375
Amyls, 222-23
Anemia, 67
Anesthesia, cocaine, *see* anesthesia,
local, 123
infiltration, 314
lack, 263
local, xviii, 31 ff., 49, 73, 80, 86-7, 97, 109, 124, 128-9, 143, 147 150, 155, 171, 182, 189, 255, 278, 282, 315-16, 318, 323, 328, 338, 346, 367, 369, 375
discovery, 284 ff., 330 ff., 334-5
world reaction, 286 ff.
Animals, coca effect, 56 ff.
experimentation, *see* experimentation, animal
Annotated Sherlock Holmes, The, 361
Anslinger, Harry, 377
Anti-Semitism, 263, 268 ff., 297-99, 303 ff., 311, 315

Aphrodisiac, 73, 80, 129, 135, 282, 329, 367
Archives of Ophthalmology, 317, 319
Arnold, Matthew, 266
Arlt, Professor, 263, 267, 385, 317
Army Medical Museum (U.S.), 368
Aschenbrandt, Theodor, 5, 10, 15, 54, 58, 61, 64, 78, 114, 279, 323
Ashton, L., 190
Asthma, 72 ff., 87, 129, 282, 329, 367
hay, 193
Astrachan, Boris, 360, 363
Atropia, *see* Atropine
Atropine, xxxvi, 190-91, 193
poisoning, 192
Auch Einer, 91
Austro-Hungarian Empire, 263
Autobiographical Study, An (Freud), 255 ff., 335, 343-44
Axenfeld, 316-17
Balfour, F.M., 263
Bamberger, 93
Barbiturates, xxxviii
Baring-Gould, William S., 360
Bartholow, R., 68, 132, 134
Bauduy, J.K., 145-46
Beard, George Miller, 341
Becker, Hortense Koller, 264 ff.
"Beitrag zur Kenntnis der Cocawirkung," 173
Belladonna, *see* Atrophine
Bellevue, 204, 224
Benecke, B., 275
Bennett, A., 54, 56
Bentley, W.H., 15 ff., 70, 72-3, 279 359, 366
Berger, Frank M., xxxiii
Berlin Medical Society, 174
Bernard, Claude, 69
Bernays, Martha, 5ff., 10, 34, 39ff., 91 ff., 153, 158, 159, 161 ff., 201, 255, 300, 307, 328, 335, 340, 343, 365
Bernfeld, Siegfried, 5, 200, 263, 293, 296-7
Betel, xxv
Bettelheim, 300, 302
Bier, August, 314
Billroth, Theodor, 157, 263 ff., 298, 314
Bingel, G.A., 65
Binz, Karl, 270
Blacks, and cocaine, xxviii
Bloom, S., 319
Boltax-Astrachan Hypothesis, 360, 363
Bosworth, 187

Boston Medical and Surgical Journal, 358
Botanical monograph, *see* Dream of the Botanical Monograph
Brahms, 265
Brasig, 212
Braun, 315
Brecher, Edward, xxxi, xxxiv
Bremer, L., 145
Brettauer, Josef, 32, 285, 290, 332
Breuer, Joseph, 7, 41, 92, 157-8, 165, 265, 279, 301, 310, 327
British Medical Association, 54
British Medical Journal, 54, 358
Brock, Professor, 162
Brockhaus, 315
Brouardel, P.C.H., 162
Brücke, Ernst, 34, 158, 256, 263 ff., 274, 322, 325, 364
Brücke Institute, 155
Brun, 330, 348
Buccola, G., xix, 59, 65, 117
Buch, Max, 102, 115, 338
Bunsen, 272
Bureau of Narcotics and Dangerous Drugs, 375 ff.
Burq, V., 98

Cachexia, 80, 87, 129, 366
  and coca, 67 ff.
Caffeine, xxv, xxxviii, 23, 58, 77, 86
Caldwell, 65
Cannabis, 58
Carey, Eugene F., 358
Castelnau, 51
Cataract, 263
Catecholamine, theory of depression, xxvi
Centralblatt, Erlenmeyer's, 172, 328
Centralblatt für die gesammte Therapie, Heitlers, 8, 97, 114, 129, 171, 173, 290, 328
Centralblatt fur Klinische Medizin, see Centralblatt für diegesammte Therapie
Centralblatt fur Nervenheilkunde, 197
Cerebral hyperemia, 369
Charcot, J.M., 161 ff., 114, 165, 296, 306-7, 333, 343
Charles, E., 64
Chenopodium quinoa, 77
Chiari, O., 173
Chicago Medical Journal and Examiner, 143

Chicago Police Department, 359
Chloral, 190
  bromide, 31
Chloroform, 190
Cholera, 162
Christison, Sir Robert, 54, 59, 61, 68, 358
Chuspa, 50
Cinchona, 191, 357
Citric acid, 77
Clemens, T., 54, 61, 64
Coca, abuse, 85
  and alcoholism, 69 ff.
  and asthma, 72, 329
  and cachexia, 52, 67 ff.
  and cocaine, xxxvii, 85
  and endurance, 42
  and general well-being, 97 ff.
  and hay fever, 120 ff.
  and indigestion, 65 ff., 87, 133, 175, 329
  and literature, 357 ff.
  and morphine addiction, 108, 173 ff., 329
  and nervous diseases, 64 ff.
  and neurasthenia, 329
  and science, 357
  and syphilis, 69
  and urination, 68
  aphrodisiac, 73, 329
  champagne, 246
  cheroots, 129 ff., 367
  cigarettes, xxviii, 246, 367
  components, 54
  cordial, xxviii, 125 ff., 367
  cost, 64, 87, 121 ff.
  cultivation, 49 ff., 241, 376
  distribution, 242
  dosage, 57, 59 ff., 63-4, 71, 123 ff., 131
  duration of effect, 61
  effect on Europeans, 61ff.
  export, 242
  fluid extract, 129 ff., 179
  history, 21 ff., 49 ff., 274
  in animals, 56 ff.
  in Europe, 53 ff., 63
  in healthy humans, 58 ff.
  in U.S., 63, 69, 72
  inhalant, 246
  local application, 73, 277, 329
  metabolism, 68
  pain-reliever, 336
  paralysis, 56
  poisoning, 56-7

preparations, 121 ff., 129
religious use, 50, 85
smoking, 133 ff.
"source of savings," 68-9
stimulant, 56, 63 ff., 86, 133 ff., 329, 367, 376
tannic acid, 77
therapeutic uses, 63 ff., 277
wine, 129 ff., 175, 179 ff., 185, 246, 369
see also cocaine, erythroxylon coca, *cocainum muriaticum,* etc.
Coca-Cola, xxxvii, 376
"Coca-Koller," 262, 290
Cocaine, abuse, xxxviii
action, 78, 113
addiction, 11, 154, 171, 173, 176, 186, 188 ff., 197 ff., 244 ff., 340, 344-5, 369
administration, 383
amounts seized, 375
and aggression, 383
and alcohol, 16 ff., 143 ff.
and alcoholism, 87
and amphetamine, 375
and asthma, 87, 367
and cachexia, 80, 87, 129, 366
and delirium tremens, 158
and depression, xxvi, 145
and diabetes, 33
and endurance, 21ff., 39
and euphoria, 366
and general well-being, 153
and hay fever, 187
and heart, 183, 185
and heart disease, 39, 181, 248
and hysteria, 181
and indigestion, 79, 129, 180, 366
and malaria, 181
and masturbation, 192
and melancholia, 145
and mercurialism, 366
and migraine, 135
and moral opinion, xxxiv ff.
and morphine, *see* morphine
and morphine addiction, *see* morphine addiction
and motor power, xxv, 98 ff., 124, 135, 244, 337
and nervous exhaustion, 39
and neurasthenia, 181, 336
and opium, 16 ff., 135, 143 ff.
and paralysis, 248, 358
and paranoia, 361
and performance, 383
and phthisis, 366

and psychiatry, 113, 340 ff., 351, 366
and psychoanalysis, 323 ff.
and pulse, 141 ff.
and racial violence, xxviii
and reaction time, 103 ff.
and seasickness, 33
and sexual activity, 251
and Sherlock Holmes, 359 ff.
and syphilis, 87, 367
and tea, 276
and temperature, 102, 141 ff.
and typhoid fever, 366
and violence, xxxvii
and virility, 10
anesthetic, 255
see also anesthesia, local
animal experiments, 54 ff., 174, 381 ff.
aphrodisiac, 80, 181, 367
carrying case, 130, 367
central activity, xviii
chemical analysis, 77
classification, 57-8
clinical use, 5 ff., 122 ff.
cost, 6, 40, 109, 117, 123 ff., 125 ff., 157, 235, 278, 287, 325, 342, 373, 378, 385
crystals, 77
danger, 172, 190, 373
definition, 373
dosage, 65, 78 ff., 87-8, 99, 114, 125, 136, 139, 144, 148, 154, 157, 172, 182 ff., 186 ff., 243, 246, 250, 296, 324-5, 337, 366, 384
dose-effect curve, 179
failure, 55, 146 ff.
formula, 54, 77
freedom from, 363
harmful effects, 157, 176, 179, 198, 239 ff., 246 ff., 325
history, 113, 191, 239
human experiments, 78, 381 ff.
illegal, 373 ff.
in England, 54, 358
in France, 55
in Peru, 85 ff.
in Russia, 55
in U.S., xxviii, 22, 55, 80, 113, 117, 284, 358, 373 ff.
individual effects, 107 ff., 115, 153, 171, 175
inhalant, 129

injection, 79, 101, 136 ff., 150, 154, 172, 174, 182 ff., 185 ff., 192, 198 ff., 219 ff., 255-6, 296, 345, 348 ff., 360, 368
internal, 109, 114, 339, 347
intoxication, 154, 158, 190, 197, 202, 249, 324, 364
isomer, 251
large doses, 184 ff.
literature, 15 ff., 54 ff., 278
local anesthesia, *see* anesthesia, local
manufacture, 121 ff., 377
medical use, 127 ff.
modern legal, 376
myths, 385
narcotic, 58, 78
nasal, 349, 351
nonmedical use, 382
objective measurements, 115, 140 ff.
overdose, 173
panacea, xviii, 128 ff.
penalties, 375 ff.
pharmaceutical opinions, 77 ff.
pharmacology, xxxiv, 323, 384
physiology, 231
physiological effects, 384
poisoning, 174
preparation, 53 ff., 59, 77, 121 ff., 129, 138 ff.
prescriptions, 378
psychosis, 342
psychotogenic, xxx
psychotropic, 358, 365
rituals of use, 385
stimulant, xxiv, 79, 128-9, 180-1, 239, 359, 366
surgical use, 9 ff., 128
synthesis, 385
therapeutic, xxviii, 87, 113, 282
time-dose-effects, 383
toxicity, 78, 98, 172, 174, 336, 345, 384
unknown facts, 381 ff.
vascular effect, 174
withdrawal, 250
see also coca, alkaloid cocaine, Freud and cocaine, etc.
Cocaine alkaloid, 129 ff.
Cocaine citrate, 124 ff., 129 ff.
"The Cocaine Episode," xxxiv, 5 ff., 322
Cocaine hydrobromate, 129 ff.
Cocaine hydrochlorate, *see* cocaine hydrochloride

Cocaine hydrochloride, 60, 86, 108, 123, 125, 129 ff., 179 ff., 181
Cocaine muriate, *see* cocaine hydrochloride
Cocaine oleate, *see* cocaine hydrochloride
Cocaine Papers, The, xvii
Cocaine salicylate, 124, 129 ff.
"Cocainism," xxxvii, 237 ff.
Cocainum muriaticum, 60 ff., 86 ff. 60 ff., 86 ff., 108, 125
see also cocaine, coca, etc.
Cocks, D.C., 150
Codeine, xxiv
Coffee, 128, 176, 186, 191
Cohn, Ludwig, 316
Collan, J., 59, 61, 69
Collected Papers (Freud), 228, 297, 349
College of Physicians, Philadelphia, 136
Collin, R., 55, 59, 73, 282, 329
Commerce Business Daily, 381
Compositae, 227
Consumption, 303
"Contribution to the Knowledge of the Effect of Cocaine, A," xxv, 337
Corning, J. Leonard, 275
Cowley, 274
"Craving for and Fear of Cocaine," xxxii, 342 ff.
Crespo, Pedro, 53, 64
Crucifers, 227
Cyclamen, 230 ff.

DaCosta, J.M., 136
Danini, 55-7
Darkshevich, L.O., 309
Daudet, Alphonse, 162
DeJussieu, A.L., 53
de la Tourette, Giles, 162, 166
de Wecker, 275
Dealer: Portrait of a Cocaine Merchant, xxxix, 373 ff.
Delirium tremens, 158, 176, 197, 343
Demarle, L.G., 51, 55, 59, 68-9, 277
Demerol, *see* meperidine
Depression, xxvi ff., 10, 281, 335, 363
see also stimulants *and* cocaine as stimulant
Detroit Medical Gazette, see Detroit Therapeutic Gazette
Detroit Therapeutic Gazette, 6, 55, 60, 70, 117, 171, 279, 325, 359, **364**, 366

Deutsche Medizinalzeitung, 172
Deutsche Medizinische Wochenschrift, 78, 323
Dextro-psicaine, 251
Diabetes, 33
Digestive system, 65 ff., 282
  See also indigestion
"Dolfi," 42-3
Donders, Professor, 263 ff., 306, 317
Doors of Perception, The xxvii
Dose-effect curve, cocaine, 179
Dowdeswell, G.F., 53-5
Doyle, Sir Arthur Conan, xxviii, 361
Dream content, 224
"Dream in Brucke's Laboratory," 350
Dream interpretation, 218, 221
"Dream of Irma's Injection," 205, 229, 349
Dream of July 23-24, 1895, 206
"Dream of the Botanical Monograph," 224 ff., 231, 223 ff., 350
Dreams, 201 ff.
Dreyfuss, 298
Drugs, euphoriant, xviii
  habit-forming, 345
  hard, 377 ff.
  psychotropic, 239 ff.
  sedative, xix
DuBois-Reymond, E., 263 ff., 267
Duel, Koller's, 269, 298 ff.
Dunquin Press, xvii
Dynamometer, 31, 98 ff., 108, 115, 124 ff., 125, 153, 283, 290, 328, 330, 336 ff.
  metric results, 99 ff.
Dysentery, 214 ff., 222
Dyspepsia, 358

Ecgonin, 77
Ecroyd, 139
Edwards, Landon B., 188
Efron, D.H., xxxiv
Ego psychology, 91
Eimer and Amend, Messrs., 288
Einstein, 270
Einthoven, Willem, 263 ff., 306
Electromagnetism, 280
Eliot, George, 300
Embryology, 272, 284
Embryology of Man and Mammals, 273
Encyclopédie Methodique Botanique, 53
Endurance, and coca, 51, 85 ff.
  and cocaine, 21 ff., 97

Engel, 283
England, *see* cocaine in England
Engle, Mrs. Bernice, 321
Erlenmeyer, A., xxxii, 172-3, 193, 342, 368-9
  cocaine criticism, 339
Erythroxylon coca, 15 ff., 49 ff., 70, 77, 127 ff., 239, 276, 286, 324
  classification, 53
  cultivation, 132
"Erythroxylon Coca as an Antidote to the Opium Habit," 19 ff.
"Erythroxylon Coca in the Opium and Alcohol Habits," 15 ff.
Ethnopharmacological Search for Psychoactive Drugs, The, xxiii
Etudes sur la coca du Pérou, 55
Euphoria, 9, 60, 97, 108, 114, 249, 324, 329, 336-7, 357, 366
Euphoriants, xxxviii, 91
Exner, Sigmund, 98, 108, 115-6, 124, 153, 157, 337
  and Fleischl, 325
Experimentation, xx ff., 376, 381 ff.
  animal, 54 ff., 72, 81, 174, 245
  dynamometer, *see* dynamometer
  objective, 97 ff.
  self-, xx ff.
"Experimentelle Untersuchung der einfachsten Psychischen Prozesse," 98

Fabritius, Professor August, 316
Faust, 235
Fauvel, Charles, 73, 275, 282, 329
Federal Narcotics Bureau, 378
Ferenczi, Sandor, xix
Final Problem, The, 361
Five Orange Pips, The, 360
Fleischl, *see* von Fleischl-Marxow, Ernst
Fliess, Wilhelm, 216, 223-27, 349
Fliessburg, 65
"Flora," 231, 234 ff.
Foreign Quarterly Review, 276
Foucar, Bradley W., 288
France, *see* cocaine in France
Franceschini, 154
Frankel, B., 174
Frank, 65
Frankl, J., 54, 65
Freedman, Daniel, xxxiv
Freud, Anna, 43, 49, 97, 113, 125, 171
Freud, Rosa, 33, 42-3, 91, 271

Freud, Sigmund
    and addiction, 346 ff.
    and America, 305
    and Martha Bernays, 39 ff., 44, 91
    and biography, 256
    and Brücke's laboratory, 364
    and Fleischl, 156 ff., *see also* von Fleischl
    and General Hospital, *see* General Hospital, Vienna
    and *Journal*, 39 ff., 41
    and Konigstein, 332
    and Koller, 269, 281, 286 ff., 300 ff., 303, 307 ff., 313 ff., 332
    see also Koller
    and local anesthesia, 293 ff.
    see also anesthesia, local
    and parents, 201
    and Sherlock Holmes, 357 ff.
    and Stricker's laboratory, 272 ff., 330
    and Wittels, 256
    Autobiographical Study, An, 255 ff.
    Autobiography, 291, 323
    cocaine evaluation, 121 ff., 329-30, 364, 367
    cocaine publications, xvii ff.
    cocaine use, 91 ff., 113, 164, 205
    contemporary comment, 78
    criticism, 322
    depression, 340-1
    dozent, 92 ff.
    dreams, 205 ff., 224 ff.
    enthusiasm for cocaine, 8ff.
    experimentation, xx, xxiv ff., 31, 33, 97 ff., 124, 153
    financial problems, 39ff., 164
    friends, 265, 280
    guilt feelings, 205 ff.
    in Paris, 162 ff., 197
    introduction to cocaine, 5 ff.
    Jewishness, 167-8
    marriage, 281, 308 ff., 311, 342-3, 351
    neurasthenia, 164
    physician, 335
    self-analysis, 349-50
    self-appraisal, 165
    self-defense, 229, 346
    self-experimentation, 65 ff., 324, 337, 336
    self-observation, 58 ff.
    sinus trouble, 352
    "Über Coca," 39ff.
    university examinations, 269 ff.

youth, 265 ff. *see also*
see also individual topics of Freud involvement
Freud's father, 155, 226, 336, 350
Fronmüller, 23, 54, 55, 78
Fuchs, Ernst, 303, 316

Gartner, J., 32, 165, 226, 231, 234, 272, 283, 330-31
Garcilasso de la Vega, 50, 241
Gardeke, 276
Gauss, 283
Gazeau, C., 55, 68-9
General Hospital, Vienna, 78, 266, 268, 280-1, 286, 290, 298-9, 303 ff., 330, 332, 340, 342, 349
"General well-being," 102 ff., 113, 133, 153, 281, 337, 341
Genus Cyclamen, The 255
Gerlach, Leo, 273
German Ophthalmological Society, 317 ff.
Gesellschaft der Ärzte, 7, 32, 34, 285, 287, 294, 295, 310, 315, 332
Gilman, Alfred, xvii
Glaucoma, 225
Goethe, 235
Gold chloride, 5
Goodman, Louis, xvii
Gosse, 55
Graetz, 280
Graetz, Jr., 280
Grant, General, 192
Graves's Disease, 176
Guttmacher, Hermann, 121

Haller, C., 23
Hallucinations, 246, 279, 342
Halsted, William, xxxi, 199, 369
Hamburger, Carl, 314
Hamlet, 201, 231
Hammond, William A., xxviii, xxxii, 171, 173, 175-6, 179 ff., 198 344, 368
Hanor, Ritter von, 271
"Hard drugs," 377 ff.
    see also drugs
Hardy, Thomas, 263
Harris, Alexander, 191
Harvard University, 316
Hay asthma, *see* Hay fever
Hay fever, 134 ff., 187, 193, 369
Hay Fever Association, 193, 369

Heart, 183, 185
Heart disease, 39, 134, 176, 181, 248
Heitler, 8, 97, 114, 290, 328
Helmholtz, 34, 263 ff., 296, 317
Hering, E., 270, 280
Heroin, xxxii, xxxiii, 375 ff.
Hertwig, Oskar, 273
Herzig, 43, 98, 124, 153, 337
History of the Jews, 280
Hitler, Adolf, 312, 317
Hofmann, Albert, xx
Hogarth, 245
Hole, 67
Holmes, Sherlock, xxix, 357 ff.
   and cocaine, 359 ff., 363, 370
   and opium, 360
   melancholia, 360
   mental process, 364
   morphine use, 359
Holmstedt, Bo. xxiii
Howe, Lucien, 316
Humboldt, 51
Hutchinson, 137
Huxley, Aldous, xxvii
Hydrobromic acid, 77
Hydrochloric acid, 77, 85, 86
Hydrophobia, 155
Hygrin, 77
Hypnotism, 198, 351, 365
Hypodermic, *see* injection
Hysteria, 181, 186, 189, 198, 206, 209, 222, 309-10, 369

Impotence, 73, 181, 359
Index Catalogue, 324
Indiana University, 377
Indigestion, 79, 133, 175, 195, 329, 366
Infiltration anesthesia, 314
Inhalant, coca, 246
Injection, *see* cocaine, injection
Institute of Pathological Anatomy, 31, 226
International Anesthesia Society, 316
Interpretation of Dreams, The, xvii, 200, 205 ff., 216, 230, 297, 325, 335, 348, 351
Iodoform, 136
"Irene," 361
"Irma," 206, 208 ff., 222 ff.

Jacobson, E., xxvi
Jaffe, Jerome, xxxvii
Jefferson Medical College, 134, 136
Jelliffe, Smith E., 323, 330
Jellinek, 109, 287, 314
Jewishness, 165-6, 266, 297, 302, 317

Johns Hopkins School of Medicine, xxxi
Johnston, 22
Jones, Ernest, xxv, xxxiv, 5 ff., 31 ff., 153, 263, 293, 296-7, 322, 342
Journal of the American Medical Association, 363
Journal of Nervous and Mental Diseases, 368
Journal of Therapy, see Centralblatt für die gesammte Therapie
Journey of the Frigate "Novara," 52
Julian, Father Antonio, 53, 65
Jurist, 136-38
Jussie, 77
Justice Department (U.S.), 375 ff.

Klinische Monatsblätter für Augenheilkunde, Zeherden, 143
Knapp, Arnold, 317
Knapp, Hermann, 147-8 167, 197, 278, 288, 317
Kolliker, R.A. Von, 263 ff., 312
Konigstein, Leopold, 10, 32, 34, 97, 109, 123, 154-55, 225, 226, 228, 232, 234, 255-6, 300, 304, 328, 332 ff., 349
   and Freud's father, 336
   and Koller, 124, 293 ff., 333
Kohn, Ignatz, 311
Kokoschka, Oskar, 263
Koller, Carl, 31 ff., 34, 80 ff., 97, 109, 123, 153, 155, 167, 171, 200, 225-6, 255-6, 263, 298, 344, 367
   and America, 312-13
   and embryology, 272 ff.
   and Fleischl, 325, 342
   and Freud, 32, 278, 281
   and Freud's father, 336
   and Königstein, 333
   and ophthalmology, 273 ff.
   discoverer of cocaine, 291
   duel, 298 ff.
   emigration, 311 ff.
   fame, 264 ff.
   in New York, 302
   neglect, 315 ff.
   neurasthenia, 308
   personality, 319
   "Preliminary Communication," 32, 332
   recognition, 316
   research, 318
   University of Vienna, 267
   youth, 266

Koller, Leopold, 266
Korsakov's Psychosis, 248
Kussmaul medal, 316

"L., Frau," 234
Lamarck, 53, 77
Lancet, The, 154, 286, 361
Landauer, R., 24
Laws, colonial, 376
  modern drug, 376 ff.
Leake, Chauncey, 273, 314
Leared, Arthur, 358
Leber, Thomas, 317
Leo XIII (Pope), xxxvii
Lenau, 266
Leopold, 212 ff.
Lepine, Raphaël, 162
LePlat, 303
Lewin, Louis, xxiv, xviii, xxxii, xxxvii, xxxviii, 179, 239, 132 ff.
Life and Work of Sigmund Freud, The, 5 ff., 31 ff., 322
Lincoln, Abraham, 368
Lindesmith, Alfred R., 377
Lippmann, 55, 68
Litten, 174
llicta, 50, 132, 241
  chemical analysis, 51
LLipta, see llicta
Lluta, see llicta
Loos, Adolf, 263
Lossen, 53-4, 77
Louisville Medical News, 19, 70
Ludwig, 267, 272
Lustgarten, 270, 280, 300, 302, 310
  and Koller, 269
Lysergic acid diethylamide, xx ff.

"M., Dr.," 210 ff., 222 ff.
Mach, Ernest, 263
Macht, David, xviii
Maher, John T., 376
Maier, 323, 330
Malaria, 181, 357
Mama Cuca, 241
Man with the Twisted Lip, The, 360
Manco Capac, 8, 50
Manic-depressive disorder, 360, 363
Mantegazza, Paolo, 9, 21 ff., 51 ff., 58 ff., 277, 283, 357-8, 365
Mariani, Angelo, 275
Mariani's Wine, xxxvii
Marijuana, 376 ff.
Markham, 52-3, 72, 77
Martins, 51, 65
Marvaud, 55, 59, 68, 73

Mason, 61, 68
Masturbation, 192
"Mathilde," 212 ff.
Mauthner, Ludwig, 204, 267
Maximilian, Emperor, 265
McBean, S., 67
Medical Congress, Copenhagen, 171
Medical News, 136
Medical Record, 147, 187, 275, 277, 285 ff., 296
Medical Society of Virginia, 369
Medico-Chirurgisches Centralblatt, 154
Melancholia, xix, 9, 145, 176, 186, 360, 366, 369
Meller, J., 316
Mental illness, and drugs, xix
Meperidine, xxxiii
Meprobamate, xxxiii
Merck Company, xxvi, 6, 24, 33, 55, 58, 63, 85, 121, 125, 138 ff., 144, 154, 171, 255, 289 ff., 323, 338-9, 365, 367, 377
Merck, E., 77, 143
Merck, Sharpe and Dohme, 77
Mercurialism, 358-9, 366
Mescaline, xxvii, xxxviii
Metabolism, coca, 68
Metzger, 308
Meynert, 93, 267, 321, 335
Michel, Professor, 312
Migraine, 135
Mill, John Stuart, 266
Miltown, *see* meprobamate
Missing Three-quarter, The, 360
Monardes, Nicholas, 53, 77, 357
Moore, Thomas J., 191
Moore, W. Oliver, 275, 287
Moreau de Tours, J.J., xix, xxii
Moreno y Maïz, T., 23, 55-6, 61, 63, 69, 277, 283
Moriarty, Professor, 362 ff.
Morphine, xxiv, xxxii, 9, 15, 31, 39, 79-80, 87, 129, 136, 215, 273, 343 ff., 366, 377
  addiction, 52, 69 ff., 108, 113, 117, 154, 171 ff., 186, 192, 197-8, 244 ff., 274, 279, 281-2, 325 ff., 329, 338, 340, 342, 350, 364, 367-8
  and Sherlock Holmes, 359
  fatal dose, 144
  withdrawal, 40
Morrison, Samuel B., 191
Morse, 281
Morselli, E., xix, 59, 65, 117
Mortimer, W. Golden, xxxvii

Morton, 278
Motor power, 98 ff., 108, 116 ff., 135, 294, 337
see also cocaine, and motor power
Munich, 218
Muriatic acid, see hydrochloric acid
Musto, David, xxviii, xxix
Myths, of cocaine use, 385

Narcotic Addiction Research Center, xxiv
Narcotics, 57-8, 78, 274
National Dispensatory, 132
National Institute on Drug Abuse, xxxix, 381 ff.
National Institute of Mental Health, xviii
Nausea, 179
Nazism, 314 ff., 317 ff.
Nederlandsche Gasthuis voor Oooglijder, Utrecht, 306
Nervous exhaustion, 39
Nervous system, 56
Neudörfer, J., 54, 64
Neue Freie Presse, 154
Neus Wiener Abendblatt, 298
Neurasthenia, 9, 64, 181, 198, 308, 336, 340 ff., 366
Neuroamoebimeter, 98, 108, 115, 124, 153, 337
Neurological Institute, 339
Neurosis, 198, 351
New York Academy of Medicine, 316
New York Eye and Ear Infirmary, 150
New York Medical Journal, 146, 287
New York Medical Record, 147-8
see also *Medical Record*
New York Neurological Society, 175
Niemann, Albert, 8, 23, 53, 77, 113, 276, 283, 328, 357
Nikolsky, 55-6
Nordenson, Eric, 312, 317
Nothnagel, H., 33, 92, 165, 282
Novara, 53, 113, 121, 276, 328
Novocain, 375,
Noyes, Henry D., 285, 287-88

Obersteiner, Heinrich, 157, 164, 171-2, 197, 200, 327, 334, 338 ff., 342,
Oedipus, 201
Oersted, Hans Christian, 280
Old Story of My Farming Days, An, 212

"On Coca," xix, 114, 154, 171, 173
see also *Über Coca*
"On the Employment of Cocaine in Neuroses and Psychoses," 197
Ophthalmological Congress, Heidelberg, 32, 97, 255, 285, 290, 317, 332
Ophthalmology, 10, 31 ff., 80 ff., 87, 113, 167, 273 ff., 306, 312, 314
Ophthalmoscope, 34
Opium, 15-16, 58, 80, 117, 128, 135, 143 ff., 189 ff., 359-60, 370, 377
addiction, 245
Origins of Psychoanalysis, The, 224, 227
Osler, Sir William, xxxi
Otto, 56, 206 ff., 223 ff.,

Pagvalin, 69
Palmer, E.R., 19, 70-71
Paneth, Joseph, 39, 42, 280, 300, 349-50
Pankow, 108
Paralysis, 125, 358
coca, 56
cocaine, 123, 248
Paranoia, xix, 362 ff.
Parapraxis, 334, 347 ff., 351
Paret, Peter, 322
Parke, Davis Company, xxvi, 16, 71. 125, 127 ff., 134, 338, 367
Pasteur, 162
"Pauli," 43
Peck, E.S., 148
Peckham, 67
Penfield, Sir Wilder, xxxi
Pennsylvania Hospital, 139, 141
Perimeter, 309-10
Perles, von Moritz, 114
Peru: History of Coca, xxxvii
Peyote, xxvii
Phantastica, xviii, xxiv, 239 ff.
Pharmacological Basis of Therapeutics, The, xvii, xxxiv, xxxvii, 375
Pharmacological Institute, Würzburg, 277
Pharmacology, history of, 323, 334
Phenothiazine, xxxviii
Philadelphia Hospital, 137
Phthisis, 67, 366
see also tuberculosis
Physiological Club, 33, 154

"Physiological Effect and Significance of Cocaine Muriate on the Human Organism, The," 21 ff., 323
Physiological Institute, 349
Pizarro, Francesco, 239, 274
Plenk, 311
Poeppig, 52, 55, 77, 276
Poison experiments, 330
Poisoning, coca, 56-7
Poizat, C.H., 72
Pollak, Josef, 66, 71
Pollak, S., 84
Powarin, 102
"Preliminary Communication" (Koller), 32
Prescott, 274
  cocaine warning, 276
Procaine, 375
Progrès Medicale, Le, 288
Propionic acid, 208, 215
Propylaea, 222
Propyls, 222-23
Psychiatric Association, *see* Psychiatric Society
Psychiatric Society, 113, 154, 296, 339, 348
Psychiatrisches Verein, *see* Psychiatric Society
Psychiatry, 64, 79, 113, 116 ff., 282, 340 ff., 366
Psychic debility, 64
Psychic reaction time, *see* reaction time
Psychoanalysis, 91, 279, 323, 346 ff.
  drugs in, 352
Psychopharmacology, xvii ff., xx
Psychosis, cocaine, 342
  drug-induced, xxxvi
  drug model, xix
  intoxication, 197
Psychotherapy, 251
Pulse, 141 ff.
Pusher, 373 ff.

Quinine, 128

Rank, 176
Ranke, 338 ff.
Rapid eye movement, sleep, 205
Reactiontime, 98 ff., 337
Reichenbach Falls, 361
Reiss, 23, 55, 59

Reuss, Professor M. von, 33, 307
Reuter, Fritz, 212
Ricchetti, 161 ff.
Richardson ether spray, 273
Richter, 108, 117, 338 ff.
Riley, F.C., 146
Ring, Frank W., 187
Ringtheater, 298
Ritchie, J.M., xvii
Ritter von Basch, Samuel, 265
Rituals, in cocaine use, 385
River, E.C., 149
Roberts, Milton Josiah, 193
Robinson, W.L., 187, 193
Rohe, 191
Roosa, J.B. St. John, 192
Rosanes, I., 280, 305, 310
  and Koller, 269
Rossbach, M.J., 21, 283
  and Koller, 295
Rossier, G., 55, 59
Rowe, E.W., 190
Russia, *see* cocaine in Russia

Saale, S.S., 312
Sachs, 323
St. Louis Courier of Medicine, 146
St. Louis Medical and Surgical Journal, The, xvii, 157, 325
St. Louis Medico-Chirurgical Society, 146
St. Vincent's Hospital, 145
Salpêtrière, 166
Salicylic acid, 77
Scandal in Bohemia, A, 360-1
Schenck, 146, 160
Scherzer, 8, 53, 121, 276
Schildbach, 22
Schleich, 314
Schmeichler, R.A., 311
Schnabel, 280, 310
Schnitzler, Arthur, 198
Schönberg, Alois, 39
Schonberg, Arnold, 263
Scholz, Professor, 199, 349
Schrady, G.F., 277
Schrotter, 287
Schroff, C., xxiv, 54 ff., 78, 98, 276, 283, 295, 328, 358, 366
Schwarz, 270
Schrivener, J.H., 51, 65
Self-experimentation, 9, 58 ff., 133, 176, 179, 182 ff., 324, 337, 357, 366

Self-observation, 98
Semaine Médicale, 286
Sex, etiology of neuroses, 200
Sexual activity, 73, 223, 251
Shakespeare, 350
"Sherlock Holmes and Sigmund Freud," xxix
Shields, Charles M., 193
Sieveking, E.H. 358
Sigmund, Karl, 271
Sign of Four, The, xxix, 360
Silverman, M., 323, 327, 342
Slaughter, R.M., 190
Smidt, 172, 338 ff.
Snellen, Professor, 263 ff., 306
Society of Physicians, Budapest, 316
"Some Observations on the Use of the Hydrocholrate of Cocaine, etc.," 136 ff.
"Source of savings," 68-9, 72
Spina, 272, 330
Squibb, E.R., 138, 287-9
Standhartner, Dr. Josef, 301
Stedem, Mr., 138
Stein, Larry, xxxiv
Stepan Chemical Company, 377
Stevens, George T., 148
Stevens, Mr., 134
Stewenson, 52
Stimmel, H.F., 359
Stimulants, 16, 56, 63, 79, 86, 125-9, 133 ff., 180-1, 239, 282, 329, 359, 366-67, 376
Stockwell, G. Archie, 358, 365-66
Strachey, James, xvii
Strand, The, 359
Strauss, 162
Stricker, Professor, 31, 226, 271 ff., 286
  Stricker's laboratory, 272 ff., 283, 330
Sulle virtu igieniche e medicinali della coca, 357
Supplier, 373 ff.
Surgeon General's Office (Washington, D.C.), 324
Synthesis, of cocaine, 385
Syphilis, 69, 87, 137, 366

Tarkhanov, 5, 56-7
Tartaric acid, 77
Taylor, Hugh M., 188 ff., 191
Taylor, R.W., 69
Tea, 128, 176, 186

Temperature, 141 ff.
Theine, 23, 77, 86
Theobromin, 77
Thomas, Carl, 266
Thurber, Whyland and Company, 180
Tobacco, 187
Toffano, Emile, 163
Tonra, 51, 241
Trimethylamin, 216 ff., 223
Trommsdorf, 65
Tschudi, *see* von Tschudi
Tuberculosis, 137, 213, 359
  see also phthisis
Typhoid fever, 67, 366

"Über Coca," xvii 15 ff., 41, 49 ff., 225, 282, 290, 296, 328, 330, 348, 365
  Addenda, 107 ff.
  American abstract, 85 ff.
  differing versions, 107
  English translation, 338
  monograph, 338
  publication date, 334 ff.
Uber Morphiumsucht, 197
Unanuè, H., 23, 52, 69
Unconscious, 232
U.S., *see* cocaine in U.S.
U.S. Army, 179
U.S. Dispensatory, 132
University College, 54, 358
Upshur, John N., 190
Urea, 8
Urination, 68
Ut mine Stromtid, 212

Vash, George, 364
Vienna, 1880's, 265
Viennese Medical Society, 276
Vin Mariani, 275
Virginia Medical Monthly, 179
Virility, 10
Vischer, Friedrich Theodor, 91
Vogl, Professor August, 49, 276, 325
Voltaire, 307
Vom Scheidt, Jurgen, xviii, 91
Von Anrep, B., xx, 21, 23, 54, 56-7, 62, 72, 277, 282, 286, 295
Von Beneden, Edouard, 273
Von Bibra, E.F., 21-3, 51
Von Fleischl-Marxow, Ernst, 6, 7, 9, 33, 39 ff., 78, 85, 87, 92, 144,

154 ff., 198-99, 202, 215, 274, 279, 281, 305, 325 ff., 342, 347, 349-50, 365, 367 ff.
and cocaine, 157 ff.
and morphine, 156
cocaine intoxication, 160
Von Gaedeke, 22
Von Gorup, 22
Von Graefe, 317
Von Meyen, 52
Von Rokitansky, 279
Von Tschudi, 23, 51, 53, 72, 77
Von Voit, 68-9

Wagenmann, 317
Wagner von Jauregg, Julius, 32, 256, 265, 272, 294, 334
Wahler, Emil, 280
Walker, L.P., 150
Walle, 172, 197, 338 ff.
Watson, John, 359 ff.
Weber, 281
Weddell, 52
Weinlechner, Joseph, 92, 301-2
Welch, William Henry, xxxi
Well-being, general, *see* general well-being
Weston, Mr., 54, 133
Widder, 303, 310-11
Wiener Medizinische Presse, 121, 294
Wiener Medizinische Wochenschrift, 108, 121, 153, 173, 198, 289, 332
Wilder, 60
Winn, J.F., 191
Winston, B.L., 188
Wish-fulfillment, 219
Wittels, Fritz, 35, 200, 255, 323, 334, 348-9
Wittgenstein, Ludwig, 263
Wöhler, 8, 53, 113, 121, 276, 283, 328
Woelfler, Anton, 314
Wood, 132
Woodley, Richard, xxxix
World War II, 269

Ypadú, 241
Yellow Face, The, 360

Zeitschrift fur Therapie, 118
Zinner, Friedrich, 298 ff.
Zuckerkandl, Otto, 270